T0383307

Cutting-Edge Topics in Pediatric Anesthesia

Guest Editors

ARJUNAN GANESH, MBBS
RONALD LITMAN, DO

ANESTHESIOLOGY CLINICS

www.anesthesiology.theclinics.com

Consulting Editor
LEE A. FLEISHER, MD, FACC

June 2009 • Volume 27 • Number 2

SAUNDERS an imprint of ELSEVIER, Inc.

W.B. SAUNDERS COMPANY
A Division of Elsevier Inc.

1600 John F. Kennedy Boulevard, Suite 1800 • Philadelphia, PA 19103-2899

http://www.theclinics.com

ANESTHESIOLOGY CLINICS Volume 27, Number 2
June 2009 ISSN 1932-2275, ISBN-13: 978-1-4377-0950-6, ISBN-10: 1-4377-0950-8

Editor: Rachel Glover
Developmental Editor: Donald Mumford

Anesthesiology Clinics (ISSN 1932-2275) is published quarterly by Elsevier Inc., 360 Park Avenue South, New York, NY 10010-1710. Months of issue are March, June, September, and December. Application to mail at periodicals postage rates is pending at New York, NY and at additional mailing offices. Subscription prices are $122.00 per year (US student/resident), $244.00 per year (US individuals), $298.00 per year (Canadian individuals), $372.00 per year (US institutions), $461.00 per year (Canadian institutions), $172.00 per year (Canadian and foreign student/resident), $338.00 per year (foreign individuals), and $461.00 per year (foreign institutions). To receive student and resident rate, orders must be accompanied by name of affiliated institution, date of term, and the *signature* of program/residency coordinator on institutions letterhead. Orders will be billed at individual rate until proof of status is received. Foreign air speed delivery is included in all *Clinics'* subscription prices. All prices are subject to change without notice. POSTMASTER: Send address changes to *Anesthesiology Clinics,* Elsevier Health Sciences Division, Subscription Customer Service, 3251 Riverport Lane, Maryland Heights, MO 63043. Customer Service (orders, claims, online, change of address): Elsevier Health Sciences Division, Subscription Customer Service, 3251 Riverport Lane, Maryland Heights, MO 63043. Tel:1-800-654-2452 (U.S. and Canada); 314-447-8871 (outside U.S. and Canada). Fax: 314-447-8029. E-mail: journalscustomerservice-usa@elsevier.com (for print support); journalsonlinesupport-usa@elsevier.com (for online support).

Reprints. For copies of 100 or more of articles in this publication, please contact the Commercial Reprints Department, Elsevier Inc., 360 Park Avenue South, New York, NY 10010-1710. Tel.: 212-633-3812; Fax: 212-462-1935; E-mail: reprints@elsevier.com.

Anesthesiology Clinics, is also published in Spanish by McGraw-Hill Inter-americana Editores S. A., P.O. Box 5-237, 06500 Mexico D. F., Mexico.

Anesthesiology *Clinics,* is covered in *MEDLINE/PubMed (Index Medicus), Current Contents/Clinical Medicine, Excerpta Medica, ISI/BIOMED,* and *Chemical Abstracts.*

Printed and bound by CPI Group (UK) Ltd, Croydon, CR0 4YY

Transferred to Digital Print 2011

Contributors

CONSULTING EDITOR

LEE A. FLEISHER, MD, FACC
Robert D. Dripps Professor and Chair of Anesthesiology and Critical Care, University of Pennsylvania School of Medicine, Philadelphia, Pennsylvania

GUEST EDITORS

ARJUNAN GANESH, MBBS
Assistant Professor, Department of Anesthesiology and Critical Care Medicine, The Children's Hospital of Philadelphia; Assistant Professor of Anesthesiology, University of Pennsylvania School of Medicine, Philadelphia, Pennsylvania

RONALD LITMAN, DO
Professor of Anesthesiology and Pediatrics, University of Pennsylvania School of Medicine; Department of Anesthesiology and Critical Care, Children's Hospital of Philadelphia, Philadelphia, Pennsylvania

AUTHORS

PHILIP D. BAILEY, Jr, DO
Assistant Professor, Division of Cardiothoracic Anesthesiology, Department of Anesthesiology and Critical Care Medicine, The Children's Hospital of Philadelphia, Philadelphia, Pennsylvania

LAURA K. DIAZ, MD
Assistant Professor, Division of Cardiothoracic Anesthesiology, Department of Anesthesiology and Critical Care Medicine, The Children's Hospital of Philadelphia, University of Pennsylvania School of Medicine, Philadelphia, Pennsylvania

MICHAEL EISSES, MD
Assistant Professor, Department of Anesthesiology and Pain Medicine, University of Washington; Attending Physician in Pediatric Anesthesia, Seattle Children's Hospital, Seattle, Washington

JOHN FIADJOE, MD
Clinical Assistant Professor of Anesthesiology, Department of Anesthesiology and Critical Care Medicine, Children's Hospital of Philadelphia, University of Pennsylvania, Philadelphia, Pennsylvania

PAUL G. FIRTH, MBChB
Instructor in Anesthesia, Harvard Medical School; Attending Anesthesiologist, Department of Anesthesia and Critical Care, Massachusetts General Hospital, Boston, Massachusetts.

ARJUNAN GANESH, MBBS
Assistant Professor, Department of Anesthesiology and Critical Care Medicine, The Children's Hospital of Philadelphia; Assistant Professor of Anesthesiology, University of Pennsylvania School of Medicine, Philadelphia, Pennsylvania

HARSHAD G. GURNANEY, MBBS, MPH
Assistant Professor, Department of Anesthesiology and Critical Care Medicine, The Children's Hospital of Philadelphia; University of Pennsylvania School of Medicine, Philadelphia, Pennsylvania

JIMMY W. HUH, MD
Associate Professor of Anesthesiology, Critical Care and Pediatrics, Department of Anesthesiology and Critical Care Medicine, Children's Hospital of Philadelphia, University of Pennsylvania School of Medicine, Philadelphia, Pennsylvania

DAVID R. JOBES, MD
Professor, Division of Cardiothoracic Anesthesiology, Department of Anesthesiology and Critical Care Medicine, The Children's Hospital of Philadelphia, Philadelphia, Pennsylvania

LISA JONES, CRNA
Division of Cardiothoracic Anesthesiology, Department of Anesthesiology and Critical Care Medicine, The Children's Hospital of Philadelphia, University of Pennsylvania School of Medicine, Philadelphia, Pennsylvania; Clinical Associate, University of Pennsylvania School of Nursing Science, Philadelphia, Pennsylvania

F. WICKHAM KRAEMER, MD
Assistant Professor of Anesthesiology, University of Pennsylvania, School of Medicine, Department of Anesthesiology and Critical Care; Attending Anesthesiologist, Department of Anesthesiology and Critical Care Medicine, Children's Hospital of Philadelphia, Philadelphia, Pennsylvania

MARY ELLEN McCANN, MD, MPH, FAAP
Assistant Professor, Department of Anaesthesia (Pediatrics), Harvard Medical School; Senior Associate, Department of Anesthesiology, Perioperative and Pain Medicine, Children's Hospital Boston, Boston, Massachusetts

VIVEK MOITRA, MD
Assistant Professor, Division of Critical Care, Department of Anesthesiology, College of Physicians and Surgeons of Columbia University, New York, New York

RAMESH RAGHUPATHI, PhD
Associate Professor, Department of Neurobiology and Anatomy, Drexel University College of Medicine, Philadelphia, Pennsylvania

MICHAEL RICHARDS, BM, MRCP, FRCA
Assistant Professor, Department of Anesthesiology and Pain Medicine, University of Washington; Attending Physician in Pediatric Anesthesia, Seattle Children's Hospital, Seattle, Washington

JOHN B. ROSE, MD
Associate Professor of Anesthesiology and Pediatrics, University of Pennsylvania, School
of Medicine, Department of Anesthesiology and Critical Care; Clinical Director, Pain
Management Service, Department of Anesthesiology and Critical Care Medicine,
Children's Hospital of Philadelphia, Philadelphia, Pennsylvania

STANLEY H. ROSENBAUM, MD
Professor of Anesthesiology, Internal Medicine, Surgery; and Director, Section
of Perioperative and Adult Anesthesia; and Vice Chairman for Academic Affairs,
Department of Anesthesiology, Yale School of Medicine, New Haven, Connecticut.

ROBERT N. SLADEN, MB, ChB, MRCP, FRCP, FCCM
Professor and Vice Chair, Chief, Division of Critical Care, Department of Anesthesiology,
College of Physicians and Surgeons of Columbia University, New York, New York

SULPICIO G. SORIANO, MD, FAAP
Associate Professor, Department of Anaesthesia (Pediatrics), Harvard Medical School;
Children's Hospital Boston Endowed Chair in Pediatric Neuroanesthesia; and Senior
Associate in Anesthesiology, Department of Anesthesiology, Perioperative and Pain
Medicine, Children's Hospital Boston, Boston, Massachusetts

PAUL STRICKER, MD
Assistant Professor of Anesthesiology, Department of Anesthesiology and Critical Care
Medicine, Children's Hospital of Philadelphia, University of Pennsylvania, Philadelphia,
Pennsylvania

SHILPA VERMA, MBBS
Pediatric Anesthesia Fellow, Department of Anesthesiology and Pain Medicine, University
of Washington, Seattle, Washington; Seattle Children's Hospital, Seattle, Washington

Contents

Erratum xi

Foreword xiii

Lee A. Fleisher

Preface xv

Arjunan Ganesh and Ronald Litman

Pediatric Difficult Airway Management: Current Devices and Techniques 185

John Fiadjoe and Paul Stricker

> The anesthesiologist confronting the difficult pediatric airway is presented with a unique set of challenges. Adult difficult airway management techniques, such as awake or invasive approaches to airway management, often cannot be applied to children because of inadequate cooperation. Consequently, awake intubation in pediatrics is uncommon; most intubations are performed under general anesthesia or deep sedation. From a physiologic perspective, children have higher rates of oxygen consumption, significantly shortening the period of apnea that can be safely tolerated. Normal developmental anatomic differences of the pediatric airway and the presence of craniofacial dysmorphisms, presents additional challenges to tracheal intubation.

Ultrasound Guidance for Pediatric Peripheral Nerve Blockade 197

Arjunan Ganesh and Harshad G. Gurnaney

> There is an increasing trend in the use of peripheral nerve blockade for postoperative analgesia in children, and the use of ultrasound guidance to perform peripheral nerve blocks is gaining popularity. A thorough knowledge of anatomy will help in performing the appropriate block, and will also aid in better use and understanding of ultrasound guidance. In this article, we briefly review the use of ultrasound guidance to perform common upper and lower extremity and truncal blocks.

New Concepts in Treatment of Pediatric Traumatic Brain Injury 213

Jimmy W. Huh and Ramesh Raghupathi

> Emerging evidence suggests unique age-dependent responses following pediatric traumatic brain injury. The anesthesiologist plays a pivotal role in the acute treatment of the head-injured pediatric patient. This review provides important updates on the pathophysiology, diagnosis, and age-appropriate acute management of infants and children with severe traumatic brain injury. Areas of important clinical and basic science investigations germane to the anesthesiologist, such as the role of anesthetics and apoptosis in the developing brain, are discussed.

Pharmacologic Management of Acute Pediatric Pain   241

F. Wickham Kraemer and John B. Rose

> The accurate assessment and effective treatment of acute pain in children
> in the hospital setting is a high priority. During the past 2 to 3 decades, pe-
> diatric pain management has gained tremendous knowledge with respect
> to the understanding of developmental neurobiology, developmental phar-
> macology the use of analgesics in children, the use of regional techniques
> in children, and of the psychological needs of children in pain. A wide
> range of medications is available to treat a variety of pain types. This article
> provides an overview of the most common analgesic medications and
> techniques used to treat acute pain in children.

Is Anesthesia Bad for the Newborn Brain?   269

Mary Ellen McCann and Sulpicio G. Soriano

> Although certain data suggest that common general anesthetics may be
> neurotoxic to immature animals, there are also data suggesting that these
> same anesthetics may be neuroprotective against hypoxicischemic injury,
> and that inadequate analgesia during painful procedures may lead to in-
> creased neuronal cell death in animals and long-term behavioral changes
> in humans. The challenge for the pediatric anesthesia community is to de-
> sign and implement studies in human infants to ascertain the safety of gen-
> eral anesthesia. In this article, the authors review the relevant preclinical
> and clinical data that are currently available on this topic.

The Fontan Patient   285

Philip D. Bailey, Jr. and David R. Jobes

> Improved surgical and medical management has led to an increase in sur-
> vival after staged univentricular palliative procedures. Subsequently, this
> improved survival has led to an increase in the number of patients who
> will present for noncardiac surgical interventions with Fontan physiology.
> A comprehensive understanding of normal Fontan physiology and the per-
> turbations that the proposed surgical procedure will likely have is necessary
> to care for and design a comprehensive anesthetic plan that takes into ac-
> count the effects of anesthetic agents, ventilation strategies, cardiovascular
> drugs, and various other perioperative factors. Applying the knowledge pre-
> sented in this article should enable the anesthesiologist with the necessary
> principles to care for the patient with Fontan physiology.

Sedating the Child with Congenital Heart Disease   301

Laura K. Diaz and Lisa Jones

> The number of pediatric patients requiring sedation for procedures per-
> formed outside the operating room environment continues to grow yearly,
> as does the number of patients surviving to adulthood with the residua
> and sequelae of congenital heart disease. Ongoing efforts to develop guide-
> lines to enhance the safety of these pediatric sedative encounters have re-
> sulted in great strides in the prevention of adverse events. In addition, the
> Society for Pediatric Sedation, associated with the Pediatric Sedation Re-
> search Consortium, provides an important forum for practitioner education
> and the promotion of safe care for infants and children undergoing sedative

experiences. Care of the subset of patients with congenital heart disease or pulmonary hypertension remains especially demanding. The additional safety challenges posed by remote locations make the highest level of vigilance essential when planning and performing sedation for these children.

Anesthesia and Hemoglobinopathies   321

Paul G. Firth

Hemoglobinopathies are diseases involving abnormalities of the structure or production of hemoglobin. Examples include sickle cell disease, the thalassemias, and rare hemoglobin variants producing cyanosis. Recent advances in the understanding of the consequences of hemoglobin dysfunction on nitric oxide signaling have led to a reassessment of the pathophysiology of sickle cell disease and thalassemia. Chronic vascular inflammation and damage is now recognized as playing an important role in disease expression. Hemoglobinopathies may present to the anesthesiologist as the primary cause of a surgical procedure, as an incidental complicating factor of a surgical patient, or with a problem arising from the disease itself. This article reviews the common types of hemoglobinopathies, presents a basic summary of the pathophysiology relevant to anesthesia, and outlines current perioperative management.

Blood Conservation Strategies in Pediatric Anesthesia   337

Shilpa Verma, Michael Eisses and Michael Richards

Management of bleeding in the neonate, infant, or child presents its own set of dilemmas and challenges. One of the primary problems is the lack of good scientific evidence regarding the best management strategies for children rather than for adults. The key to success in the predicament is firstly to ensure that the physician has a clear understanding of the underlying normal physiology of the young child's hematologic status. Then by adding knowledge of the abnormal pathology that is being presented, the physician can at least understand what anomalies he or she is facing. Once all the available information concerning the patient's clinical condition and the options available has been well digested, a multidisciplinary approach allows the optimal use of all available resources. Good teamwork, understanding, and communication between all vested parties allows for a synergistic relationship to enhance patient care and give the best available end result.

Bonus Article: Monitoring Endocrine Function   353

Vivek Moitra and Robert N. Sladen
Edited by Stanley H. Rosenbaum

This article reviews current knowledge concerning the monitoring of endocrine function in patients in the clinical setting. Monitoring techniques are discussed and literature is reviewed regarding diabetes mellitus, thyroid, and parathyroid disorders, pheochromocytoma, adrenal insufficiency, and carcinoid tumors.

Index   365

FORTHCOMING ISSUES

September 2009
Problems with Geriatric Anesthesia Patients
Jeffrey H. Silverstein, MD, *Guest Editor*

December 2009
Preoperative Medical Consultation: A Multidisciplinary Approach
Lee A. Fleisher, MD and
Stanley H. Rosenbaum, MD, *Guest Editors*

RECENT ISSUES

March 2009
Anesthesia Outside the Operating Room
Wendy L. Gross, MD, MHCM and
Barbara Gold, MD, *Guest Editors*

December 2008
Value-Based Anesthesia
Alex Macario, MD, MBA, *Guest Editor*

September 2008
Cardiac Anesthesia: Today and Tomorrow
Davy C.H. Cheng, MD, MSc, FRCPC, FCAHS,
Guest Editor

RELATED INTEREST

Pediatric Clinics of North America, March 2008 (Volume 92, Issue 2)
Pediatric Quality
Leonard Feld, MD and Shabnam Jain, MD, *Guest Editors*

THE CLINICS ARE NOW AVAILABLE ONLINE!

Access your subscription at:
www.theclinics.com

Erratum

Intraoperative Management: Peripheral Vascular Surgery

Richard P. Serianni, MD[a],*, Cynthia H. Shields, MD[b],
Dale F. Szpisjak, MD, MPH[b], Paul D. Mongan, MD[b]

In the June 2004 issue of the *Anesthesiology Clinics of North America* (Volume 22, Issue 2), the name of Dale F. Szpisjak, MD, MPH was misspelled in the table of contents, in the contributors list, and on the title page of the article.

[a] Department of Anesthesiology, National Naval Medical Center Bethesda, 8901 Jones Bride Road, Bethesda, MD 20814, USA
[b] Department of Anesthesia, Uniformed Services University of the Health Sciences, 4301 Jones Bridge Road, Bethesda, MD 20814, USA
* Corresponding author.
E-mail address: rpserianni@bethesda.navy.mil (R.P. Serianni).

Anesthesiology Clin 27 (2009) xi
doi:10.1016/j.anclin.2009.07.001
1932-2275/09/$ – see front matter

Foreword

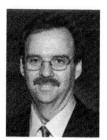

Lee A. Fleisher, MD, FACC
Consulting Editor

As surgery and the condition of patients who undergo surgery become more complex, hospitals specifically devoted to care for these patients have developed. One of the first such types of hospitals were the children's hospitals. These specialized hospitals allow for the translation of the latest science into clinical care. Yet it is important to recognize that most routine anesthesia care for pediatric patients is performed in general hospitals by non–specialty trained anesthesiologists. As new knowledge is produced, it is important to diffuse it to the larger population. This issue of *Anesthesiology Clinics* is devoted to disseminating lessons learned from and practices developed in several major referral pediatric hospitals.

To accomplish these goals, I was fortunate to have two outstanding editors from the Department of Anesthesiology and Critical Care at the Children's Hospital of Philadelphia. Dr Litman is Professor of Anesthesiology and Critical Care at the University of Pennsylvania School of Medicine and Director of Clinical Research and Director of Fellow Education at The Children's Hospital of Philadelphia. He has been active in the American Academy of Pediatrics, the American Society of Anesthesiologists, and the Society of Pediatric Sedation. He investigates, lectures, and writes extensively on issues of pediatric sedation. Dr Ganesh is Assistant Professor of Anesthesiology and Critical Care at the University Of Pennsylvania School Of Medicine. He is a member of the World Health Organization Expanded Review Panel on guidelines for pain management. His research, lectures, and writing focus on regional anesthesia. Together, they have assembled an outstanding group of authors to disseminate the newest information.

Lee A. Fleisher, MD, FACC
Department of Anesthesia
University of Pennsylvania School of Medicine
3400 Spruce Street
Dulles 680
Philadelphia, PA 19104, USA

E-mail address:
fleishel@uphs.upenn.edu (L.A. Fleisher)

Anesthesiology Clin 27 (2009) xiii
doi:10.1016/j.anclin.2009.07.013   anesthesiology.theclinics.com
1932-2275/09/$ – see front matter © 2009 Elsevier Inc. All rights reserved.

Preface

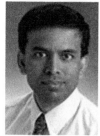 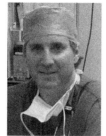

Arjunan Ganesh, MBBS   Ronald Litman, DO
Guest Editors

Many thousands of times each day, practitioners of pediatric anesthesia perform routine anesthetics safely with an inconspicuous and remarkable consistency. However, unless one pays careful attention to the published literature and scientific meeting abstracts, the progress behind the clinical scenes can be easily missed. These subtle advances and evolving controversies in pediatric anesthesia are the main focus of this thrilling issue of *Anesthesiology Clinics*. Our goal was to provide readers with updates in areas where clinical and basic science research have led to changes in clinical practice or areas of continuing research that have generated new and provocative results. In choosing the topics, one of our primary goals was to update not only specialists in pediatric anesthesia but also practitioners who anesthetize pediatric patients only occasionally.

Many of the articles are written by authors based at our institution, The Children's Hospital of Philadelphia. Dr. Fiadjoe, one of our difficult-airway experts, provides an update on the various new devices for managing the difficult pediatric airway and Dr. Ganesh, an internationally known expert in the field of regional anesthesia and one of the coeditors of this issue, has written a primer on the use of ultrasound when performing peripheral nerve blocks in children. Drs. Huh and Raghupathi, whose research careers are based on finding novel treatments for pediatric traumatic brain injury, provide an update in that evolving field, and two of our pain experts, Drs. Kraemer and Rose, provide a broad overview of current thinking in acute pediatric pain management. We also tapped into the expertise of our world-renowned cardiac anesthesia team. Drs. Bailey and Jobes decipher the complex management of the child with Fontan anatomy and physiology, and Dr. Diaz and Ms. Jones provide pearls on sedating children who have congenital heart disease. Experts on additional controversial areas were found in other prestigious institutions. Drs. Soriano and McCann from Boston Children's Hospital lend their expertise on a current controversy—the neurotoxicity of anesthetics in newborns—and Dr. Firth of Massachusetts General Hospital provides an overview on the anesthetic management of children with hemoglobinopathies, in particular, sickle cell disease. Finally, Dr. Richards and his team from

Anesthesiology Clin 27 (2009) xv–xvi
doi:10.1016/j.anclin.2009.07.003
1932-2275/09/$ – see front matter © 2009 Elsevier Inc. All rights reserved.

Seattle Children's Hospital provide us a fresh perspective on strategies for blood conservation in children.

The editors would like to thank all the contributors for their outstanding efforts to bring this issue to fruition. We would also like to thank Ms. Glover at Elsevier for her tireless assistance and patience while putting this issue together.

Arjunan Ganesh, MBBS
Department of Anesthesiology and Critical Care
The Children's Hospital of Philadelphia
34th Street and Civic Center Boulevard
Philadelphia, PA 19104, USA

Ronald Litman, DO
Department of Anesthesiology and Critical Care
The Children's Hospital of Philadelphia
34th Street and Civic Center Boulevard
Philadelphia, PA 19104, USA

E-mail addresses:
ganesha@email.chop.edu (A. Ganesh)
litmanr@email.chop.edu (R. Litman)

Pediatric Difficult Airway Management: Current Devices and Techniques

John Fiadjoe, MD*, Paul Stricker, MD

KEYWORDS

- Pediatric difficult airway management
- Pediatric video laryngoscopy • Fiberoptic intubation
- Optical stylets • Pediatric laryngeal mask

The anesthesiologist confronting the difficult pediatric airway is presented with a unique set of challenges. Adult difficult airway management techniques, such as awake or invasive approaches to airway management, often cannot be applied to children because of inadequate cooperation. Consequently, awake intubation in pediatrics is uncommon; most intubations are performed under general anesthesia or deep sedation. From a physiologic perspective, children, have higher rates of oxygen consumption, significantly shortening the period of apnea that can be safely tolerated. Normal developmental anatomic differences of the pediatric airway and the presence of craniofacial dysmorphisms, presents additional challenges to tracheal intubation.

Planning and preparation is the most important factor for successful airway management in these children. The authors have a standardized setup for the care of these patients. This setup consists of equipment and drugs, typically a lighted stylet for use if visualization is obscured, a laryngeal mask, a flexible fiberoptic bronchoscope, an antisialogogue, a topical anesthetic, an IV anesthetic (typically propofol), and a muscle relaxant. In the past, equipment available to care for these children was limited. With recent advances in video technology have come many new tools for pediatric airway management. Presented here is an overview and discussion of some of the devices and techniques address some of the challenges faced in caring for this population.

OPTICAL STYLETS

Optical stylets embody a combination of the form of a lighted stylet and the optics of a flexible fiberoptic bronchoscope. Many practitioners find navigation of these

Department of Anesthesiology and Critical Care Medicine, Children's Hospital of Philadelphia, University of Pennsylvania, 34th and Civic Center Boulevard, Philadelphia, PA 19104, USA
* Corresponding author.
E-mail address: fiadjoej@email.chop.edu (J. Fiadjoe).

Anesthesiology Clin 27 (2009) 185–195
doi:10.1016/j.anclin.2009.06.002
1932-2275/09/$ – see front matter © 2009 Elsevier Inc. All rights reserved.

anesthesiology.theclinics.com

relatively rigid stylets more intuitive than the flexible bronchoscope. There is a short learning curve, and their rigidity facilitates control of the stylet tip and allows for the displacement of soft tissue.[1] One advantage optical stylets have over flexible fiberoptic intubation is the ability to visualize the passage of the tip of the tracheal tube into the trachea. With flexible fiberoptic intubation, the advancement of the tracheal tube is not visualized, and any resistance to advancement of the tube into the trachea is usually managed blindly. Optical stylets allow the operator to place the tube into the trachea under direct vision because the optical vantage point is within the endotracheal tube, proximal to its distal tip.

Optical stylets are useful in the management of the pediatric difficult airway.[1–3] There is, however, a learning curve of approximately 20 intubations before the technique becomes facile. When using an optical stylet in a difficult intubation, a useful maneuver is to perform direct laryngoscopy with a standard blade, while using the stylet to navigate under the epiglottis.[4]

The Shikani Optical Stylet

The Shikani optical stylet (SOS; Clarus Medical, Minneapolis, Minnesota) is a J-shaped malleable stylet with a central optical channel that ends in an eyepiece (**Fig. 1**). A video camera can be attached to the eyepiece to display the image from the distal tip on a monitor. The SOS is placed inside an appropriately sized and lubricated endotracheal tube with the tip maintained just proximal to the endotracheal tube tip. The view through the eyepiece of an ideally positioned endotracheal tube should reveal a small rim of the endotracheal tube tip in front of the stylet. The SOS is malleable and can be configured to an individual patient's anatomy. The authors use two techniques when using the device: a two-practitioner technique or a single-practitioner technique. For the single-practitioner technique, the SOS is held in the dominant hand of the operator. Jaw thrust is performed with the nondominant hand and the tip of the SOS is placed along the curvature of the tongue in the midline. The ideal view through the eyepiece should reveal the base of the tongue in the upper half of the image and the space below the tongue in the lower half. Success with the optical stylet requires maintenance of this view as one advances the device along the curvature of the tongue into the hypopharynx. If this maneuver is correctly performed, the uvula should come into view as the stylet is advanced; this is a good indicator of midline insertion. Further advancement should reveal the epiglottis and the glottic opening. The SOS can be placed just past the vocal cords and the tube advanced into the trachea under direct vision. Some practitioners prefer a left molar approach when using the SOS; a higher success rate with this method has been reported for novice users.[5]

With the two-practitioner technique, the SOS is held with two hands, while the second practitioner performs jaw thrust and pulls the tongue forward to create space

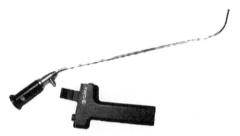

Fig. 1. Shikani optical stylet.

for the stylet. The two-handed technique may provide better control of the stylet tip. The SOS can also be used in combination with a laryngoscope, where the laryngoscope elevates the tongue and widens the hypopharyngeal space. The SOS is then placed below the epiglottis to visualize the glottic opening. Similar intubation times and success rate are reported using the SOS alone or in conjunction with a laryngoscope.

The SOS is a useful adjunct in the management of routine and difficult pediatric intubations. It is an uncomplicated tool that is easily learned, portable, and simple to prepare. Disadvantages include a short optical depth of field and the potential for impaired visualization from fogging and secretions.

Bonfils Endoscope

The Bonfils endoscope (Karl Storz Endoscopy, Tuttlingen, Germany) is a rigid stylet with a 40° anterior curve (**Fig. 2**).[6] It was originally designed more than 20 years ago and recently modified for pediatric use.[7] The rigid, nonmalleable shaft houses a fiberoptic channel that delivers a higher quality image than the SOS. The Bonfils is manufactured with two configurations—one with an eyepiece that can be mounted with a video camera and a second without an eyepiece that attaches to a Storz Direct Coupled Interface (DCI) camera (Karl Storz GmbH, Tuttlingen, Germany). The Bonfils is loaded and prepared in a similar fashion to the SOS. The manufacturer recommends a retromolar approach to intubation. However, the authors reserve this approach for cases in which the midline approach is unsuccessful. They have found a high success rate with the midline approach in infants and neonates. The SOS and Bonfils have ports for insufflating oxygen during intubation attempts. The authors avoid using these ports for this purpose in neonates and small children because of the risk of pneumothorax.[8,9] Because of the small infant and neonatal airway size, a pathway for oxygen egress is not assured when the stylet is in the trachea. Older children may tolerate low flows of oxygen during intubation. The manufacturer of the Bonfils recommends oxygen flows less than 3 L/min to minimize secretions on the optical lens. Successful use of the Bonfils was limited by secretions during elective use in a randomized pediatric study.[10] Suctioning the mouth and pharynx before intubation attempts and administering an antisialogogue can help prevent this problem. Additional measures to improve success rate include the application of jaw thrust by an assistant and the adjunctive use of a laryngoscope.

VIDEO/OPTICAL LARYNGOSCOPES

Video laryngoscopes of several designs are manufactured for use in children. Currently available designs include video laryngoscopes that integrate a camera into a laryngoscope blade, such as the GlideScope (Verathon, Bothwell, Washington) and Storz video laryngoscope (Karl Storz GmbH, Tuttlingen, Germany). Other devices are constructed using prisms and mirrors, such as the Airtraq optical laryngoscope (Prodol Meditec SA, Vizcaya, Spain) and the Truview EVO2 (Truphatek

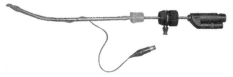

Fig. 2. Bonfils endoscope.

International, Netanya, Israel). The GlideScope, Storz video laryngoscope, Airtraq, and Truview EVO2 are currently available in sizes appropriate for pediatric patients of all ages. Each of these devices has design characteristics that make them advantageous for routine and difficult airway management.

Despite the apparent similarity to intubation of direct laryngoscopy, a different skill set is required for tracheal intubation using video guidance. The blade of the device is inserted in the midline or slightly to the left of midline in the oropharynx. The tongue, uvula, tongue base, epiglottis, and glottic opening are visualized in succession with proper advancement. The authors prefer to place the blade tip in the vallecula and reserve directly elevating the epiglottis for cases where glottic exposure is poor, with the blade tip in the vallecula. Once an optimal view is obtained, a preconfigured styletted tube is placed just lateral to or along the shaft of the video blade; the styletted tube is placed in the oropharynx under direct vision until the tube comes into view on the video monitor. Visualization of tube insertion into the pharynx reduces the chance of injury to the pharyngeal mucosa from a misguided tube that is blindly inserted.[11–16] The integration of a tracheal tube channel in the Airtraq directs the tube to the tip of the scope and circumvents this potential problem.

For anesthesiologists who are universally experienced with direct laryngoscopy, video laryngoscopy is an attractive modality for difficult intubation because of its similarity to intubation with a standard laryngoscope. Video laryngoscopy is not a panacea for difficult airway management, and several limitations have been noted. Firstly, some mouth opening is required to insert any of these devices—enough to allow passage of the device. Secondly, while nasotracheal intubation can be performed, these devices are primarily designed for orotracheal intubation with the exception of the Airtraq. Some problems seen with use of these devices include difficulty with tracheal tube placement despite an excellent view of the glottic opening, trauma to upper airway structures related to blind passage of the styletted tube into the pharynx, and poor visualization related to blood and secretions.

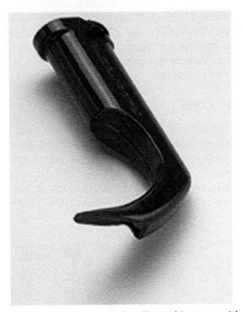

Fig. 3. GVL 2. (*Courtesy of* Verathon, Inc., Bothwell, Washington; with permission.)

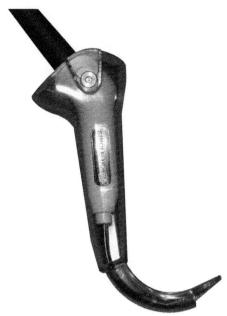

Fig. 4. GlideScope Cobalt.

GlideScope

The GlideScope integrates a high-resolution video camera into the tip of a plastic laryngoscope blade. The pediatric blade (GlideScope video laryngoscope [GVL] 2) features a curved blade with a 40° angulated tip (**Fig. 3**). The image from the tip of the GlideScope is displayed on a portable video screen. The tip of the device is heated to prevent fogging during use. Success with the GVL 2 is variable, with difficult visualization reported in neonates and infants.[17] The GVL 2 seems to be more appropriate for children older than 2 years.[18] The GlideScope Cobalt (**Fig. 4**) represents a new design. It has a thinner profile, allowing for easy placement in the smallest neonates, and a more anterior tip angle, which provides an improved wide-angle glottic view. A reusable video baton (**Fig. 5**) is inserted into a disposable plastic blade for intubation. Early clinical experience with this new version has been favorable; however, there are no clinical studies regarding its efficacy.

Storz Video Laryngoscope

The Storz DCI video laryngoscope (**Fig. 6**) is a rigid blade that integrates fiberoptics and a lens into the light source of Miller- and Macintosh-type blades. There are currently 4 blade designs: Macintosh 3 and Miller 0, 1, and 3. The blade connects to a device-specific camera that transmits the image to a video monitor. One advantage of these video laryngoscope blades is that they can be used for direct

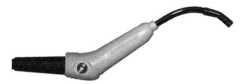

Fig. 5. GlideScope Cobalt reusable video baton.

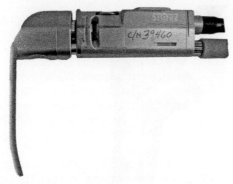

Fig. 6. The Storz Miller 1 video laryngoscope.

laryngoscopy. If the direct laryngoscopy view is poor, the operator can convert to using the video monitor view. This is particularly useful in children who are suspected, but not known, to be difficult to intubate by direct laryngoscopy. Unlike many other video systems, the Storz Miller 1 video laryngoscope allows documentation of the direct laryngoscopy grade before intubating using video guidance. The Storz Miller 1 video laryngoscope has been shown to improve laryngoscopy grade and intubation success in a difficult airway manikin model providing a one grade improvement over the direct laryngoscopy view.[19] The Storz video laryngoscope is a useful adjunct in the management of the difficult infant airway; the authors have successfully used it to rescue several infants in whom direct laryngoscopy failed.

Airtraq

The Airtraq is a single-use indirect laryngoscope that incorporates a guide channel for the endotracheal tube into the curve of the device. A magnified wide-angle image is transmitted from the distal tip using a series of prisms and mirrors to a viewfinder. The Airtraq incorporates an antifog system that requires a 30- to 45-second warm-up time. The tip of the Airtraq is placed in the vallecula; however, it is sometimes necessary to elevate the epiglottis to obtain an optimal view. The guidance of the endotracheal tube using the Airtraq is different from the video laryngoscopes without a channel; it requires the manipulation of the entire device to center the glottic opening and allow the advancement of the endotracheal tube. The Airtraq is available in pediatric and infant sizes (**Fig. 7**); a model of this device is available with the posterior wall of the endotracheal tube channel removed to enable use of this device for nasotracheal intubation.

Truview EVO2

The Truview EVO2 (**Fig. 8**) is a rigid laryngoscope with an angulated tip that uses a series of prisms to transmit the image from the distal tip to an eyepiece.[20] The device

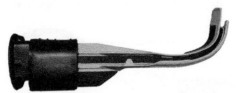

Fig. 7. Airtraq optical laryngoscope with size table. (*Courtesy of* Truphatek Ltd., Netanya, Israel; with permission.)

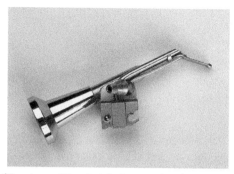

Fig. 8. Truview EVO2. (*Courtesy of* Truphatek, International, Netanya, Israel.)

tip is angulated 46° anteriorly from the direct line of sight, and the device provides a wide-angle magnified view. The Truview infant blade has been compared with the Miller laryngoscope blade in a prospective randomized trial; similar intubation times and better laryngeal views were found with the Truview.[21]

LARYNGEAL MASKS

Laryngeal masks continue to have an important place in the management of the challenging pediatric airway. They are useful as ventilation adjuncts and as conduits for tracheal intubation, particularly in patients with craniofacial dysmorphisms. Since the development of the classic laryngeal mask airway, there has been a proliferation of new supralaryngeal airway devices for use in adults and children. Although some models fail to offer significant design improvements, others have improved on the original design by Dr. Brain, making specific modifications to facilitate pediatric use. Laryngeal masks remain a critically important adjunct in the airway management of infants and neonates.

Some laryngeal masks incorporate the means to allow verification of correct positioning of the device and the ability to decompress the gastrointestinal tract via a gastric access channel. The LMA ProSeal (LMA North America, Inc, San Diego, California) is currently the only laryngeal mask incorporating a gastric channel that is available in all pediatric sizes.

A limitation of many infant-sized laryngeal masks when used as conduits to fiberoptic intubation is the inability to pass the pilot balloon of a cuffed tracheal tube through the airway tube of the laryngeal mask. The use of cuffed tubes in pediatric airway

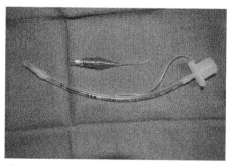

Fig. 9. Tracheal tube with cut pilot balloon.

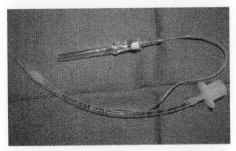

Fig. 10. IV catheter inserted into cut end of pilot balloon inflation line.

management is often advantageous; advantages include reduction in operating room pollution, reduction in the number of tracheal tube exchanges, and improved ventilation in children with reduced lung compliance. For many infants and children, initial placement of a cuffed tube when using a laryngeal mask as a conduit to intubation is advantageous because the additional step of replacing an uncuffed tube that is too small is avoided. Avoiding such extra steps is desirable because they are points at which a secured airway can be lost. If a cuffed tube is desired, several additional steps are required. The pilot balloon can be cut and discarded, thereby facilitating passage of the cuffed treacheal tube through the laryngeal mask. It can then be reconstructed by firmly inserting an appropriately sized intravenous (IV) catheter into the cut end of the tubing, retracting the needle, and applying a one-way Luer lock valve port adapter to the end of the IV catheter. This allows a manometer to be attached to the one-way valve for cuff inflation and measurement of the cuff pressure (**Figs. 9–11**). A less desirable alternative is to place an uncuffed endotracheal tube and then perform an endotracheal tube exchange to a cuffed tube. In the most dysmorphic children, a tube exchange may be very difficult, and the short tracheal length makes the margins for dislodgement of the tube exchanger very small.

Air-Q

The air-Q (Mercury Medical, Clearwater, Florida; **Figs. 12** and **13**) is a curved laryngeal mask. It has unique characteristics that facilitate fiberoptic intubation with cuffed endotracheal tubes in infants and neonates without the need to perform additional maneuvers. The airway tube is wide enough to accommodate the pilot balloon of standard endotracheal tubes and the length is shortened to facilitate the removal of the mask after tracheal intubation. The 15-mm adapter on the airway tube is detachable, thereby facilitating fiberoptic intubation through the device. As with other laryngeal masks, it is easy to insert and position, and full glottic visualization is typical when using the air-Q as a conduit for fiberoptic intubation in patients of all ages. The

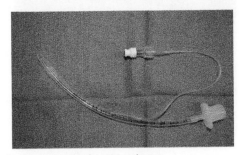

Fig. 11. Needle-free valve port attached to IV catheter.

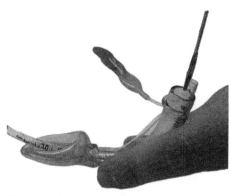

Fig. 12. Air-Q airway with tracheal tube in situ stabilized by laryngeal forceps.

manufacturer supplies a stabilizer bar, which is a long plastic rod with a triangulated tip that wedges securely into the end of the endotracheal tube. This stabilizer bar is used to stabilize the endotracheal tube as the air-Q is removed. The air-Q is a useful adjunct in the armamentarium of the pediatric anesthesiologist, and it addresses several challenging issues in the use of laryngeal masks as intubation conduits in the smallest patients.

FLEXIBLE SCOPES

The flexible fiberoptic scope remains the gold standard for the management of the difficult airway. Recent technological advances have allowed the introduction of charge-coupled devices into these scopes, thereby providing an image quality comparable to that seen with rigid bronchoscopes. These high-definition scopes are limited in size, the smallest being approximately 2.7 mm. The authors have a methodical approach to fiberoptic intubation in children, with a primary plan and several backup plans. An inhaled induction of anesthesia is typically performed, and an antisialogogue is administered after obtaining IV access. The airway is then anesthetized with a topical local anesthetic (typically lidocaine) after an adequate anesthetic depth is obtained. Adequate anesthetic depth can be confirmed by the lack of movement to a sustained jaw thrust for 5 seconds. Oxymetazoline is applied to the nares bilaterally and a fiberoptic examination of both nares performed to assess patency. A modified nasal trumpet (**Fig. 14**) facilitates the maintenance of anesthetic depth and oxygenation during fiberoptic intubation in children. The modified nasal trumpet has a 15-mm tracheal tube adapter placed into the flared end (see **Fig. 14**).

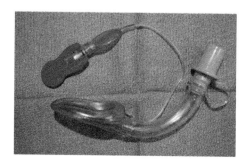

Fig. 13. Air-Q.

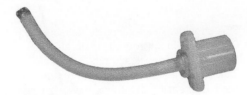

Fig. 14. Modified nasal trumpet.

Provided there is no nasal obstruction, a lubricated modified nasal trumpet is placed into one nare and then connected to the anesthesia circuit. An inhaled anesthetic and oxygen are administered via the trumpet as the child spontaneously ventilates. Fiberoptic intubation can then be performed through the oropharynx or controlateral nare.

SUMMARY

Difficult intubation remains a significant cause of morbidity in pediatric airway management. All practitioners are encouraged to develop a systematic approach to the care of these patients. Many of the outlined devices and techniques may facilitate intubation in this patient population; however, mastery of all or several of these devices is impractical. The authors recommend that all practitioners maintain skill in fiberoptic intubation and two additional devices. This skill development can only come about by frequent use of these techniques in patients with normal airways.

REFERENCES

1. Shukry M, Hanson R, Koveleskie J, et al. Management of the difficult pediatric airway with Shikani Optical Stylet. Paediatr Anaesth 2005;15:342–5.
2. Mihai R, Blair E, Kay H, et al. A quantitative review and meta-analysis of performance of non-standard laryngoscopes and rigid fibreoptic intubation aids. Anaesthesia 2008;63:745–60.
3. Pfitzner L, Cooper MG, Ho D. The Shikani Seeing Stylet for difficult intubation in children: initial experience. Anaesth Intensive Care 2002;30:462–6.
4. Aucoin S, Vlatten A, Hackmann T. Difficult airway management with the Bonfils fiberscope in a child with Hurler syndrome. Paediatr Anaesth 2009;19:421–2.
5. Yao YT, Jia NG, Li CH, et al. Comparison of endotracheal intubation with the Shikani Optical Stylet using the left molar approach and direct laryngoscopy. Chin Med J 2008;121:1324–7.
6. Halligan M, Charters P. A clinical evaluation of the Bonfils Intubation Fibrescope. Anaesthesia 2003;58:1087–91.
7. Wong P. Intubation times for using the Bonfils intubation fibrescope. Br J Anaesth 2003;91:757 [author reply 757–8].
8. Hemmerling T, Bracco D. Subcutaneous cervical and facial emphysema with the use of the Bonfils fiberscope and high-flow oxygen insufflation. Anesth Analg 2008;106:260–2.
9. Sorbello M, Paratore A, Morello G, et al. Bonfils fiberscope: better preoxygenate rather than oxygenate! Anesth Analg 2009;108:386.
10. Bein B, Wortmann F, Meybohm P, et al. Evaluation of the pediatric Bonfils fiberscope for elective endotracheal intubation. Paediatr Anaesth 2008;18:1040–4.
11. Chin KJ, Arango MF, Paez AF, et al. Palatal injury associated with the GlideScope. Anaesth Intensive Care 2007;35:449–50.

12. Cooper RM. Complications associated with the use of the GlideScope videolaryngoscope. Can J Anaesth 2007;54:54–7.
13. Cross P, Cytryn J, Cheng KK. Perforation of the soft palate using the GlideScope videolaryngoscope. Can J Anaesth 2007;54:588–9.
14. Hirabayashi Y. Pharyngeal injury related to GlideScope videolaryngoscope. Otolaryngol Head Neck Surg 2007;137:175–6.
15. Hsu WT, Hsu SC, Lee YL, et al. Penetrating injury of the soft palate during GlideScope intubation. Anesth Analg 2007;104:1609–10.
16. Hsu WT, Tsao SL, Chen KY, et al. Penetrating injury of the palatoglossal arch associated with use of the GlideScope videolaryngoscope in a flame burn patient. Acta Anaesthesiol Taiwan 2008;46:39–41.
17. Trevisanuto D, Fornaro E, Verghese C. The GlideScope video laryngoscope: initial experience in five neonates. Can J Anaesth 2006;53:423–4.
18. Kim JT, Na HS, Bae JY, et al. GlideScope video laryngoscope: a randomized clinical trial in 203 paediatric patients. Br J Anaesth 2008;101:531–4.
19. Fiadjoe JE, Stricker PA, Hackell RS, et al. The efficacy of the Storz Miller 1 video laryngoscope in a simulated infant difficult intubation. Anesth Analg 2009;108:1783–6.
20. Li JB, Xiong YC, Wang XL, et al. An evaluation of the TruView EVO2 laryngoscope. Anaesthesia 2007;62:940–3.
21. Singh R, Singh P, Vajifdar H. A comparison of Truview infant EVO2 laryngoscope with the Miller blade in neonates and infants. Paediatr Anaesth 2009;19:338–42.

Ultrasound Guidance for Pediatric Peripheral Nerve Blockade

Arjunan Ganesh, MBBS[a,b,]*, Harshad G. Gurnaney, MBBS, MPH[a,b]

KEYWORDS

- Peripheral nerve block • Pediatric • Ultrasound guidance
- Regional anesthesia • Post operative analgesia

The efficacy and safety of peripheral nerve blocks (PNBs) for postoperative analgesia after orthopedic surgery has been well established in adults. Recent studies have also shown earlier functional recovery after surgery in patients treated with PNBs. In children, PNB is gaining in popularity and increasing data are emerging to show feasibility, efficacy, and safety in this population. Pediatric PNBs are usually performed under general anesthesia.

The major PNB used in children include interscalene and infraclavicular blocks for procedures on the upper extremity and lumbar plexus, and femoral and sciatic nerve blocks for lower extremity surgery. Continuous PNBs have the ability to prolong efficacy and can also be performed at home. The use of ultrasound to perform PNB has increased its success and speed of onset through permitting clear anatomic visualization of the whole process. Performance of PNB requires personnel who are trained in regional anesthesia, appropriate equipment, and education of the patient and patient's family and the nursing staff involved in the postoperative care of these patients.

PNBs in children are emerging as a safe and effective technique for postoperative analgesia after orthopedic surgery in children. Several studies in children have shown the safety, feasibility, and efficacy of PNB.[1–8] The advantages of PNB include efficient, site-specific analgesia and a decrease in the need for opioids, and consequently a decrease in opioid-related side effects.

The most common PNBs performed in children are single-injection blocks.[9] Continuous peripheral nerve blocks (CPNB) are performed when significant analgesia is

This work was supported by the Department of Anesthesiology and Critical Care at The Children's Hospital of Philadelphia, PA 19104.
[a] Department of Anesthesiology and Critical Care Medicine, The Children's Hospital of Philadelphia, 34th Street and Civic Center Boulevard, Philadelphia, PA 19104-4399, USA
[b] University of Pennsylvania School of Medicine, 3451 Walnut St, Philadelphia, PA 19104, USA
* Corresponding author. Department of Anesthesiology and Critical Care Medicine, The Children's Hospital of Philadelphia, 34th Street and Civic Center Boulevard, Philadelphia, PA 19104-4399.
E-mail address: ganesha@email.chop.edu (A. Ganesh).

required for periods exceeding 12 to 24 hours. Ultrasound guidance for PNBs is emerging as a popular technique. Use of ultrasound for PNBs has been shown to quicken onset time, improve the quality of the block,[10] and decrease the amount of local anesthetic needed.[11,12] However, complications such as intravascular injection may occur even with ultrasound guidance,[13,14] and hence other routine precautions to prevent intravascular injections must be taken.

Localizing the nerve with a nerve stimulator before injecting local anesthetic is the most widely used technique for performing PNB. Several types of nerve stimulators are available, though using only one type in a practice would be prudent. Insulated needles are used in conjunction with stimulators. For most PNB in pediatrics, a 1- or 2-in block needle is adequate. For deeper blocks (sciatic nerve block) and in larger children, a 4-in needle may be appropriate.

Using ultrasound for PNB recently has become popular. Ultrasound helps localize the neural structures and guide the needle to the intended target. Ultrasound has been shown to increase success rates, increase the speed of onset, and lower the volume of local anesthetic needed for PNB.[10,11,15] Ultrasound machines are cheaper than ever before and the technique is noninvasive, which has increased its popularity in performing PNB. However, one must be trained to use it to ensure safety and increase efficacy. The higher the frequency used, the better the resolution (the ability to distinguish two adjacent objects). However, as the frequency increases, more of the ultrasound beam is absorbed by the medium and the beam cannot penetrate far. Therefore, higher frequencies (for example, 7.5–15 MHz) are used to provide good detail of superficial structures, such as the interscalene brachial plexus and femoral nerve, whereas lower frequencies (3-7.5 MHz) are used to image deeper structures, such as the sciatic nerve and brachial plexus. However, in small children, because of their smaller size, higher frequency transducers may be used to image the sciatic nerve and infraclavicular brachial plexus.

This article discusses ultrasound-guided techniques used to perform some of the common upper and lower extremity and truncal PNBs in children.

UPPER EXTREMITY BLOCKS: INTERSCALENE, INFRACLAVICULAR, AND AXILLARY

The brachial plexus can be blocked at the interscalene, infraclavicular, or axillary area. A clear understanding of the anatomy and variations helps in selecting the ideal block for the particular procedure and in improving the success and efficacy of the block. A thorough knowledge of anatomy also helps in understanding the relationship of important surrounding structures, and potentially minimizes complications or permits early recognition of complications. In addition, practitioners performing the PNB must understand the extent of the surgical procedure to perform the appropriate blockade.

Anatomy

The brachial plexus is formed by the anterior primary rami of the lower four cervical and first thoracic spinal nerves. The upper two roots join to form the upper trunk, the middle root forms the lower trunk, and the lower two roots join to form the lower trunk. The trunks emerge between the scalenus anterior and scalenus medius muscles. Each trunk divides into anterior and posterior divisions, posterior to the clavicle. In the infraclavicular area, the posterior divisions of all three trunks join together to form the posterior cord, the anterior divisions of the upper two trunks join together for the lateral cord, and the anterior division of the lower trunk forms the medial cord. In the axilla, the cords radiate various branches, finally forming the median, radial, ulnar, musculocutaneous, and other nerves that innervate the upper extremity.

INTERSCALENE BRACHIAL PLEXUS BLOCK
Indications

An interscalene brachial plexus block is necessary when surgery is to performed on the shoulder and proximal to the elbow joint.

Technique

The interscalene brachial plexus block was first described in 1970 using the paresthesia technique.[16] This block is now more commonly performed using a nerve stimulator. However, a recent study questioned the reliability of the nerve stimulator for this particular block,[17] and the use of ultrasound guidance is increasing.

Although peripheral nerve blocks in children are commonly performed under general anesthesia, the performance of interscalene blocks under general anesthesia has raised some controversy after a report of a series spinal cord injuries.[18] Recent practice guidelines released by the American Society of Regional Anesthesia also advise against performing this block in anesthetized subjects.[19] All reported cases of spinal cord injury involved the use of neurostimulation, and whether the use of ultrasound, although seemingly logical, helps prevent this dreaded complication remains unknown.

Ultrasound Guidance

In the authors' practice, the interscalene block is routinely performed in anesthetized children, and ultrasound guidance (**Fig. 1**) is used in all cases. Interscalene blocks can be performed using only ultrasound guidance or a combination of ultrasound guidance and nerve stimulation. A high-resolution probe (≥ 10 MHz) is recommended, because the brachial plexus is superficial. The probe is placed approximately 2 cm above and parallel to the clavicle. After visualizing the brachial plexus in the interscalene groove, the needle is advanced (lateral to medial direction) in line with the ultrasound beam, thus enabling the visualization of the entire needle. If a nerve stimulator is used in conjunction, the recommendations in the previous paragraph can be followed. Also, the same caution as outlined previously must be exercised when injecting the local anesthetic. The needle may also be advanced across the beam, but makes visualization of the tip more difficult. The dose of local anesthetic given is 0.5 mL/kg of 0.2% ropivacaine.

INFRACLAVICULAR BRACHIAL PLEXUS BLOCKADE
Indications

Infraclavicular brachial plexus blockade is indicated for surgery on and distal to the elbow.

Technique (Nerve Stimulation)

Several techniques for infraclavicular brachial plexus blockade have been described.[20–24] Almost all techniques have the insertion point close to the coracoid process. This block is easier to perform with the arm abducted. The needle (22 gauge 2-in or 21 gauge 4-in insulated) is advanced toward the plexus until the cords are stimulated. Stimulation of the musculocutaneous nerve should not be accepted because this structure exits the axillary sheath early in a significant percentage of patients and injection may not result in blockade of other nerves of the brachial plexus.

Stimulation of the posterior cord or multiple cords may predict a successful infraclavicular block.[25] When stimulation is just present with the nerve stimulation approximately 0.5 mA, 0.5 to 1 mL/kg (maximum of 40 mL) of 0.15% to 0.2% ropivacaine

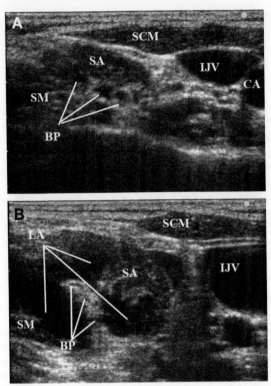

Fig. 1. Ultrasound images of interscalene block before the injection of local anesthetic (*A*) and after injection of local anesthetic (*B*). BP, brachial plexus; CA, carotid artery; IJV, internal jugular vein; LA, local anesthetic; SA, scalenus anterior; SCM, sternocleidomastoid; SM, scalenus medius.

is injected in increments after negative aspiration of blood. If resistance is encountered or blood is aspirated, the needle is withdrawn, flushed and the procedure repeated.

Ultrasound Guidance

One approach described by Sandhu and Capan[26] is the technique used by the author. With the arm abducted and after sterile preparation, the ultrasound probe is placed just inferomedial to the coracoid process to obtain a sagittal image of the axillary artery (**Fig. 2**). In young or thin children, a high-resolution probe can be used, whereas in bigger children a lower frequency probe is used to achieve greater depth of penetration. An 18-gauge Tuohy needle is advanced through the pectoralis major and minor muscles using an in-plane technique and is directed toward the posterior cord of the brachial plexus, where 0.5 mL/kg of 0.15% to 0.2% ropivacaine is injected in increments. One can also verify spread of local anesthetic around the lateral and medial cords using ultrasound. If necessary, separate injections may be made around the lateral and medial cords.

AXILLARY BRACHIAL PLEXUS BLOCK
Indications

Axillary brachial plexus block is indicated for surgery distal to the elbow.

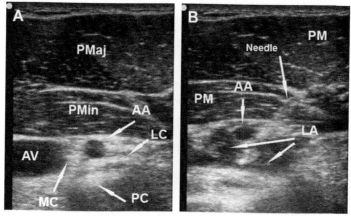

Fig. 2. Ultrasound images of the infraclavicular block, preinjection (*A*) and postinjection (*B*). AA, axillary artery; AV, axillary vein; LA, local anesthetic; LC, lateral cord; MC, medial cord; PC, posterior cord, PMaj, pectoralis major; PMin, pectoralis minor.

Technique

Multiple injection technique using the nerve stimulator is the gold standard for this block.[27] With the arm abducted and externally rotated, the axilla is prepped. The axillary artery is felt and a 24-gauge 1-in or 22-gauge 2-in insulated needle is advanced on either side of the axillary artery and the median, ulnar, and radial nerves are separately sought out and approximately 5 mL of local anesthetic is injected around each of these nerves. The musculocutaneous nerve is separately identified within the belly of the coracobrachialis using the nerve stimulator and another 5 mL of local anesthetic is injected.

Ultrasound Guidance

All four nerves can be clearly identified using a high-resolution ultrasound probe and injected under direct ultrasound guidance.[28] The position of the arm is the same as for the nerve stimulator technique. Small quantities of local anesthetic are adequate to perform this block. Needle may be advanced either using the in-plane technique or out-of-plane technique.

MEDIAN AND RADIAL NERVE BLOCK ABOVE THE ELBOW
Indications

Median and radial nerve block above the elbow is indicated for surgery to the hand.

Technique

The median (**Fig. 3A**) and radial nerves (**Fig. 3B**) can be blocked easily above the elbow with ultrasound guidance using a high-resolution probe. The median nerve lies immediately medial to the brachial artery, and the radial nerve lies adjacent to the antero-lateral aspect of the humerus. The needle may be advanced using the in-plane or out-of-plane technique.

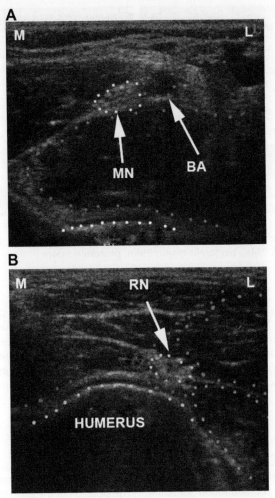

Fig. 3. Ultrasound images of the median nerve (*A*) and the radial nerve (*B*) above the elbow. BA, brachial artery; L, lateral; M, medial; MN, median nerve; RN, radial nerve.

LOWER EXTREMITY BLOCKS: LUMBAR PLEXUS, FEMORAL, AND SCIATIC

Lower extremity nerve blocks have gained popularity in recent years with the increase in lower extremity sports medicine procedures. One of the concerns with lower extremity regional anesthesia has been the inability to perform a single nerve block to provide complete postoperative anesthesia/analgesia. Another factor has been the availability of an alternate technique (ie, neuraxial anesthesia [caudal/epidural/spinal]), which is more widely performed and with which most practitioners are familiar. The use of nerve stimulation and, more recently, of ultrasound guidance has helped encourage use of PNBs for providing anesthesia and analgesia for these procedures.

Appropriate placement of these nerve blocks requires anesthesia practitioners to be familiar with the anatomy of neurovascular structures in the lower extremity and the sensory distribution of the nerves.

Lumbar Plexus Anatomy

The lumbar plexus lies within the substance of the psoas major muscle, anterior to the transverse processes of the lumbar vertebrae. The first three and a part of the fourth lumbar ventral rami form the lumbar plexus. The lumbar plexus lies between the anterior and the posterior masses of the psoas major in line with the intervertebral foramina. The branches of the plexus include the iliohypogastric, ilioinguinal, genitofemoral, lateral femoral cutaneous, femoral, and obturator nerves.[29–31]

The femoral nerve descends through the psoas major and emerges at its lateral border. Above the inguinal ligament it lies between the psoas major and iliacus muscle deep to the iliac fascia. Posterior to the inguinal ligament the femoral nerve lies in a plane deep to the fascia lata and the fascia iliaca and is lateral to the femoral artery.[32,33] As the nerve passes into the thigh, it divides into an anterior and a posterior division and quickly arborizes. The anterior division of the femoral nerve supplies the skin of the anterior and medial surface of the thigh, muscular branches to the sartorius and pectineus muscles, and an articular branch to the hip joint. The posterior division supplies cutaneous innervation to the anteromedial aspect of the lower leg down to the medial aspect of the foot and muscular branches to the quadriceps femoris and an articular branch to the knee joint.

LUMBAR PLEXUS BLOCK

The lumbar plexus provides sensory innervation to the anterior surface of the leg up to the knee and along the anteromedial aspect of the lower leg up to the medial aspect of the foot. The lumbar plexus block has been described in pediatric regional anesthesia.[30,34–36] A few studies have reported that this block provides excellent postoperative analgesia after hip and femoral shaft surgeries.

The use of ultrasound guidance to help place this nerve block has been described in children. An observational study evaluated the landmarks for placing lumbar plexus block in pediatric patients. In this study, the authors found that the point at two thirds of the distance from the midline on a line connecting the L4 vertebrae to a paramedian line through the posterior superior iliac spine to be feasible for placing a lumbar plexus block.[37]

Ultrasound Guidance

The lumbar paravertebral region should be examined in a longitudinal paravertebral plane to evaluate the transverse processes of L4 through L5. The erector spinae, quadratus lumborum, and psoas major muscles then should be evaluated in a transverse scan. In a transverse scan, the lumbar plexus appears as an ovoid structure consisting of hypoechoic dots (fascicles) within the substance of the psoas muscle.

Technique

To place a lumbar plexus block, the child is positioned in the lateral decubitus position with the nonoperative side down. Ultrasound scanning of the area using a 3 to 5 MHz curved array probe held in a paramedian longitudinal plane is performed to identify the depth and lateral edge of the transverse processes. The probe then can be rotated to a transverse plane. The lumbar plexus can be identified within the substance of the psoas muscle as a hypoechoic structure.

The ultrasound probe is then reoriented in the longitudinal paramedian plane. The nerve stimulator is set at 2 mA to identify the plexus. A 4-in insulated stimulating needle is placed perpendicular to the skin to elicit stimulation of the quadriceps femoris muscle. The needle is advanced using the in-plane approach so it can be observed at all times during advancement. After identification of the plexus, the needle position is adjusted to achieve approximately 1 mA of stimulation before the local anesthetic is injected. If long-term analgesia is required, a catheter can be placed into the region of the lumbar plexus after the local anesthetic is placed. The transverse processes serve as a good landmark to the depth of the lumbar plexus. The lumbar plexus should be no more than 2 cm deep to the transverse process of L4.[29,30,35]

Dose of Local Anesthetic

For lumbar plexus blockade, 0.5 mL/kg of 0.2% ropivacaine should be used, up to a maximum of 20 mL. Caution should be used during injection of the local anesthetic because of the potential for epidural spread. A good technique is to inject the dose in 5-mL increments with frequent aspiration and continuous hemodynamic monitoring.[32]

FEMORAL NERVE BLOCK

Femoral nerve block has been described extensively in adult regional anesthesia.[38] The feasibility of ultrasound guidance has been extensively evaluated in placing femoral nerve blocks in adult population.[11] These studies have found that the onset of sensory block and duration of postoperative analgesia is better with ultrasound guidance than with nerve stimulation.[12,39] The incidence of failed block was not seen to be significantly different in these studies. Femoral nerve block in combination with sciatic nerve block in pediatric patients using ultrasound guidance was seen to have a 30% increase in duration of postoperative analgesia.[12] In addition, a decrease was seen in the amount of local anesthetic needed in the ultrasound group compared with the nerve stimulation group.

Indications

This block is used for perioperative analgesia for femur fractures, surgery on the anterior thigh, arthroscopy of the knee, anterior cruciate ligament reconstruction, and total knee arthroplasty as part of a multimodal regimen.

Technique

The femoral nerve divides into an anterior and posterior division in the groin region. For procedures involving the knee joint, block of the posterior division is important. This portion is identified through stimulation of the quadriceps muscle using the nerve stimulator. The groin region is prepped and draped in sterile fashion. With the patient in the supine position, a linear ultrasound probe is used to perform this block. The probe (linear) is held close and parallel to the inguinal ligament, which allows the nerve to be imaged before division.

The initial mapping scan should identify the femoral nerve, artery, and vein and branches of the femoral artery by scanning in a caudal direction (superficial femoral artery).[33] The nerve is found lateral to the vessels, superficial to the iliopsoas muscles, and beneath the fascia iliaca. The nerve seems to be a hyperechoic oval structure (**Fig. 4**). The needle is advanced in the out-of-plane approach with the nerve positioned in the center of the field. Experts recommend placing the needle above the level of origin of the superficial femoral artery and at the lateral border of the nerve to decrease the risk for accidental vascular injury. The needle is placed with the nerve stimulator set at 1 mA to identify the femoral nerve. The needle position is adjusted to achieve stimulation at approximately 0.5 mA before injection of the local anesthetic for a single-injection femoral nerve block.

Dose of Local Anesthetic

For femoral nerve blockade, 0.5 to 1 mL/kg of 0.2% ropivacaine should be used, up to a maximum of 30 mL. For prolonged postoperative analgesia, a catheter (stimulating

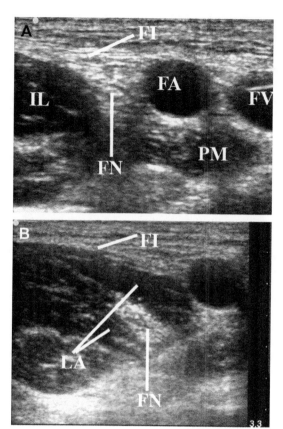

Fig. 4. Ultrasound images of the femoral nerve preinjection (*A*) and postinjection (*B*). FA, femoral artery; FN, femoral nerve; FV, femoral vein; IL, iliacus; LA, local anesthetic; PM, psoas major.

or nonstimulating) can be placed through the needle with this technique before the local anesthetic is injected.

SAPHENOUS NERVE BLOCK

Saphenous nerve block is useful as a supplement to the sciatic nerve block for foot and ankle surgery. Techniques for performing saphenous block include perifemoral approach, transsartorial approach, block at the medial femoral condyle, below-the-knee field block, and blockade at the level of the medial malleolus.[40] The transsartorial block was seen to be superior to the other techniques in a volunteer study.[40] The sartorius muscle is identified and the point of needle insertion is 3 to 4 cm superior to the superomedial aspect of the patella. This approach relies on the detection of a paresthesia in the saphenous distribution.

Sacral Plexus Regional Anesthesia

Anatomy

The sciatic nerve is formed of two components: tibial and common peroneal nerves. The L4 through L5 nerve roots and the anterior divisions of the sacral plexus (S1 through S3) form the tibial nerve, whereas the posterior divisions of the same nerve roots (L4 through S3) form the common peroneal component. The sciatic nerve exits the pelvis by way of the greater sciatic notch.

At this level, the sciatic nerve lies lateral and posterior to the ischial spine. In the thigh the nerve is posterior to the lesser trochanter of the femur on the posterior surface of the adductor magnus and deep to the biceps femoris (**Fig. 5**). In the upper part of the popliteal fossa, the sciatic nerve lies posterolateral to the popliteal vessels. The sciatic nerve divides into the two components in the popliteal fossa. The tibial branch continues along the tibialis posterior muscle, along the posterior tibial vessels. The common peroneal nerve diverges laterally in the popliteal fossa and lies subcutaneously just behind the fibular head, where it is prone to injury.[31]

SCIATIC NERVE BLOCK

Efficacy of the sciatic nerve block in providing postoperative analgesia for procedures involving the posterior aspect of the leg, lower leg, and foot has been described in children.[41,42] Although the depth of this nerve led to increased technical difficulty in using ultrasound guidance for this nerve block, recent reports in adults and children have shown its feasibility.[43–45] One prospective study in pediatric patients showed that using ultrasound guidance increased the duration of postoperative analgesia by 30%.[12] In addition, a decreased amount of local anesthetic was needed in the ultrasound group.

Other studies have shown that ultrasound guidance decreases time to completion of nerve block and also has less needle passes for block completion.[39] It also provides a real-time assessment of delivery of the local anesthetic around the nerve and helps identify needle tip dislodgement during injection.

Subgluteal Approach

The depth of this nerve from the skin in the gluteal region (6–8 cm) made high-frequency ultrasound difficult to use to localize this nerve. The more superficial location of the sciatic nerve in the subgluteal makes use of ultrasound guidance for this approach feasible (**Fig. 5**). The nerve is typically located in the space between the ischial tuberosity and the greater trochanter.[45] After identifying the bony landmarks, the nerve can be visualized as a hyperechoic flattened structure between the gluteus maximus and quadriceps femoris muscles, and lateral to the semitendinosus muscle. To differentiate it from the tendon of the biceps femoris muscle, the nerve structure can be followed down the leg as a hyperechoic bundle, but the tendon will continue

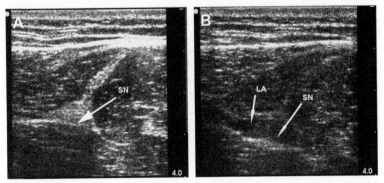

Fig. 5. Ultrasound images of the sciatic nerve preinjection (*A*) and postinjection (*B*) in the subgluteal area. LA, local anesthetic; SN, sciatic nerve.

into a muscle bundle. After the needle is placed near the sciatic nerve, stimulation is sought to confirm that the structure is the sciatic nerve. Local anesthetic is injected after the sciatic nerve is stimulated at 0.5 mA or less.

Popliteal Approach

For the posterior approach, the needle insertion is between the lateral border of the biceps femoris and medial border of the semimembranous/semitendinous tendons. For the lateral approach, the needle is inserted between the groove of the biceps femoris and the vastus lateralis on the lateral aspect of the thigh at approximately the junction of the proximal two thirds and distal one third of the thigh.

Posterior Approach

The posterior tibial component of the sciatic nerve is posterior and somewhat lateral to the popliteal artery. When scanning cephalad, this nerve is joined by the common peroneal nerve from the lateral side (**Fig. 6**). This nerve can be traced further cephalad and will maintain the hyperechoic texture. The needle entry point is as high in the popliteal fossa between the semimembranous and biceps femoris tendons medial to the biceps femoris tendon. A 21-gauge 4-inch stimulating needle is introduced perpendicular to the skin and advanced until the sciatic nerve is stimulated. The initial current from the nerve stimulator is set at 1.0 mA, 2 Hz, 0.1 ms. After either branch of the sciatic nerve is identified (ie, common peroneal nerve, which is identified by dorsiflexion or eversion of the foot or posterior tibial nerve which is identified by plantar flexion and inversion), the needle is positioned to reduce the stimulating current to 0.5 mA before the local anesthetic is injected.[46,47] Inversion response to nerve stimulation has been shown to have better clinical outcomes than plantar flexion and eversion.[48,49] In randomized prospective studies, ultrasound has been associated with a higher success rate, faster onset, and faster progression of sensorimotor block.[50,51]

Lateral approach

The needle entry point is in the groove between the vastus lateralis and the biceps femoris muscles approximately 5 to 10 cm cephalad to the lateral femoral condoyle. The needle is directed at a 30° angle posterior to the horizontal plane until stimulation

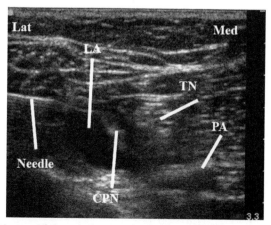

Fig. 6. Ultrasound image of the sciatic nerve in the popliteal fossa. CPN, common peroneal nerve; LA, local anesthetic; Lat, lateral; Med, medial; PA, popliteal artery; SN, sciatic nerve; TN, tibial nerve.

of either of the branches of the sciatic nerve is identified. If the stimulation cannot be elicited, the needle should be redirected with small changes in the angle by 3° to 5° anteriorly or posteriorly. The needle is positioned to reduce the stimulating current to 0.5 mA before the local anesthetic is injected.[52] In one study separate stimulation of the components of the sciatic nerve was associated with improved success rate.[53] Ultrasound guidance along with nerve stimulation was shown to improve the success rate of the lateral approach to the sciatic nerve at the mid-femoral level.[54]

Dose of Local Anesthetic

The dose of local anesthetic used for these techniques is 0.5 mL/kg of 0.15% ropivacaine, up to a maximum of 20 mL. A catheter (stimulating or nonstimulating) can be placed through the needle using either technique before local anesthetic is injected for prolonged postoperative analgesia.

TRUNK BLOCKS
Ilioinguinal and Iliohypogastric Nerve Blocks

The superficial location of these nerves makes this block amenable to the use of ultrasound guidance, and its use has also led to a dramatic decrease in the amount of local anesthetic needed to perform this block.[55,56] The anterior superior iliac spine serves as the landmark for this block, with the nerves identified as hypoechoic structures between the internal oblique and transversus abdominalis muscles. The amount of local anesthetic needed for this block is considerably less if using ultrasound guidance.[57] One study also found that blind injection of local anesthetic was often not in the correct plane.[58]

Dose of Local Anesthetic

The minimal volume necessary for ultrasound-guided ilioinguinal/iliohypogastric nerve block was found to be 0.075 mL/kg of 0.25% levobupivcaine.[55]

RECTUS SHEATH BLOCK

The rectus sheath block has been used for umbilical hernia repairs. It is a superficial field block of the intercostal nerves as they enter the posterior rectus sheath. Under ultrasound guidance, a needle is placed between the posterior rectus sheath and the rectus abdominis muscle (**Fig. 7**).[59] The procedure is performed bilaterally at the

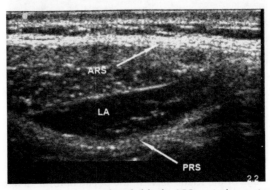

Fig. 7. Ultrasound image of the rectus sheath block. ARS, anterior rectus sheath; LA, local anesthetic; PRS, posterior rectus sheath; SN, sciatic nerve.

level of the umbilicus, with 0.25 mL/kg or less of 0.25% bupivacaine administered per side. Placing the local anesthetic close to the lateral border of the rectus abdominis muscle avoids accidental injury to the epigastric vessels.

A few studies have found this block to be useful for analgesia for umbilical hernia repair.[59,60]

LOCAL ANESTHETICS AND ADDITIVES

Ropivacaine and bupivacaine are the most commonly used local anesthetics for PNB in children. Because of its slightly better safety profile, ropivacaine is increasingly replacing bupivacaine as the preferred local anesthetic for PNB.[61,62] The authors now exclusively use ropivacaine for PNB in their practice.

In contrast with adult patients, lower concentrations of local anesthetics are sufficient in children (0.1%–0.2%), because almost all procedures are performed under general anesthesia. Using lower concentrations of local anesthetics provides adequate sensory block for postoperative analgesia and lowers the incidence of motor blockade. It also decreases the total dose administered, and consequently the potential for local anesthetic toxicity.

Several different agents have been added to local anesthetics to attempt to increase the duration and quality of analgesia, such as clonidine, which was shown to increase the duration of PNB in children.[63]

SUMMARY

The use of ultrasound guidance for PNB is increasing in popularity. A good knowledge of anatomy and adequate expertise in ultrasound will help experts perform these blocks successfully and safely with this technology.

REFERENCES

1. Dadure C, Capdevila X. Continuous peripheral nerve blocks in children. Best Pract Res Clin Anaesthesiol 2005;19:309–21.
2. Dadure C, Pirat P, Raux O, et al. Perioperative continuous peripheral nerve blocks with disposable infusion pumps in children: a prospective descriptive study. Anesth Analg 2003;97:687–90.
3. Ganesh A, Cucchiaro G. Multiple simultaneous perineural infusions for postoperative analgesia in adolescents in an outpatient setting. Br J Anaesth 2007;98: 687–9.
4. Ganesh A, Rose JB, Wells L, et al. Continuous peripheral nerve blockade for inpatient and outpatient postoperative analgesia in children. Anesth Analg 2007;105: 1234–42 [table of contents].
5. Giaufre E, Dalens B, Gombert A. Epidemiology and morbidity of regional anesthesia in children: a one-year prospective survey of the French-Language Society of Pediatric Anesthesiologists. Anesth Analg 1996;83:904–12.
6. Ludot H, Berger J, Pichenot V, et al. Continuous peripheral nerve block for postoperative pain control at home: a prospective feasibility study in children. Reg Anesth Pain Med 2008;33:52–6.
7. Rochette A, Dadure C, Raux O, et al. A review of pediatric regional anesthesia practice during a 17-year period in a single institution. Paediatr Anaesth 2007; 17:874–80.

8. van Geffen GJ, Gielen M. Ultrasound-guided subgluteal sciatic nerve blocks with stimulating catheters in children: a descriptive study. Anesth Analg 2006;103: 328–33 [table of contents].

9. Ecoffey C. Pediatric regional anesthesia—update. Curr Opin Anaesthesiol 2007; 20:232–5.

10. Marhofer P, Schrogendorfer K, Koinig H, et al. Ultrasonographic guidance improves sensory block and onset time of three-in-one blocks. Anesth Analg 1997;85:854–7.

11. Casati A, Baciarello M, Di Cianni S, et al. Effects of ultrasound guidance on the minimum effective anaesthetic volume required to block the femoral nerve. Br J Anaesth 2007;98:823–7.

12. Marhofer P, Schrogendorfer K, Wallner T, et al. Ultrasonographic guidance reduces the amount of local anesthetic for 3-in-1 blocks. Reg Anesth Pain Med 1998;23:584–8.

13. Loubert C, Williams SR, Helie F, et al. Complication during ultrasound-guided regional block: accidental intravascular injection of local anesthetic. Anesthesiology 2008;108:759–60.

14. Zetlaoui PJ, Labbe JP, Benhamou D. Ultrasound guidance for axillary plexus block does not prevent intravascular injection. Anesthesiology 2008;108:761.

15. Dingemans E, Williams SR, Arcand G, et al. Neurostimulation in ultrasound-guided infraclavicular block: a prospective randomized trial. Anesth Analg 2007;104:1275–80 [table of contents].

16. Winnie AP. Interscalene brachial plexus block. Anesth Analg 1970;49:455–66.

17. Urmey WF, Stanton J. Inability to consistently elicit a motor response following sensory paresthesia during interscalene block administration. Anesthesiology 2002;96:552–4.

18. Benumof JL. Permanent loss of cervical spinal cord function associated with interscalene block performed under general anesthesia. Anesthesiology 2000;93: 1541–4.

19. Neal JM, Bernards CM, Hadzic A, et al. ASRA practice advisory on neurologic complications in regional anesthesia and pain medicine. Reg Anesth Pain Med 2008;33:404–15.

20. Borgeat A, Ekatodramis G, Dumont C. An evaluation of the infraclavicular block via a modified approach of the Raj technique. Anesth Analg 2001;93:436–41, 434th contents page.

21. Labat G. Brachial plexus block: details of technique. Anesth Analg 1927;6:81–2.

22. Raj PP, Montgomery SJ, Nettles D, et al. Infraclavicular brachial plexus block–a new approach. Anesth Analg 1973;52:897–904.

23. Sims JK. A modification of landmarks for infraclavicular approach to brachial plexus block. Anesth Analg 1977;56:554–5.

24. Whiffler K. Coracoid block—a safe and easy technique. Br J Anaesth 1981;53:845–8.

25. Lecamwasam H, Mayfield J, Rosow L, et al. Stimulation of the posterior cord predicts successful infraclavicular block. Anesth Analg 2006;102:1564–8.

26. Sandhu NS, Capan LM. Ultrasound-guided infraclavicular brachial plexus block. Br J Anaesth 2002;89:254–9.

27. Handoll HH, Koscielniak-Nielsen ZJ. Single, double or multiple injection techniques for axillary brachial plexus block for hand, wrist or forearm surgery. Cochrane Database Syst Rev 2006;(1):CD003842.

28. Casati A, Danelli G, Baciarello M, et al. A prospective, randomized comparison between ultrasound and nerve stimulation guidance for multiple injection axillary brachial plexus block. Anesthesiology 2007;106:992–6.

29. Awad IT, Duggan EM. Posterior lumbar plexus block: anatomy, approaches, and techniques. Reg Anesth Pain Med 2005;30:143–9.
30. Capdevila X, Coimbra C, Choquet O. Approaches to the lumbar plexus: success, risks, and outcome. Reg Anesth Pain Med 2005;30:150–62.
31. Enneking FK, Chan V, Greger J, et al. Lower-extremity peripheral nerve blockade: essentials of our current understanding. Reg Anesth Pain Med 2005;30:4–35.
32. Dalens B. [Peripheral nerve block of the limbs in children]. Cah Anesthesiol 1995; 43:291–7 [in French].
33. Orebaugh SL. The femoral nerve and its relationship to the lateral circumflex femoral artery. Anesth Analg 2006;102:1859–62.
34. Chayen D, Nathan H, Chayen M. The psoas compartment block. Anesthesiology 1976;45:95–9.
35. Dalens B, Tanguy A, Vanneuville G. Lumbar plexus block in children: a comparison of two procedures in 50 patients. Anesth Analg 1988;67:750–8.
36. Parkinson SK, Mueller JB, Little WL, et al. Extent of blockade with various approaches to the lumbar plexus. Anesth Analg 1989;68:243–8.
37. Capdevila X, Macaire P, Dadure C, et al. Continuous psoas compartment block for postoperative analgesia after total hip arthroplasty: new landmarks, technical guidelines, and clinical evaluation. Anesth Analg 2002;94:1606–13 [table of contents].
38. Vloka JD, Hadzic A, Drobnik L, et al. Anatomical landmarks for femoral nerve block: a comparison of four needle insertion sites. Anesth Analg 1999;89: 1467–70.
39. Orebaugh SL, Williams BA, Kentor ML. Ultrasound guidance with nerve stimulation reduces the time necessary for resident peripheral nerve blockade. Reg Anesth Pain Med 2007;32:448–54.
40. Benzon HT, Sharma S, Calimaran A. Comparison of the different approaches to saphenous nerve block. Anesthesiology 2005;102:633–8.
41. Oberndorfer U, Marhofer P, Bosenberg A, et al. Ultrasonographic guidance for sciatic and femoral nerve blocks in children. Br J Anaesth 2007;98:797–801.
42. Gurnaney H, Ganesh A, Cucchiaro G. The relationship between current intensity for nerve stimulation and success of peripheral nerve blocks performed in pediatric patients under general anesthesia. Anesth Analg 2007;105:1605–9 [table of contents].
43. Gray AT, Collins AB, Schafhalter-Zoppoth I. Sciatic nerve block in a child: a sonographic approach. Anesth Analg 2003;97:1300–2.
44. Dufour E, Quennesson P, Van Robais AL, et al. Combined ultrasound and neurostimulation guidance for popliteal sciatic nerve block: a prospective, randomized comparison with neurostimulation alone. Anesth Analg 2008;106:1553–8 [table of contents].
45. Karmakar MK, Kwok WH, Ho AM, et al. Ultrasound-guided sciatic nerve block: description of a new approach at the subgluteal space. Br J Anaesth 2007;98: 390–5.
46. Singelyn FJ, Gouverneur JM, Gribomont BF. Popliteal sciatic nerve block aided by a nerve stimulator: a reliable technique for foot and ankle surgery. Reg Anesth 1991;16:278–81.
47. Konrad C, Johr M. Blockade of the sciatic nerve in the popliteal fossa: a system for standardization in children. Anesth Analg 1998;87:1256–8.
48. Sukhani R, Nader A, Candido KD, et al. Nerve stimulator-assisted evoked motor response predicts the latency and success of a single-injection sciatic block. Anesth Analg 2004;99:584–8 [table of contents].

49. Borgeat A, Blumenthal S, Karovic D, et al. Clinical evaluation of a modified posterior anatomical approach to performing the popliteal block. Reg Anesth Pain Med 2004;29:290–6.
50. Perlas A, Brull R, Chan VW, et al. Ultrasound guidance improves the success of sciatic nerve block at the popliteal fossa. Reg Anesth Pain Med 2008;33:259–65.
51. Danelli G, Fanelli A, Ghisi D, et al. Ultrasound vs nerve stimulation multiple injection technique for posterior popliteal sciatic nerve block. Anaesthesia 2009;64: 638–42.
52. Hadzic A, Vloka JD. A comparison of the posterior versus lateral approaches to the block of the sciatic nerve in the popliteal fossa. Anesthesiology 1998;88: 1480–6.
53. Paqueron X, Bouaziz H, Macalou D, et al. The lateral approach to the sciatic nerve at the popliteal fossa: one or two injections? Anesth Analg 1999;89:1221–5.
54. Domingo-Triado V, Selfa S, Martinez F, et al. Ultrasound guidance for lateral mid-femoral sciatic nerve block: a prospective, comparative, randomized study. Anesth Analg 2007;104:1270–4 [table of contents].
55. Willschke H, Bosenberg A, Marhofer P, et al. Ultrasonographic-guided ilioinguinal/iliohypogastric nerve block in pediatric anesthesia: what is the optimal volume? Anesth Analg 2006;102:1680–4.
56. Willschke H, Marhofer P, Bosenberg A, et al. Ultrasonography for ilioinguinal/iliohypogastric nerve blocks in children. Br J Anaesth 2005;95:226–30.
57. Weintraud M, Lundblad M, Kettner SC, et al. Ultrasound versus landmark-based technique for ilioinguinal-iliohypogastric nerve blockade in children: the implications on plasma levels of ropivacaine. Anesth Analg 2009;108:1488–92.
58. Weintraud M, Marhofer P, Bosenberg A, et al. Ilioinguinal/iliohypogastric blocks in children: where do we administer the local anesthetic without direct visualization? Anesth Analg 2008;106:89–93 [table of contents].
59. Willschke H, Bosenberg A, Marhofer P, et al. Ultrasonography-guided rectus sheath block in paediatric anaesthesia—a new approach to an old technique. Br J Anaesth 2006;97:244–9.
60. Ferguson S, Thomas V, Lewis I. The rectus sheath block in paediatric anaesthesia: new indications for an old technique? Paediatr Anaesth 1996;6:463–6.
61. Buckenmaier CC III, Bleckner LL. Anaesthetic agents for advanced regional anaesthesia: a North American perspective. Drugs 2005;65:745–59.
62. Graf BM. The cardiotoxicity of local anesthetics: the place of ropivacaine. Curr Top Med Chem 2001;1:207–14.
63. Cucchiaro G, Ganesh A. The effects of clonidine on postoperative analgesia after peripheral nerve blockade in children. Anesth Analg 2007;104:532–7.

New Concepts in Treatment of Pediatric Traumatic Brain Injury

Jimmy W. Huh, MD[a],*, Ramesh Raghupathi, PhD[b]

KEYWORDS

- Traumatic brain injury • Pediatric • Child • Guidelines
- Treatment • Anesthetics

Since the publication in 2003 of the first version of the guidelines for the medical management of severe traumatic brain injury (TBI) in infants, children, and adolescents,[1] there has been increasing clinical and basic science research to better understand the pathophysiologic responses associated with pediatric TBI. Evidence is beginning to accumulate that the traumatized pediatric brain may have unique responses that are distinct from the traumatized adult brain. Even within the immature brain, there seem to be age-dependent responses following trauma. As anesthesiologists play an important role in resuscitating infants and children with severe TBI in the emergency room and operating room, it is integral that they understand the injury patterns, pathophysiology, recent advances in diagnostic modalities, and different therapeutic options. In this article a review of the recent studies relevant to these important issues in pediatric TBI is presented. Areas for future investigation, such as neuromonitoring and the effects of anesthetics on the developing brain, are also discussed.

INJURY PATTERNS

Age-dependent injury patterns occur following pediatric TBI.[2] In infants and young children, inflicted or nonaccidental TBI is a major cause of brain injury and often is associated with repetitive injury.[3,4] Accidental TBIs in this age group are mainly due

Dr. Huh is supported by NIH NS053651, Clinical & Translational Research Center (MO1-RR00240), and the Endowed Chair of Critical Care Medicine at Children's Hospital of Philadelphia. Dr. Raghupathi is supported by NIH HD41699 and a VA Merit Review grant.

[a] Critical Care and Pediatrics, Department of Anesthesiology and Critical Care Medicine, Children's Hospital of Philadelphia, University of Pennsylvania School of Medicine, Critical Care Office, 7 South Tower, Room 7C26, 34th Street & Civic Center Boulevard, Philadelphia, PA 19104-4399, USA

[b] Department of Neurobiology and Anatomy, Drexel University College of Medicine, 2900 Queen Lane, Philadelphia, PA 19129, USA

* Corresponding author.

E-mail address: huh@email.chop.edu (J. W. Huh).

to motor vehicle accidents and falls. By toddler age, falls are the predominant injury mechanism, but abuse must also be considered if the history is not consistent with the injury pattern. Among motor vehicle-related injuries in toddlers, pedestrian versus vehicle crashes are more common than motor vehicle occupant injuries.[5,6] In school-aged children, falls requiring hospitalization decrease with age, whereas there is an increase in injuries associated with bicycle crashes. In adolescents, there is a dramatic increase in TBI due to motor vehicle accidents and sports-related repetitive injury, with violence being an unfortunate common cause.[7]

Age-dependent pathology following pediatric TBI is also common. In infants and young children, diffuse injury, such as diffuse cerebral swelling, and subdural hematomas are more common than focal injury, such as contusions.[8,9] Hypoxia-ischemia seems to be more common in infants and young children sustaining nonaccidental than accidental TBI.[10,11]

PATHOPHYSIOLOGY: IMMEDIATE (PRIMARY) AND DELAYED (SECONDARY) INJURY

Immediate or primary brain injury results from the initial forces generated following trauma. Focal injuries such as contusions and hematomas are generated by contact, linear forces when the head is struck by a moving object. Inertial, angular forces produced by acceleration-deceleration can lead to immediate physical shearing or tearing of axons termed "primary" axotomy. Following primary brain injury, two forms of secondary brain injury can occur. The first form of secondary brain injury, such as hypoxemia, hypotension, intracranial hypertension, hypercarbia, hyper- or hypoglycemia, electrolyte abnormalities, enlarging hematomas, coagulopathy, seizures, and hyperthermia are potentially avoidable or treatable.[1] The primary goal in the acute management of the severely head-injured pediatric patient is to prevent or ameliorate these factors that promote secondary brain injury.

The other form of secondary brain injury involves an endogenous cascade of cellular and biochemical events in the brain that occurs within minutes and continues for months after the primary brain injury, leading to ongoing or "secondary" traumatic axonal injury (TAI) and neuronal cell damage (delayed brain injury), and ultimately, neuronal cell death.[12] Intense research continues in the ultimate hope of discovering novel therapies to halt the progression or to inhibit these mechanisms for which there is no current therapy. Some of these important mechanisms associated with secondary brain injury are discussed later in this article. For a more detailed review of these and other mechanisms associated with secondary brain injury the reader is referred to an excellent article by Kochanek and colleagues.[13]

NECROSIS AND APOPTOSIS

Following head trauma, the release of excessive amounts of the excitatory amino acid glutamate, termed "excitotoxicity," is believed to occur, which can lead to neuronal injury in two phases. The first phase is characterized by sodium-dependent neuronal swelling, followed by delayed, calcium-dependent neuronal degeneration.[14] These effects are mediated through ionophore-linked receptors such as N-methyl-D-aspartate (NMDA), kainite, and α-amino-3-hydroxy-5-methyl-4-isoxazolepropionic acid (AMPA) (glutamate receptors), and metabotropic receptors, which are receptors linked to second-messenger systems. Activation of these receptors allows calcium influx through receptor-gated or voltage-gated channels, or through the release of intracellular calcium stores. This increase in intracellular calcium is then associated with activation of proteases, lipases, and endonucleases, that can lead to neuronal degeneration and necrotic cell death. Consistent with excitotoxic-mediated neuronal cell death, recent research has shown that calcium-activated proteases, calpains, may participate in neuronal cell loss in the injured cortex following TBI in the immature rat.[15] In addition, experimental pediatric TBI has been shown to alter NMDA receptor subunit composition.[16]

In contrast to necrotic cell death that is marked by neuronal cell swelling, apoptotic cell death is marked by DNA fragmentation and the formation of apoptotic cell bodies associated with neuronal cell shrinkage. Apoptosis requires a cascade of intracellular events for completion of "programmed cell death," and is initiated by intracellular or extracellular signals. Intracellular signals are initiated in the mitochondria as a result of depletion of ATP (dATP), oxidative stress, or calcium flux.[17] Mitochondrial dysfunction leads to cytochrome *c* release in the cytosol, which in the presence of apoptotic-protease activating factor (APAF-1) and dATP activates the initiator protease caspase-9.[18] Caspase-9 then activates the effector protease caspase-3, which ultimately causes apoptosis.[19] Extracellular signaling occurs by way of the tumor necrosis factor (TNF) superfamily of cell surface death receptors, which include TNFR-1 and Fas/Apo1/CD95.[20] Receptor ligand binding of TNFR-1-TNF-α or Fas-Fas L promotes "death domains" which activate caspase-8, ultimately leading to caspase-3 activation and apoptotic cell death.[21] Because differentiating necrotic versus apoptotic cell death is sometimes difficult in TBI, cells that die can be characterized as a morphologic continuum ranging from necrosis to apoptosis.[22]

There seems to be an age-dependent response in relation to excitotoxicity and apoptosis. Animal studies have shown that the developing neuron is more susceptible to excitotoxic injury than the mature neuron, probably because more calcium is transmitted through the NMDA-mediated calcium channel in the immature brain.[23] However, following TBI, calcium accumulation in the injured brain was more extensive and appeared for a longer duration in the mature animal than in the immature animal.[24] This difference may have been because the immature animals were less severely injured as no neuronal cell death was observed, whereas delayed cell death was present in the traumatized mature animals. This result suggests that in addition to age, injury severity may play an important role in the extent of excitotoxicity. Additional studies are needed to look at the effects of injury severity in the developing brain. Other animal studies have shown that the administration of NMDA or excitotoxic antagonists following TBI in immature and mature rats decreased excitotoxic-mediated neuronal death; however, apoptotic cell death increased in immature rats.[25,26] The increased propensity of the developing brain for posttraumatic apoptotic cell death is a key area for further research.

To date, no novel antiexcitotoxic agents have been shown to be successful in clinical trials of TBI. However, this failure may be due to many causes including incorrect dosing, delayed treatment, and failure to administer injury-specific and mechanism-specific treatments. Many investigators believe that further research is still needed to better understand the role of excitotoxicity and apoptosis following TBI at different developmental stages of the brain.

CEREBRAL SWELLING

Diffuse cerebral swelling following pediatric TBI is an important contributor to intracranial hypertension, which can result in ischemia and herniation. Some studies suggest that diffuse cerebral swelling is more common in children than in adults.[8] Cerebral swelling is believed to result from osmolar shifts, edema at the cellular level (cytotoxic or cellular edema), and blood-brain barrier breakdown (vasogenic edema). Furthermore, cerebral swelling is believed to be worsened with hypoxia and hypoperfusion.

Osmolar shifts occur primarily in areas of necrosis whereby osmolar load increases with the degradation of neurons. As reperfusion occurs, water is drawn into the area secondary to the high osmolar load and the surrounding neurons become edematous. Cellular swelling independent of osmolar load primarily occurs in astrocyte foot processes and is believed to be brought on by excitotoxicity and uptake of glutamate. Glutamate uptake is coupled to sodium-potassium adenosine triphosphatase (ATPase), with sodium and water being accumulated in astrocytes.[27] Recent experimental data also suggest the role of endogenous water channels, called aquaporins, present in the astrocyte that may participate in brain edema.[28] Clinical studies suggest that cellular edema, and not hyperemia or vasogenic edema, may be the major component of cerebral swelling.[29,30] Further studies to better understand the mechanisms associated with diffuse cerebral swelling are strongly warranted.

CEREBRAL BLOOD FLOW AND AUTOREGULATION

Early important studies in cerebral blood flow (CBF) suggested that hyperemia was the mechanism underlying secondary diffuse cerebral swelling in pediatric TBI.[31,32] However, the values of "hyperemia" were based on referencing the head-injured children's CBF to that of normal young adults, whose CBF values are lower than that of normal children.[33] Reanalysis of the published pediatric TBI CBF studies compared with the age-dependent changes of CBF in normal children have suggested that hyperemia does not play a large role following severe pediatric TBI.[30] Other data suggest that posttraumatic hypoperfusion was more common and a global decreased CBF (<20 mL/100 g/min) in the initial first day following TBI in infants and children was associated with poor outcome.[34]

Recent studies have demonstrated impaired cerebral autoregulation in infants and children following TBI. Using transcranial Doppler imaging, impaired cerebral autoregulation early after severe pediatric TBI was associated with poor outcome.[35] In a subsequent study, all of the children with nonaccidental TBI had impaired cerebral autoregulation in both hemispheres and poor outcome.[36] Furthermore, age younger than 4 years old was a risk factor for impaired autoregulation, independent of TBI severity.[37]

Following experimental pediatric TBI, age-dependent changes in CBF have been described. Younger age was associated with more prolonged decreases in CBF and sustained hypotension compared with older animals following diffuse pediatric TBI.[38,39] In contrast, following focal (contusive) injury, the older animals exhibited the most pronounced decrease in CBF.[40] This suggests that besides age, the pathologic type of TBI may also contribute to CBF alterations. Mechanisms that may underlie posttraumatic hypoperfusion include direct damage to cerebral blood vessels and reduced levels of vasodilators, including nitric oxide, cyclic guanosine 3',5'-monophosphate (cGMP), cyclic adenosine 3',5'-monophosphate (cAMP), and prostaglandins, which are believed to contribute to decreased CBF.[41–43] In a similar way increased levels of vasoconstrictors, such as endothelin-1, are also implicated in cerebral blood flow alterations.[44] NMDA and endogenous opioids (NOC/OFQ) recently were also found to participate in age-dependent impairment of cerebrovascular reactivity in the youngest animals following diffuse TBI.[45]

TRAUMATIC AXONAL INJURY

A common pathologic condition observed in infants and young children in accidental and nonaccidental TBI is diffuse or TAI. TAI involves widespread damage to axons in the white matter of the brain, most commonly in the corpus callosum, basal ganglia, and periventricular white matter.[46] Hypoxic-ischemic injury, calcium and ionic flux dysregulation, and mitochondrial and cytoskeletal dysfunction are believed to play important roles in axonal injury.[47] TAI is believed to be a major cause of morbidity in pediatric TBI.[48–50] Using recent advances in MRI to detect axonal injury, such as susceptibility-weighted and diffusion tensor imaging, more extensive TAI in pediatric TBI patients was associated with worse outcomes.[51]

Whereas immediate or "primary" axotomy or immediate physical tearing of the axon can occur following TBI, TAI is believed to primarily occur by a delayed process called "secondary" axotomy.[52] This suggests an extended window of opportunity for therapeutic intervention to stop this delayed and ongoing axonal degeneration, in the ultimate hope of improving outcome. Animal data suggest that the younger brain may be more vulnerable to widespread TAI with equivalent injury severity than the adult brain.[53] A clinically relevant animal model of pediatric TBI has recently been developed that exhibits diffuse TAI and ongoing axonal degeneration associated with chronic cognitive dysfunction.[54] Ongoing research on better understanding the mechanisms associated with TAI and chronic cognitive dysfunction in the traumatized developing brain may lead to novel therapies in the future.

EMERGENCY DEPARTMENT EVALUATION

On arrival of a head-injured pediatric patient in the emergency department (ED), information on the timing and mechanism of injury and resuscitative efforts from emergency medical personnel and witnesses at the scene are vital. The use of the "AMPLE" mnemonic (Allergies, Medications currently used, Past illnesses, Last meal, and Events/environment related to the injury) may be useful to quickly acquire the necessary information to improve understanding the pediatric patient's current physiologic state.[55] Initial symptoms on presentation have been found to have little or no correlation with injury severity following pediatric TBI, and the anesthesiologist must rely on repeated physical examinations and vital signs.[56]

Physical Examination

The anesthesiologist is an expert in quickly assessing the "ABCs" (Airway, Breathing, Circulation). He or she must also be adept at quickly assessing and reassessing the patient's neurologic status, while simultaneously evaluating for life-threatening signs and symptoms of intracranial hypertension or impending herniation, such as altered level of consciousness, pupillary dysfunction, lateralizing extremity weakness, Cushing's triad (hypertension, bradycardia, and irregular respirations), or other herniation syndromes (**Table 1**). The patient should have rapid assessment and reassessments of vital signs including heart rate, respiratory rate, blood pressure, pulse oximetry, and temperature. The head and spine should be examined for any external evidence of injury such as scalp lacerations and skull depressions, which warrants concern for an underlying skull fracture and severe intracranial injury. In the infant, a bulging fontanelle may be a sign of increased intracranial pressure (ICP).[57] Mastoid ("Battle's sign") and peri-orbital ("raccoon eyes") bruising due to dissection of blood, hemotympanum, and clear rhinorrhea are all signs of possible basilar skull fracture.

A quick, but detailed and easily reproducible neurologic assessment should be performed and documented. Whereas the Glasgow Coma Scale (GCS) for older children and adults is the most widely used method to quantify initial neurologic assessment,[58] the Children's Coma Scale is most often used in infants and younger children (**Table 2**).[59] With regard to TBI, a GCS score of 13 to 15 is mild, 9 to 12 is moderate, and 3 to 8 is severe. It is critical that the GCS be recorded on the initial medical record and

Table 1
Herniation syndromes

	Eye Findings	Gross Motor	Respiration
Uncal (lateral transtentorial)	Ipsilateral fixed pupillary dilatation and ptosis	Contralateral hemiparesis	Irregular
Diencephalic	Small midpoint pupils, but reactive to light	Decorticate posturing, hypertonia	Cheyne-Stokes (episodes of apnea and tachypnea)
Midbrain	Midpoint fixed pupils	Decerebrate posturing	Hyperventilation
Medullary	Dilated and fixed pupils	No response to pain	Irregular or gasping

reassessed regularly to detect changes in GCS over time. For example, a child suffering a head injury may arrive in the ED with an initial GCS of 14 but it then can rapidly decrease over time, secondary to an expanding epidural hematoma and impending herniation.

The pupillary examination is of paramount importance when assessing the neurologic status of the head-injured child. The size, shape, and reactivity to light provide vital insight into the balance of sympathetic and parasympathetic influences. An enlarged unreactive pupil (mydriasis) can be secondary to dysfunction or injury to the oculomotor nerve (cranial nerve III) and can be associated with disorders of oculomotor muscle and ptosis.[57] Uncal (lateral transtentorial) herniation or a lesion along the course of the oculomotor nerve may cause unilateral mydriasis and ptosis. Direct trauma to the eye may cause injury to the iris and result in mydriasis without

Table 2
Modified children's coma scale

Eye opening	
Spontaneous	4
To speech	3
To pain	2
None	1
Verbal	
Coos, babbles	5
Irritable	4
Cries to pain	3
Moans to pain	2
None	1
Motor	
Normal spontaneous movements	6
Withdraws to touch	5
Withdraws to pain	4
Abnormal flexion	3
Abnormal extension	2
Flaccid	1

oculomotor dysfunction. Bilateral mydriasis can be the result of ingestions (anticholinergics) or administration of atropine or adrenergic agonists such as epinephrine during resuscitation. A small pupil (miosis) is usually secondary to dysfunction of sympathetic innervation. Because the efferent sympathetic fibers travel along the carotid artery, injury to the neck or skull base must also be considered in the pediatric TBI patient.

Evaluation of eye movements and brain stem reflexes can help localize the intracranial lesion. Dysfunction of all the three cranial nerves in eye movement (oculomotor, trochlear, and abducens nerves) can be the result of injury to the ipsilateral cavernous sinus. Cough and gag reflexes detect glossopharygneal and vagus nerve function. Abnormalities in respiratory pattern may also assist in localizing brain injury and herniation syndromes (**Table 1**). Deep tendon reflexes (DTR) are typically exaggerated in head-injured patents due to the lack of cortical inhibition. However, decreased DTR may suggest a spinal cord injury. Babinski response, characterized by extension of the great toe and abduction of the remaining toes, is an abnormal finding in children older than 6 months of age when the plantar reflex is tested.

Diagnostic Studies

The mainstay of the initial radiologic evaluation of the severely head-injured pediatric patient is CT imaging; but before transport to the CT scanner "the ABCs must always be addressed," and appropriate monitoring must be instituted and blood samples sent. For intubated patients, continuous capnometry is vital for titrating treatment of intracranial hypertension.

A chemistry panel should be sent to assess electrolyte abnormalities and renal function, especially if hyperosmolar therapy may be instituted.[60] Liver enzymes and pancreatic function should also be evaluated for possible blunt trauma, especially if nonaccidental trauma is suspected. Complete blood count (CBC) to evaluate for anemia and especially thrombocytopenia in the presence of intracranial bleeding is imperative. Tests for coagulopathy and a type and screen should be sent. In one prospective observational study, 22% of children with severe head injury had laboratory evidence of disseminated intravascular coagulation.[61] Furthermore, a normal coagulation profile and platelet count on presentation does not rule out the possibility of coagulopathy or thrombocytopenia developing over time.[62] In the adolescent population, a toxicology screen should also be considered.

Cervical spine films should be obtained, as well as chest radiographs for intubated patients to evaluate for right main stem intubations or pneumothorax. Other radiographs should be performed based on the results of the secondary survey. If there is no clear history or mechanism of accidental trauma, especially in infants and young children, further investigation for other occult injuries such as abdominal injuries, skeletal injuries, and retinal hemorrhages (which are commonly associated with nonaccidental TBI or shaken-baby or shaken-impact syndrome) should be sought.[3] However, this workup should not take precedence over life-threatening issues such as hypoxemia, hypotension, and intracranial hypertension.

CT scan is the imaging modality of choice and can rapidly detect intracranial hematoma, intraparenchymal contusion, skull fracture, and cerebral edema, as well as transependymal flow and obliteration of the basal cisterns, which are concerns for elevated ICP. Certain findings on early CT scan have been associated with outcome.[63,64] The basal cisterns are evaluated at the level of the mid brain; compressed or absent cisterns increase the risk of intracranial hypertension and are associated with poor outcome.[65] The presence of midline shift at the foramen of Monroe is also inversely related to prognosis.[63,65] The presence of traumatic subarachnoid hemorrhage increases mortality and its presence in the basal cisterns is also a predictor of poor outcome.[63,65] MRI, especially susceptibility-weighted and diffusion tensor imaging, has demonstrated superiority on detecting traumatic axonal injury and its correlation with long-term outcome.[51,66] Due to the length of time required for image acquisition and limited physiologic monitoring in the MRI suite, this imaging modality is of limited value in the initial evaluation of the critically ill pediatric TBI patient. However, an ongoing study is evaluating a quick-brain MRI to enhance image quality in areas such as the posterior fossa without the potential risk of radiation associated with CT.[67]

THERAPEUTIC OPTIONS: THE "INITIAL GOLDEN MINUTES" OF PEDIATRIC TRAUMATIC BRAIN INJURY
Airway, Breathing, and Circulation

Hypoxemia and hypotension are to be avoided or treated to prevent or minimize secondary brain injury from hypoxic-ischemic brain damage, which may promote diffuse cerebral swelling and intracranial hypertension. Criteria for tracheal intubation include hypoxemia not resolved with supplemental oxygen, apnea, hypercarbia ($PaCO_2$ >45 mm Hg), GCS of 8 or less, a decrease in GCS of greater than three independent of the initial GCS, anisocoria greater than 1 mm, cervical spine injury compromising ventilation, loss of pharyngeal reflex, and any clinical evidence of a herniation syndrome or Cushing's triad.[57]

All patients should be assumed to have a full stomach and cervical spine injury, so the intubation should be carried out using a cerebroprotective, rapid-sequence induction whenever possible. Bag-valve-mask (BVM) ventilation should not be done unless the patient has signs and symptoms of impending herniation, apnea, or hypoxemia.[57] Vigilant care of the cervical spine is especially advised during BVM ventilation due to an increased risk for cervical spine injury.[68] A second person's sole responsibility is to maintain the child's neck in the neutral position by mild axial traction during airway maneuvers. Cricoid pressure should be applied by a third individual. Orotracheal intubation by direct laryngoscopy is the preferred method; nasotracheal intubation should be avoided, due to the possibility of direct intracranial damage in a patient with a basilar skull fracture and also because nasotracheal intubation may require excessive movement of the cervical spine. After successful tracheal intubation, oxygen saturation of 100%, normocarbia (35–39 mm Hg) and no hyperventilation, confirmed by arterial blood gas and trended with an end-tidal CO_2, and a chest radiograph showing the tracheal tube in good position above the carina (as right main stem tracheal intubation is common) should be confirmed.

Unless the patient has signs or symptoms of herniation, prophylactic hyperventilation ($PaCO_2$ <35 mm Hg) should be avoided. Hyperventilation causes cerebral vasoconstriction, which decreases CBF and subsequent cerebral blood volume that will lower ICP, but ischemia can also occur.[69] Furthermore, respiratory alkalosis caused by hyperventilation makes it more difficult to release oxygen to the brain, by shifting the hemoglobin-oxygen curve to the left.

Because endotracheal intubation is a noxious stimulus and can increase ICP, appropriate medications should be used during rapid-sequence induction. The hemodynamic and neurologic status of the patient dictates the choice of drugs used. For the patient in cardiopulmonary arrest, no medications are needed for tracheal intubation. All other patients should usually receive lidocaine (1–1.5 mg/kg) intravenously (IV) before intubation to help blunt the increase in ICP that occurs during direct laryngoscopy.[70] For the hemodynamically unstable patient, the combination of lidocaine, etomidate (0.2–0.6 mg/kg), and neuromuscular blockade with rocuronium (1 mg/kg) or vecuronium (0.3 mg/kg) intravenously is a popular choice. An alternative is the combination of lidocaine, fentanyl (2–4 μg/kg), and rocuronium or vecuronium. In the hemodynamically stable patient, either of the above combinations with the fast-acting benzodiazepine, midazolam (0.1–0.2 mg/kg) can be added. Another alternative in the hemodynamically stable patient is the combination of thiopental (3–5 mg/kg), lidocaine, and rocuronium or vecuronium. Thiopental and etomidate are ultrafast-acting and quickly reduce cerebral metabolism, which ameliorates the increased ICP associated with direct laryngoscopy. In addition the short-acting narcotic fentanyl, when used with lidocaine, can decrease the catecholamine release associated with direct laryngoscopy.[57] The endotracheal tube should be secured with tape, but this adhesive tape should not pass around the neck as venous return from the brain can be obstructed and potentially elevate ICP. The neck should be immobilized in an appropriately pediatric-sized collar.

Assessment and reassessment of the patient's circulatory status (central and peripheral pulse quality, capillary refill, heart rate, blood pressure) is critical as hypotension after pediatric TBI is associated with increases in morbidity and mortality.[1,71,72] The most common cause for compensated or early shock (tachycardia with normal blood pressure) and uncompensated or late shock (low blood pressure) in the trauma patient is hypovolemic (ie, hemorrhagic) shock. In severe TBI, rapid intravenous fluid resuscitation is the goal for hypovolemic shock. Isotonic solutions, such as 0.9% NaCl solution or packed red blood cells (for hemorrhagic shock) can be administered, but hypotonic fluids should not be used in the initial resuscitation of these patients. Although not yet studied in a clinical trial, resuscitation with hypertonic saline (3% saline) in a severe pediatric TBI patient with initial signs and symptoms of hypovolemic shock and intracranial hypertension may be considered (further discussed in the "Intracranial hypertension management: first-tier therapies" section).

Special consideration must be given to spinal (neurogenic) shock, especially with suspected cervical-thoracic spine injuries, in addition to hypovolemic or hemorrhagic shock as the cause of hypotension. These patients may be bradycardic with shock. Bradycardia and shock must be treated accordingly with isotonic fluid/blood resuscitation to ensure adequate circulation and prevent further ischemia. In spinal shock, α-adrenergic agonists, such as intravenous phenylephrine, are also needed to treat the vasodilatation that results from injury to the sympathetic outflow tract.

Prophylactic brain-specific interventions (such as hyperventilation and hyperosmolar therapy with mannitol or 3% saline) in the absence of signs and symptoms of herniation or other neurologic deterioration currently are not recommended. However, in the presence of signs and symptoms of herniation, such as Cushing's triad (irregular respirations, bradycardia, and systemic hypertension), pupillary dysfunction, lateralizing extremity weakness, or extensor posturing, emergency treatment is needed.

Herniation

While the ABCs are being addressed, signs and symptoms of impending herniation, such as Cushing's triad or one of the herniation syndromes, must also be immediately treated. Early consultation with a neurosurgeon is important. Hyperventilation with 100% oxygen can be life-saving in the setting of impending herniation, such as in a child who has a rapidly expanding epidural hematoma with pupillary dilatation, bradycardia, systemic hypertension, and extensor posturing. Elevating the head to 30° increases venous drainage and lowers ICP.[73] Furthermore, the head should be midline to prevent obstruction of venous return from the brain. If these maneuvers do not relieve the signs and symptoms of herniation, such as by improvement in pupillary response or resolution of Cushing's triad, hyperosmolar therapy (mannitol, 3% saline) should be instituted (further discussed in the "Intracranial hypertension management: first-tier therapies" section). In addition, short-acting medications such as thiopental (3–5 mg/kg) can be administered emergently in this setting.[57] During this time the patient usually goes to the CT scanner or directly to the operating room with the neurosurgeon, as the definitive therapy for a rapidly expanding epidural hematoma with herniation symptoms is surgery. Besides expanding mass lesions, diffuse cerebral swelling may also lead to herniation. As a result, secondary causes of brain injury such as hypoxemia, hypercarbia, hypotension, excessive fluid administration, or seizures can precipitate herniation and therefore must be avoided or immediately treated.

PEDIATRIC TRAUMATIC BRAIN INJURY GUIDELINES AND BEYOND

The "Guidelines for the acute medical management of severe TBI in infants, children, and adolescents" are summarized in **Figs. 1** and **2**.[1] Although they are informative and helpful, most of the recommendations are at the "Option" level or are "Class III" evidence. As the number of evidence-based pediatric studies were lacking, the authors of these guidelines made many recommendations after reaching a consensus based on published adult guidelines. Still, this seminal publication has been an important step toward a better understanding of pediatric TBI and is helping to increase the number of clinical and experimental pediatric TBI studies.

INTRACRANIAL HYPERTENSION MANAGEMENT: FIRST-TIER THERAPIES

Once the initial resuscitation with the ABCs, herniation, and expanding intracranial masses have been medically and surgically addressed, further management is aimed at preventing or treating causes of secondary brain injury (such as hypoxemia, hypotension, intracranial hypertension, hypercarbia, hyper- or hypoglycemia, electrolyte abnormalities, enlarging hematomas, coagulopathy, seizures, and hyperthermia).

One of the most important consequences of secondary brain injury is the development of intracranial hypertension. First described in the Monroe-Kellie doctrine, the intracranial vault is a fixed volume of brain, cerebrospinal fluid (CSF), and blood.[57] An enlarging space-occupying lesion, such as an expanding epidural hematoma or worsening cerebral edema, will not initially cause intracranial hypertension, as the initial compensatory mechanisms of displacement of CSF to the spinal canal and venous blood to the jugular veins prevent elevated ICP. However, once these compensatory mechanisms are exhausted, even a small increase in the size of the hematoma or cerebral edema will lead to increased ICP, which will compromise cerebral perfusion. This increase will then lead to brain ischemia and further edema, and ultimately lead to brain herniation.

Cerebral autoregulation and cerebral perfusion pressure is another important concept. Under normal conditions, cerebral autoregulation provides constant CBF over a wide range of cerebral perfusion pressures and is "coupled" to the metabolic demands of the brain. Cerebral perfusion pressure (CPP) is defined as the difference between mean systemic arterial blood pressure (MAP) minus the greater of the ICP or central venous pressure (CVP) (or CPP = MAP – ICP or CVP).[57] After TBI, cerebral autoregulation can become "uncoupled" from the metabolic demands of the brain and alterations in CPP (due to either rising ICP or changing MAP) may result in fluctuations of CBF, which can lead to cerebral ischemia or hyperemia. For example, a study using xenon CBF-CT studies in children after TBI demonstrated marked reductions in CBF

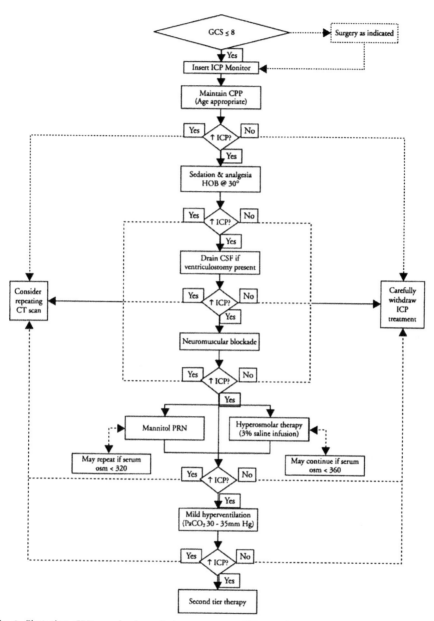

Fig. 1. First tier. CPP, cerebral perfusion pressure; CSF, cerebrospinal fluid; CT, computed tomography; GCS, Glasgow coma scale; HOB, head of bed; ICP, intracranial pressure; PRN, as needed. (*Reprinted from* Adelson PD, Bratton SL, Carney NA, et al. Critical pathway for the treatment of established intracranial hypertension in pediatric traumatic brain injury. Pediatr Crit Care Med 2003;4(3 suppl):S66; with permission.)

within the first 24 hours after injury, which was associated with poor outcome, whereas the children with high CBF 24 hours after the injury exhibited improved outcome.[34] However, because this type of study cannot measure minute-to-minute assessment of CBF changes, and due to the potential risk of transporting and of performing

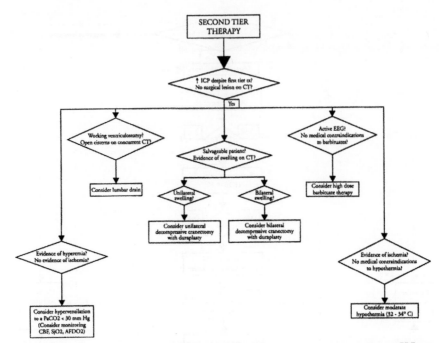

Fig. 2. Second tier. AJDO2, arterial-jugular venous difference in oxygen content; CBF, cerebral blood flow; CT, computed tomography; EEG, electroencephalogram; ICP, intracranial pressure; SjO2, jugular venous oxygen saturation. (*Reprinted from* Adelson PD, Bratton SL, Carney NA, et al. Critical pathway for the treatment of established intracranial hypertension in pediatric traumatic brain injury. Pediatr Crit Care Med 2003;4(3 suppl):S67; with permission.)

prolonged studies in critically ill patients, most institutions continuously measure CPP to "estimate CBF."

A flow diagram showing a general approach to first-tier treatments for established intracranial hypertension in pediatric TBI was provided in the 2003 Guidelines (**Fig. 1**).[1] As discussed fully later, first-tier therapies include maintaining age-appropriate CPP, head position, sedation, analgesia, neuromuscular blockade, ventricular CSF drainage, hyperosmolar therapy, and mild hyperventilation. In general, an ICP monitor is placed by the neurosurgeon in children with an initial GCS of eight or less, after initial stabilization and resuscitation for treatment of potential intracranial hypertension. If the ventricles are not compressed due to severe cerebral swelling, ICP monitoring by a ventricular catheter allows a potential therapeutic option of CSF drainage. Because clinical signs and symptoms of herniation are late signs of intracranial hypertension, the use of ICP monitors allows early detection of intracranial hypertension before signs and symptoms of herniation are observed.[74] However, ICP monitors can cause hemorrhage and infection. Coagulopathy needs to be corrected before ICP monitor placement, and some centers use prophylactic antibiotics.

Intracranial Pressure and Cerebral Perfusion Pressure

Treatment of intracranial hypertension should begin at an ICP of 20 mm Hg or less, as most pediatric TBI studies show poor outcome with ICP 20 mm Hg or more, and aggressive treatment of intracranial hypertension is associated with improved outcomes in some studies.[75–78] However, further studies need to be done to determine an age-appropriate treatment for intracranial hypertension. In infants and young children, the threshold for "intracranial hypertension" treatment may be an ICP less than 20 mm Hg (because the MAP is lower) to optimize CPP (MAP minus ICP).

The optimal or "age-appropriate" CPP for pediatric TBI is currently unknown and there is no evidence that targeting a specific CPP for a specific age of the pediatric patient improves outcome. However, there are pediatric TBI studies showing that CPP ranging from 40 to 65 mm Hg are associated with favorable outcome and a CPP less than 40 mm Hg is associated with poor outcome.[79–81] As a result, the 2003 pediatric recommendations are that a CPP greater than 40 mm Hg and an "age-related continuum" of CPP from 40 to 65 mm Hg in infants to adolescents be maintained.[1] In a recent study, CPP values of 53 mm Hg for 2 to 6 years old, 63 mm Hg for 7 to 10 years old, and 66 mm Hg for 11 to 16 years old were suggested to represent minimum values for favorable outcome.[82] However, this study was limited by the following: only the initial 6 hours of CPP data were analyzed, the specificity of the study was only 50%, and no infants and children younger than 2 years old were included. Further studies are paramount to determine the "age-appropriate" CPP.

According to the formula for CPP, lowering the ICP or raising the MAP will increase CPP. Most treatments are aimed at lowering ICP, maintaining normal MAP, and euvolemia. If the treatments fail to lower ICP, vasopressors are commonly added to increase the CPP by augmenting the MAP; this mechanism works if autoregulation is intact. Otherwise, as the MAP is increased the ICP will also increase and there is no net augmentation in CPP. If the child is hypotensive, isotonic fluid boluses or vasopressors can be administered to augment the MAP in the hope of improving CPP. In a recent pilot study comparing "CPP-targeted therapy" (CPP >60 mm Hg for children less than 2 years old; CPP >70 mm Hg for children at least 2 years old) to "ICP-targeted therapy" (ICP <20 mm Hg; CPP >50 mm Hg) in children with severe TBI, the "CPP-targeted" group revealed a trend toward improved outcome (P=.08).[83] However, this study was limited by a small number of patients: 12 patients in the "CPP" group and 5 patients in the "ICP" group. Furthermore, the "ICP" group was also a "CPP" group as they had to maintain a minimum CPP of greater than 50 mm Hg. In another study, aggressive treatment to lower ICP to 20 mm Hg or less using systemic antihypertensive agents and aggressive maintenance of normovolemia (the "Lund concept") revealed favorable outcomes.[84] One major concern of the "Lund concept" is the potential for hypotension, which can promote secondary brain injury and worsen outcome.[1,71,72]

Head Position

In adults after severe TBI, the head elevated at 30° reduced ICP without decreasing CPP.[73] Whereas no pediatric studies are known, the same degree of head elevation with midline position to promote venous drainage is currently recommended in the pediatric guidelines. In some centers, practitioners avoid placing a central venous catheter in the internal jugular vein to maximize venous drainage from the brain. In addition, minimal mean airway pressure from positive pressure ventilation is used to adequately ventilate and oxygenate the tracheally intubated patient to prevent impedance of venous return and to maximize venous drainage from the brain.

Sedation, Analgesia, and Neuromuscular Blockade

If there is continued ICP elevation, sedation, analgesia, and neuromuscular blockade can be administered.

It is well known that anxiety, stress, and pain can increase cerebral metabolic demands, which can pathologically increase cerebral blood volume and increase ICP. Narcotics, benzodiazepines, or barbiturates are commonly used. There are virtually no randomized, controlled studies on varying the use of sedatives in pediatric patients with severe TBI. As a result, the choice of sedatives is left up to the "treating physician," according to the guidelines.[1] However, the goal should be to use the minimum amount to lower ICP without causing side effects such as hypotension. In addition, potentially noxious stimulus such as endotracheal tube suctioning should be pretreated with sedation or analgesics, and lidocaine (1 mg/kg IV) should be considered to blunt increases in ICP.

Two drugs that are worth mentioning are ketamine and propofol. Ketamine is a potent cerebrovasodilator and increases CBF.[85] Ketamine markedly increases ICP, which can be reduced, but not prevented, by hyperventilation.[86,87] Whereas some recent clinical adult TBI studies have argued that ketamine may be safe,[88–90] there are no data on ketamine in clinical pediatric TBI. Though controversial, ketamine is believed to be contraindicated in patients with increased ICP.[91] In our institution, ketamine is NOT administered to pediatric TBI patients. Several non-TBI and one TBI case report have reported metabolic acidosis and death in pediatric patients on prolonged (24 h) continuous infusion of propofol.[92–94] Based on recommendations of the Food and Drug Administration, "continuous infusion of propofol is not recommended in the treatment of pediatric traumatic brain injury" in the pediatric guidelines.[1]

Neuromuscular blocking agents are believed to reduce ICP by reducing airway and intrathoracic pressure with improved cerebral venous outflow and by preventing shivering, posturing, or ventilator-patient asynchrony.[95] Risks of neuromuscular blockade include hypoxemia and hypercarbia due to inadvertent extubation, masking of seizures, nosocomial pneumonia (shown in adults with severe TBI), immobilization stress due to inadequate sedation and analgesia, increased length of stay in the intensive care unit, and critical illness myopathy.[95] The loss of clinical examination should be of less concern if ICP monitoring is used, as increases in ICP usually occur before changes in clinical examination.

Overall, it is clear that a paucity of data exists on the use of sedatives, analgesics, and neuromuscular blocking agents in pediatric TBI patients. This is an area of research that has tremendous potential.

Ventricular Cerebrospinal Fluid Drainage

The intracranial volume decreases by removing CSF, which may decrease ICP in a patient with intracranial hypertension. If a child with severe TBI requires ICP monitoring in our center, the neurosurgeon is encouraged to place a ventricular ICP monitor, unless contraindications such as coagulopathy or small ventricles due to diffuse cerebral edema make catheter placement difficult. In a recent study, continuous CSF drainage was associated with lower mean ICP, lower concentrations of CSF markers of neuronal and glial injury, and increased CSF volume drained compared with intermittent CSF drainage.[96] Further study is warranted to find out if prolonged continuous CSF drainage may affect electrolyte balance or intravascular volume status. One potential concern of continuous CSF drainage is that ICP can only be monitored intermittently, not continuously. Whether either mode of CSF drainage improves outcome would be an important subject of future study.

Hyperosmolar Therapy

The blood-brain barrier is nearly impermeable to mannitol and sodium. Whereas mannitol has been traditionally administered, hypertonic saline (3% saline) is also gaining favor. There is no literature to support the superiority of one over the other in severe pediatric TBI. Mannitol reduces ICP by two mechanisms. Mannitol rapidly reduces blood viscosity, which promotes reflex vasoconstriction of the arterioles by autoregulation, and decreases cerebral blood volume and ICP. This mechanism is rapid but transient, lasting about 75 minutes and requiring an intact autoregulation.[97,98] The second mechanism by which mannitol reduces ICP is through an osmotic effect: it increases serum osmolality, causing the shift of water from the brain cell to the intravascular space, and decreases cellular or cytotoxic edema. Whereas this effect is slower in onset (more than 15–30 minutes), the osmotic effect lasts up to 6 hours. This effect also requires an intact blood-brain barrier, and there are concerns that if the blood-brain barrier is not intact, mannitol may accumulate in injured brain regions and cause a shift from the intravascular space to the brain parenchyma and worsen ICP. However, this side effect is reported to be more likely when mannitol is present in the circulation for extended periods of time, supporting the use of intermittent boluses.[99,100] Furthermore, mannitol is a potent osmotic diuretic and may precipitate hypotension and renal failure if the patient becomes hypovolemic and the serum osmolality is greater than 320 mOsm/L.[1,101] Mannitol is administered in intravenous bolus doses of 0.25 g/kg to 1 g/kg.[1]

Hypertonic saline has been gaining favor recently as hyperosmolar therapy in pediatric head-injured patients with signs and symptoms of herniation. The main mechanism of action is the osmotic effect, similar to mannitol. The main theoretical advantage over mannitol is that hypertonic saline can be administered in a hemodynamically unstable patient with impending herniation, as hypertonic saline is believed to preserve intravascular volume status.[102–104] Hypertonic saline exhibits several other theoretical benefits such as restoration of normal cellular resting membrane potential and cell volume, inhibition of inflammation, stimulation of atrial natriuretic peptide release, and enhancement of cardiac output.[104–106] Hypertonic saline, as 3% saline, has recently become the most popular concentration used in the setting of TBI. It can be administered as a bolus intravenous dose; though not well studied, 1 to 6 mL/kg IV has become a popular bolus dose (unpublished observations). Doses as high as 10 mL/kg IV bolus have been reported in the literature.[107] In our pediatric institution, 2 to 6 mL/kg as an initial bolus dose is commonly used. Continuous infusions of 0.1 to 1 mL/kg/h titrated to maintain ICP at less than 20 mm Hg have also been reported.[108,109] Whereas the guidelines state that 3% saline will not precipitate renal failure as long as serum osmolality is less than 360 mOsm/L,[1] caution should be exercised if the serum osmolality approaches 320 mOsm/L as there may be an increased risk of renal insufficiency.[60] Another potential concern with the use of hypertonic saline is central pontine (demyelination of the pons) or extrapontine myelinosis (demyelination of the thalamus, basal ganglia, and cerebellum) that occurs with hypernatremia or rapid increase in serum Na,[110] although this has not been clinically reported. A further theoretical concern with the use of hypertonic saline is subarachnoid hemorrhage due to rapid shrinking of the brain associated with mechanical tearing of the bridging vessels; this too has not been clinically reported. Rebound intracranial hypertension has been described clinically with the use of hypertonic saline bolus administration or after stopping continuous infusion.[108,111]

Future studies are needed to compare mannitol administration with hypertonic saline, particularly studies evaluating optimal dosing and evaluating long-term outcome.

Hyperventilation

Hyperventilation is one of the fastest methods to lower ICP and is the best initial medical therapy with a child in impending herniation. However, without signs of herniation, mild or prophylactic hyperventilation ($PaCO_2$ <35 mm Hg) in children should be avoided. Mild hyperventilation ($PaCO_2$ 30–35 mm Hg) may be considered as a first-tier option for longer periods of intracranial hypertension refractory to all the above measures (sedation, analgesia, neuromuscular blockade, CSF drainage, and hyperosmolar therapy).[1] This rationale is based on studies that CBF may be decreased early following pediatric TBI and may be associated with poor outcome, and that prophylactic hyperventilation may cause further ischemia.[69] However, no studies on the use of hyperventilation and long-term outcomes exist in the pediatric population following TBI.

INTRACRANIAL HYPERTENSION MANAGEMENT: SECOND-TIER THERAPIES

Refractory intracranial hypertension occurs in as much as 42% of cases of severe pediatric TBI and is associated with mortality rates of between 29% and 100%.[112–115] At this point, a repeat CT scan should be performed to rule out a surgical cause for persistent, refractory intracranial hypertension. If there is no surgical lesion, the 2003 guideline recommends second-tier therapies (**Fig. 2**), which include aggressive hyperventilation, barbiturates, hypothermia, decompressive craniectomy, and lumbar CSF drainage.[1]

Hyperventilation

Aggressive hyperventilation ($PaCO_2$ <30 mm Hg) may be considered as a "second-tier" option in the setting of refractory intracranial hypertension. Cerebral blood flow, jugular venous oxygen saturation, or brain tissue oxygen monitoring to help identify cerebral ischemia is suggested.[116,117]

Barbiturates

As the use of aggressive hyperventilation for treatment of refractory intracranial hypertension has become less popular, other therapies such as barbiturates are being used. Barbiturates reduce ICP by decreasing the cerebral metabolic rate.[118–120] An electroencephalogram (EEG) should be used to assess the cerebral metabolic response to barbiturate treatment. Either a continuous infusion or frequent dosing is used. Pentobarbital or thiopental is often administered to achieve burst suppression on the EEG. However, the minimum dose should be administered as smaller doses that are associated with EEG activity may still decrease ICP and higher doses can lead to decreased cardiac output, decreased systemic vascular resistance, and hypotension.[113] If high-dose barbiturate therapy is used to treat refractory intracranial hypertension, then appropriate hemodynamic monitoring and cardiovascular support must be provided.

Further studies need to address optimal dosing to prevent unwanted side effects such as hypotension and the long-term effects of barbiturate therapy.

Decompressive Craniectomy

The main goal of decompressive craniectomy is to control ICP and maintain CPP, and prevent herniation in the face of refractory cerebral swelling. This surgical option may be particularly appropriate in patients who have a potentially recoverable brain injury. These patients have no episodes of sustained ICP of more than 40 mm Hg before surgery and exhibit a GCS greater than three at some point subsequent to injury. Other indications for decompressive craniectomy include secondary clinical deterioration or evolving cerebral herniation syndrome within 48 hours of injury.[1] A randomized trial of early decompressive craniectomy in children with TBI and sustained intracranial hypertension revealed that 54% of the surgically treated patients versus only 14% of the medically treated group had favorable outcome.[121] Other small case series and retrospective reviews have also reported benefits.[122–125] Furthermore, decompressive craniectomy may be considered in the treatment of severe TBI and refractory intracranial hypertension in infants and young children with nonaccidental head trauma or shaken-impact syndrome, as these patients had improved survival and neurologic outcomes compared with those undergoing medical management alone.[126]

However, there are concerns that this procedure may exacerbate hemorrhage and cerebral edema formation. In a recent study, decompressive craniectomy was associated with an increased incidence of posttraumatic hydrocephalus, wound complications, and epilepsy in children with severe TBI.[127] Further studies are warranted on the timing, efficacy, safety, and the type of decompressive craniectomy (unilateral vs bilateral), and the effects on long-term outcome.

Hypothermia

Posttraumatic hyperthermia is defined as a core body temperature greater than 38.5°C. Whereas hypothermia is defined as a temperature of less than 35°C In animal studies of experimental TBI, hyperthermia has been shown to exacerbate neuronal cell death. However, therapeutic hypothermia was found to be neuroprotective by ameliorating mechanisms of secondary brain injury, such as decreasing cerebral metabolism, inflammation, lipid peroxidation, and excitotoxicity.[128] In one recent study early hyperthermia (within 24 hours of admission) occurred in 29.9% of pediatric TBI patients and was associated with poor outcome.[129] Whereas most agree that hyperthermia should be avoided in children with severe TBI, the role of hypothermia is unclear. A phase II clinical trial showed that 48 hours of moderate hypothermia (32–34°C) initiated within 6 to 24 hours of acute TBI in pediatric patients reduces ICP and was "safe," although there was a higher incidence of arrhythmias (reversed with fluid administration or rewarming) and rebound ICP elevation after rewarming.[130] This rebound ICP elevation after rewarming was also observed in another study.[131] A multicenter, international (Canada, UK, and New Zealand) study of children with severe TBI randomized to hypothermia therapy (32.5°C for 24 hours) initiated within 8 hours after injury or to normothermia (37°C) was conducted recently.[132] The study reported a worsening trend with hypothermia therapy: 31% of the patients in the hypothermia group had an unfavorable outcome, compared with 22% in the normothermia group. Another multicenter, clinical trial is currently ongoing in the United States with earlier randomization to hypothermia (within 6 hours) after injury and longer duration of hypothermia (48 hours).

Until further clinical studies are completed, avoidance of hyperthermia is prudent. However, before hypothermia can become a standard of care for pediatric TBI patients, further issues need to be addressed, such as: (1) the degree of hypothermia: is mild (35°C) hypothermia just as effective as moderate hypothermia?, (2) the onset of hypothermia, (3) the duration of hypothermia, (4) the rate of rewarming after hypothermia, (5) the effect of hypothermia on drug metabolism, and (6) potential complications associated with hypothermia, such as increased bleeding risk, arrhythmias, and increased susceptibility to infection.

Seizure

Seizures should be aggressively treated as they can cause hyperthermia and intracranial hypertension. Whereas prophylactic anticonvulsants may be considered a treatment option to prevent early posttraumatic seizures (occurring within 7 days following injury) in infants and young children, prophylactic anticonvulsants are not recommended for preventing late posttraumatic seizures (occurring after 7 days) as this has not been shown to improve outcome.[133,134] Future studies with newer anticonvulsants, such as levetiracetam and topiramate, are warranted.[135]

Lumbar CSF Drainage

Although not commonly used, lumbar CSF drainage has been shown to be successful in treating refractory intracranial hypertension following pediatric TBI.[136] However, to avoid the risk of herniation the child must already have a functional ventriculostomy drain and open basal cisterns, and no mass effect or shift on concurrent CT.

FUTURE DIRECTIONS
Neuromonitoring

An area of considerable clinical interest since publication of the guidelines is the use of protein biomarkers in the diagnosis and prognosis of pediatric TBI. One study revealed that in children with accidental TBI, early (within 12 hours) elevated serum levels of S100β, a marker of astrocyte injury or death, were associated with poor outcome.[137] A recent study also revealed that S100β was elevated early after children sustained accidental TBI but also in children who sustained nonaccidental (inflicted) TBI or hypoxic-ischemic encephalopathy (HIE).[138] In addition, peak levels of serum neuron-specific enolase (NSE), a marker of neuronal injury or death, occurred early (within 12 hours) after accidental pediatric TBI whereas peak levels of NSE were delayed (as much as 3–5 days) in children with nonaccidental TBI or HIE. Furthermore, serum levels of myelin basic protein (MBP), a marker of white matter injury, revealed a delayed increase after accidental and nonaccidental TBI, but not in the HIE group. These data suggest that the biochemical response of the developing brain to nonaccidental TBI is distinct from the response to accidental TBI and shares similarities with hypoxic-ischemic brain injury. Studies have also shown CSF biomarkers to be valuable in assessing pathologic mechanisms associated with pediatric TBI, such as excitotoxicity, apoptosis, and oxidative stress.[139–141] The potential use of urine biomarkers in pediatric TBI has recently been evaluated. Because serum S100β has a short half-life that may limit its usefulness in detecting injury, a recent study revealed that urine S100β levels were elevated in children with TBI.[142] Whereas further studies need to address the sensitivity and specificity of serum and urine biomarkers, including the possibility of a nonneuronal origin for some of these biomarkers, the sampling error of hemolyzed specimens as NSE is present in red blood cells,[143] how the CSF biomarkers are obtained (continuous vs intermittent drainage) which can affect the protein biomarker levels,[96] and whether the CSF values truly correlate with the brain tissue or interstitial concentration, the use of biomarkers may potentially become an invaluable asset for monitoring the pediatric TBI patient.

In recent years intraparenchymal ICP devices have been modified to also measure the partial pressure of oxygen within the brain interstitial space (PbO_2) to monitor for cerebral hypoxia (<15 mm Hg).[144] In a recent prospective study in adult TBI patients, the use of ICP- and PbO_2-guided monitoring and therapy (ICP <20 mm Hg, CPP >60 mm Hg, and PbO_2 >25 mm Hg) significantly decreased the mortality rate from 44% to 25% compared with historical controls in using ICP monitoring and therapy alone.[144] Whereas the major limitation of this study was of the use of "historical controls," the potential advantage of PbO_2 monitoring and therapy mandates further evaluation. Whereas there is less published literature on the use of PbO_2 in children with TBI, one study revealed that PbO_2 was decreased when ICP was increased or CPP was decreased; surprisingly, there were episodes of low PbO_2 despite normal ICP and

CPP.[117] Another pediatric TBI study revealed that PbO_2 was increased in survivors.[145] One major limitation of the PbO_2 monitor is that it may represent only local, but not global assessment of brain oxygenation. Further studies clearly need to be conducted to answer questions such as: (1) where should the location of this monitor be placed: in the "uninjured" area versus "the injured" or "peri-injured" area?; (2) does optimizing PbO_2 improve outcome in a head-injured pediatric patient?

Other neuromonitoring modalities, such as magnetic resonance spectroscopy (MRS) and cerebral microdialysis, may become an important area of investigation to better understand the metabolic demands of the head-injured child. The major disadvantage of MRS is that it provides information only at a particular point in time; there is also a potential risk in transporting a critically ill patient to and from the MRS scanner. Limitations of cerebral microdialysis are the invasiveness needed to monitor the brain metabolism and, similar to the PbO_2 monitor, the question of where to place the microdialysis catheter in the brain.

Effects of Anesthetics on the Developing Brain

It is arguable that nothing has garnered more investigation and discussion among anesthesiologists than the effects of anesthetics on the developing brain. There is increasing animal data demonstrating that the administration of NMDA-antagonist or γ-aminobutyrate (GABA)-agonist anesthetics (isoflurane, nitrous oxide, ketamine, benzodiazepines, barbiturates) in the neonatal brain lead to a marked increase in apoptotic cell death, with some studies also demonstrating cognitive dysfunction.[146–151] Following TBI in neonatal rats, the administration of NMDA antagonists also increased apoptotic cell death.[25] Because the neonatal brain requires excitatory-mediated neurotransmission for normal development and activity, it is not surprising that the indiscriminate inhibition of the normal excitotoxicity-mediated events during a critical period may interfere with normal brain maturation. However, other animal data suggest beneficial effects of antiexcitotoxic agents. Following hypoxia-ischemia in neonatal rodents, administration of isoflurane was found to be neuroprotective.[152–154] Following deep hypothermic circulatory arrest or low-flow cardiopulmonary bypass in newborn pigs, administration of desflurane also improved neurologic outcome.[155,156]

It is obvious that further research is of paramount importance regarding the role of anesthetics and apoptosis in the developing brain. For example, there may be an age-dependent response to anesthetics: the vulnerability to anesthesia-induced apoptosis quickly diminishes with increasing age in the developing rodent brain.[157,158] Following experimental TBI, whereas NMDA antagonists promoted apoptosis in the neonatal rodent brain,[25] the administration of isoflurane (an NMDA antagonist) provided neuroprotection in the adult rodent brain.[159] Furthermore, whereas animal data suggest that anesthetics clearly promote apoptosis, it is unknown whether this is beneficial or harmful; are anesthetics promoting cell death in healthy neurons or are anesthetics accelerating cell death in neurons that were supposed to die anyway? Another area of research is looking at different combinations of medications and their effects on apoptosis and long-term neurologic outcome: is administration of an NMDA-antagonist medication with a GABA-agonist agent worse or better than administering 2 NMDA-antagonist or 2 GABA-agonist agents to induce anesthesia?

Most importantly, caution should be advised when extrapolating animal data to human data. Whereas there are anecdotal cases of temporary neurologic dysfunction after early exposure to anesthetics, most pediatric patients are safely anesthetized and there are no published data on anesthetics causing long-term neurologic problems or structural brain abnormalities in infants and children.[158] That said, further investigation is a must on the role of anesthetics on the developing brain in the laboratory and in the pediatric population.

SUMMARY

The publication of the 2003 pediatric TBI guidelines have served as an impetus for new studies that have led to an improved understanding of the unique age-dependent responses following pediatric TBI. Whereas ongoing research to better understand the unique injury patterns, pathophysiology, therapeutic options, neuromonitoring, and the effects of anesthetics on different developmental stages of the head-injured pediatric TBI is important, it is clear that management in the "initial golden minutes" is critical to improving outcomes. Avoiding or rapidly correcting hypotension and hypoxemia, and other causes of secondary brain injury such as intracranial hypertension, cannot be overemphasized. Anesthesiologists must recognize the signs and symptoms of severe pediatric TBI and initiate appropriate therapeutic interventions.

REFERENCES

1. Adelson PD, Bratton SL, Carney NA, et al. Guidelines for the acute medical management of severe traumatic brain injury in infants, children, and adolescents. Pediatr Crit Care Med 2003;4:S1–75.
2. Schneier AJ, Shields BJ, Hostetler SG, et al. Incidence of pediatric traumatic brain injury and associated hospital resource utilization in the United States. Pediatrics 2006;118:483–92.
3. Duhaime AC, Christian CW, Rorke LB, et al. Nonaccidental head injury in infants-the "shaken-baby syndrome". N Engl J Med 1998;338:1822–9.
4. Ewing-Cobbs L, Prasad M, Kramer L, et al. Acute neuroradiologic findings in young children with inflicted or noninflicted traumatic brain injury. Childs Nerv Syst 2000;16:25–33.
5. Agran PF, Anderson C, Winn D, et al. Rates of pediatric injuries by 3-month intervals for children 0 to 3 years of age. Pediatrics 2003;111:e683–92.
6. Durkin MS, Laraque D, Lubman I, et al. Epidemiology and prevention of traffic injuries to urban children and adolescents. Pediatrics 1999;103:1–8.
7. Langlois JA, Rutland-Brown W, Thomas KE. The incidence of traumatic brain injury among children in the United States: differences by race. J Head Trauma Rehabil 2005;20:229–38.
8. Aldrich EF, Eisenberg HM, Saydjari C, et al. Diffuse brain swelling in severely head-injured children. A report from the NIH Traumatic Coma Data Bank. J Neurosurg 1992;76:450–4.
9. Duhaime AC, Durham S. Traumatic brain injury in infants: the phenomenon of subdural hemorrhage with hemispheric hypodensity "Big Black Brain". Prog Brain Res 2007;161:293–302.
10. Suh DY, Davis PC, Hopkins KL, et al. Nonaccidental pediatric head injury: diffusion-weighted imaging findings. Neurosurgery 2001;49(2):309–20.
11. Ichord RN, Naim M, Pollock AN, et al. Hypoxic-ischemic injury complicates inflicted and accidental traumatic brain injury in young children: the role of diffusion-weighted imaging. J Neurotrauma 2007;24:106–18.
12. Lenzlinger PM, Saatman K, Raghupathi R, et al. Overview of basic mechanisms underlying neuropathological consequences of head trauma. In: Miller, Hayes, editors. Head trauma- basic, preclinical, and clinical directions. New Jersey: Wiley-Liss; 2001. p. 3–36.

13. Kochanek PM, Bayir H, Jenkins LW, et al. Molecular biology of brain injury. In: Nichols D, editor. Rogers' textbook of pediatric intensive care. 4th edition. Pennsylvania: Lippincott Williams & Wilkins; 2008. p. 826–45.
14. Choi DW. Ionic dependence of glutamate neurotoxicity. J Neurosci 1987;7: 369–79.
15. Huh JW, Franklin MA, Widing AG, et al. Regionally distinct patterns of calpain activation and traumatic axonal injury following contusive brain injury in immature rats. Dev Neurosci 2006;28:466–76.
16. Giza CC, Maria NS, Hovda DA. N-Methyl-D-aspartate receptor subunit changes after traumatic injury to the developing brain. J Neurotrauma 2006;23:950–61.
17. Zamzami N, Susin SA, Marchetti P, et al. Mitochondrial control of nuclear apoptosis. J Exp Med 1996;183:1533–44.
18. Li P, Nihawan D, Budihardjo I, et al. Cytochrome c and dATP-dependent formation of Apaf-1/caspase-9 complex initiates an apoptotic protease cascade. Cell 1997;91:479–89.
19. Clark RSB, Kochanek PM, Watkins SC, et al. Caspase-3 mediated neuronal death after traumatic brain injury in rats. J Neurochem 2000;74:740–53.
20. Ashkenazi A, Dixit VM. Death receptors: signaling and modulation. Science 1998;281:1305–8.
21. Raghupathi R, Graham DI, McIntosh TK. Apoptosis after traumatic brain injury. J Neurotrauma 2000;17:927–38.
22. Rink AD, Fung KM, Trojanowski JQ, et al. Evidence of apoptotic cell death after experimental traumatic brain injury in the rat. Am J Pathol 1995;147:1575–83.
23. McDonald JW, Silverstein FS, Johnston MV. Neurotoxicity of N-methyl-D-aspartate is markedly enhanced in developing rat central nervous system. Brain Res 1988;459:200–3.
24. Osteen CL, Moore AH, Prins ML, et al. Age-dependency of 45calcium accumulation following lateral fluid percussion: acute and delayed patterns. J Neurotrauma 2001;18:141–62.
25. Pohl D, Bittigau P, Ishimaru MJ, et al. N-Methyl-D-aspartate antagonists and apoptotic cell death triggered by head trauma in developing rat brain. Proc Natl Acad Sci U S A 1999;96:2508–13.
26. Sun FY, Faden AI. Neuroprotective effects of 619C89, a use-dependent sodium channel blocker, in rat traumatic brain injury. Brain Res 1995;673: 133–40.
27. Kochanek PM, Clark RSB, Ruppel RA, et al. Biochemical, cellular, and molecular mechanisms in the evolution of secondary damage after severe traumatic brain injury in infants and children: lessons learned from the bedside. Pediatr Crit Care Med 2000;1:4–19.
28. Oshio K, Watanabe H, Song Y, et al. Reduced cerebrospinal fluid production and intracranial pressure in mice lacking choroid plexus water channel Aquaporin-1. FASEB J 2005;19:76–8.
29. Barzo P, Marmarou A, Fatouros P, et al. Contribution of vasogenic and cellular edema to traumatic brain swelling measured by diffusion-weighted imaging. J Neurosurg 1997;87:900–7.
30. Zwienenberg M, Muizelaar JP. Severe pediatric head injury: the role of hyperemia revisited. J Neurotrauma 1999;16:937–43.
31. Bruce DA, Alavi A, Bilaniuk L, et al. Diffuse cerebral swelling following head injuries in children: the syndrome of "malignant brain edema". J Neurosurg 1981;54:170–8.

32. Muizelaar JP, Marmarou A, DeSalles AA, et al. Cerebral blood flow and metabolism in severely head-injured children. Part 1: relationship with GCS score, outcome, ICP, and PVI. J Neurosurg 1989;71:63–71.

33. Suzuki K. The changes of regional cerebral blood flow with advancing age in normal children. Nagoya Med J 1990;34:159–70.

34. Adelson PD, Clyde B, Kochanek PM, et al. Cerebrovascular response in infants and young children following severe traumatic brain injury: a preliminary report. Pediatr Neurosurg 1997;26:200–7.

35. Vavilala MS, Muangman S, Tontisirin N, et al. Impaired cerebral autoregulation and 6-month outcome in children with severe traumatic brain injury: preliminary findings. Dev Neurosci 2006;28:348–53.

36. Vavilala MS, Muangman S, Waitayawinyu P, et al. Neurointensive care; impaired cerebral autoregulation in infants and young children early after inflicted traumatic brain injury: a preliminary report. J Neurotrauma 2007;24:87–96.

37. Freeman SS, Udomphorn Y, Armstead WM, et al. Young age as a risk factor for impaired cerebral autoregulation after moderate to severe pediatric traumatic brain injury. Anesthesiology 2008;108:588–95.

38. Prins ML, Lee SM, Cheng CLY, et al. Fluid percussion brain injury in the developing and adult rat: a comparative study of mortality, morphology, intracranial pressure and mean arterial blood pressure. Brain Res Dev Brain Res 1996;95:272–82.

39. Armstead WM, Kurth CD. Different cerebral hemodynamic responses following fluid-percussion brain injury in the newborn and juvenile pig. J Neurotrauma 1994;11:487–97.

40. Durham SR, Raghupathi R, Helfaer MA, et al. Age-related differences in acute physiologic response to focal traumatic brain injury in piglets. Pediatr Neurosurg 2000;33:76–82.

41. Armstead WM. Cerebral hemodynamics after traumatic brain injury of immature brain. Exp Toxicol Pathol 1999;51:137–42.

42. Armstead WM. Age-dependent impairment of K_{ATP} channel function following brain injury. J Neurotrauma 1999;16:391–402.

43. Armstead WM. Brain injury impairs prostaglandin cerebrovasodilation. J Neurotrauma 1998;15:721–9.

44. Armstead WM. Role of endothelin-1 in age-dependent cerebrovascular hypotensive responses after brain injury. Am J Physiol 1999;277:H1884–94.

45. Armstead WM. Age and cerebral circulation. Pathophysiology 2005;12:5–15.

46. Adams JH, Graham DI, Murray LS, et al. Diffuse axonal injury due to nonmissile head injury in humans: an analysis of 45 cases. Ann Neurol 1982;12:557–63.

47. Povlishock JT, Christian CW. The pathobiology of traumatically induced axonal injury in animals and humans: a review of current thoughts. In: Bandak FA, Eppinger RH, Ommaya AK, editors. Traumatic brain injury: bioscience and mechanics. New York: Mary Ann Liebert; 1996. p. 51–60.

48. Chiaretti A, Visocchi M, Viola L, et al. [Diffuse axonal lesions in childhood]. Pediatr Med Chir 1998;20:393–7 [in Italian].

49. Tong KA, Ashwal S, Holshouser BA, et al. Diffuse axonal injury in children: clinical correlation with hemorrhagic lesions. Ann Neurol 2004;56:36–50.

50. Shannon P, Smith CR, Deck J, et al. Axonal injury and the neuropathology of shaken baby syndrome. Acta Neuropathol 1998;95:625–31.

51. Ashwal S, Holshouser BA, Tong KA. Use of advanced neuroimaging techniques in the evaluation of pediatric traumatic brain injury. Dev Neurosci 2006;28:309–26.

52. Povlishock JT, Christman CW. The pathobiology of traumatically induced axonal injury in animals and humans: a review of current thoughts. J Neurotrauma 1995; 12:555–64.
53. Raghupathi R, Margulies SS. Traumatic axonal injury after closed head injury in the neonatal pig. J Neurotrauma 2002;19:843–53.
54. Huh JW, Widing AG, Raghupathi R. Midline brain injury in the immature rat induces sustained cognitive deficits, bihemispheric axonal injury and neurodegeneration. Exp Neurol 2008;213:84–92.
55. ATLS: advanced trauma life support for doctors. 7th edition. Chicago: American College of Surgeons; 2004.
56. Falk AC, Cederfjall C, Von WL, et al. Management and classification of children with head injury. Childs Nerv Syst 2005;21:430–6.
57. Kochanek PM, Forbes ME, Ruppel RA, et al. Severe traumatic brain injury in infants and children. In: Fuhrman BP, Zimmerman JJ, editors. Pediatric critical care. Philadelphia: Mosby; 2006. p. 1595–617.
58. Teasdale G, Jennett B. Assessment of coma and impaired consciousness. A practical scale. Lancet 1974;2:81–4.
59. Reilly PL, Simpson DA, Sprod R, et al. Assessing the conscious level in infants and young children: a paediatric version of the Glasgow Coma Scale. Childs Nerv Syst 1988;4:30–3.
60. Dominguez TE, Priestley MA, Huh JW. Caution should be exercised when maintaining a serum sodium level >160 meq/L. Crit Care Med 2004;32:1438–9.
61. Chiaretti A, Pezzotti P, Mestrovic J, et al. The influence of hemocoagulative disorders on the outcome of children with head injury. Pediatr Neurosurg 2001;34: 131–7.
62. Carrick MM, Tyroch AH, Youens CA, et al. Subsequent development of thrombocytopenia and coagulopathy in moderate and severe head injury: support for serial laboratory examination. J Trauma 2005;58:725–9.
63. Hiler M, Czosnyka M, Hutchinson P, et al. Predictive value of initial computerized tomography scan, intracranial pressure, and state of autoregulation in patients with traumatic brain injury. J Neurosurg 2006;104:731–7.
64. Pillai S, Praharaj SS, Mohanty A, et al. Prognostic factors in children with severe diffuse brain injuries: a study of 74 patients. Pediatr Neurosurg 2001;34:98–103.
65. Maas AI, Steyerberg EW, Butcher I, et al. Prognostic value of computerized tomography scan characteristics in traumatic brain injury: results from the IMPACT study. J Neurotrauma 2007;24:303–14.
66. Wilde EA, Chu Z, Bigler ED, et al. Diffusion tensor imaging in the corpus callosum in children after moderate to severe traumatic brain injury. J Neurotrauma 2006;23: 1412–26.
67. Missios S, Quebada PB, Forero JA, et al. Quick-brain magnetic resonance imaging for nonhydrocephalus indications. J Neurosurg Pediatr 2008;2:438–44.
68. Hauswald M, Sklar DP, Tandberg D, et al. Cervical spine movement during airway management: cinefluoroscopic appraisal in human cadavers. Am J Emerg Med 1991;9:535–8.
69. Skippen P, Seear M, Poskitt K, et al. Effect of hyperventilation on regional cerebral blood flow in head-injured children. Crit Care Med 1997;25:1402–9.
70. Lev R, Rosen P. Prophylactic lidocaine use preintubation: a review. J Emerg Med 1994;12:499–506.
71. Coates BM, Vavilala MS, Mack CD, et al. Influence of definition and location of hypotension on outcome following severe pediatric traumatic brain injury. Crit Care Med 2005;33:2645–50.

72. Ducrocq SC, Meyer PG, Orliaguet GA, et al. Epidemiology and early predictive factors of mortality and outcome in children with traumatic severe brain injury: experience of a French pediatric trauma center. Pediatr Crit Care Med 2006;7: 461–7.

73. Feldman Z, Kanter MJ, Robertson CS, et al. Effect of head elevation on intracranial pressure, cerebral perfusion pressure, and cerebral blood flow in head-injured patients. J Neurosurg 1992;76:207–11.

74. Lundberg N. Continuous recording and control of ventricular fluid pressure in neurosurgical practice. Acta Psychiatr Scand Suppl 1960;36:1–193.

75. Pfenninger J, Kaiser G, Lutschg J, et al. Treatment and outcome of the severely head injured child. Intensive Care Med 1983;9:13–6.

76. Esparza J, Portillo J, Sarabia M, et al. Outcome in children with severe head injuries. Childs Nerv Syst 1985;1:109–14.

77. Sharples PM, Stuart AG, Matthews DS, et al. Cerebral blood flow and metabolism in children with severe head injury. Part 1: relation to age, Glasgow coma score, outcome, intracranial pressure, and time after injury. J Neurol Neurosurg Psychiatry 1995;58:145–52.

78. Shapiro K, Marmarou A. Clinical applications of the pressure-volume index in treatment of pediatric head injuries. J Neurosurg 1982;56:819–25.

79. Elias-Jones AC, Punt JA, Turnbull AE, et al. Management and outcome of severe head injuries in the Trent region 1985–90. Arch Dis Child 1992;67:1430–5.

80. Downard C, Hulka F, Mullins RJ, et al. Relationship of cerebral perfusion pressure and survival in pediatric brain-injured patients. J Trauma 2000;49:654–8.

81. Barzilay Z, Augarten A, Sagy M, et al. Variables affecting outcome from severe brain injury in children. Intensive Care Med 1988;14:417–21.

82. Chambers IR, Stobbart L, Jones PA, et al. Age-related differences in intracranial pressure and cerebral perfusion pressure in the first 6 hours of monitoring after children's head injury: association with outcome. Childs Nerv Syst 2005;21: 195–9.

83. Prabhakaran P, Reddy AT, Oakes WJ, et al. A pilot trial comparing cerebral perfusion pressure-targeted therapy to intracranial pressure-targeted therapy in children with severe traumatic brain injury. J Neurosurg 2004;100:454–9.

84. Wahlstrom MR, Olivecrona M, Koskinen LO, et al. Severe traumatic brain injury in pediatric patients: treatment and outcome using an intracranial pressure targeted therapy—the Lund concept. Intensive Care Med 2005;31:832–9.

85. Takeshita H, Okuda Y, Sari A. The effects of ketamine on cerebral circulation and metabolism in man. Anesthesiology 1972;36:69–75.

86. Gardner AE, Dannemiller FJ, Dean D. Intracranial cerebrospinal fluid pressure in man during ketamine anesthesia. Anesth Analg 1972;51:741–5.

87. Wyte SR, Shapiro HM, Turner P, et al. Ketamine-induced intracranial hypertension. Anesthesiology 1972;36:174–6.

88. Schmittner MD, Vajkoczy SL, Horn P, et al. Effects of fentanyl and S(+)-ketamine on cerebral hemodynamics, gastrointestinal motility, and need of vasopressors in patients with intracranial pathologies: a pilot study. J Neurosurg Anesthesiol 2007;19:257–62.

89. Bourgoin A, Albanese J, Leone M, et al. Effects of sufentanil or ketamine administered in target-controlled infusion on the cerebral hemodynamics of severely brain-injured patients. Crit Care Med 2005;33:1109–13.

90. Sehdev RS, Symmons DA, Kindl K. Ketamine for rapid sequence induction in patients with head injury in the emergency department. Emerg Med Australas 2006;18:37–44.

91. Silvay G. Ketamine. Mt Sinai J Med 1983;50:300–4.
92. Bray RJ. Propofol infusion syndrome in children. Paediatr Anaesth 1998;8: 491–9.
93. Parke TJ, Stevens JE, Rice AS, et al. Metabolic acidosis and fatal myocardial failure after propofol infusion in children: five case reports. BMJ 1992;305:613–6.
94. Canivet JL, Gustad K, Leclercq P, et al. Massive ketonuria during sedation with propofol in a 12 year old girl with severe head trauma. Acta Anaesthesiol Belg 1994;45:19–22.
95. Hsiang JK, Chesnut RM, Crisp CB, et al. Early, routine paralysis for intracranial pressure control in severe head injury: is it necessary? Crit Care Med 1994;22: 1471–6.
96. Shore PM, Thomas NJ, Clark RS, et al. Continuous versus intermittent cerebro-spinal fluid drainage after severe traumatic brain injury in children: effect on biochemical markers. J Neurotrauma 2004;21:1113–22.
97. Muizelaar JP, Lutz HA III, Becker DP. Effect of mannitol on ICP and CBF and correlation with pressure autoregulation in severely head-injured patients. J Neurosurg 1984;61:700–6.
98. Muizelaar JP, Wei EP, Kontos HA, et al. Mannitol causes compensatory cerebral vasoconstriction and vasodilation in response to blood viscosity changes. J Neurosurg 1983;59:822–8.
99. James HE. Methodology for the control of intracranial pressure with hypertonic mannitol. Acta Neurochir (Wien) 1980;51:161–72.
100. Kaufmann AM, Cardoso ER. Aggravation of vasogenic cerebral edema by multiple-dose mannitol. J Neurosurg 1992;77:584–9.
101. Feig PU, McCurdy DK. The hypertonic state. N Engl J Med 1977;297:1444–54.
102. Shackford SR, Bourguignon PR, Wald SL, et al. Hypertonic saline resuscitation of patients with head injury: a prospective, randomized clinical trial. J Trauma 1998;44:50–8.
103. Walsh JC, Zhuang J, Shackford SR. A comparison of hypertonic to isotonic fluid in the resuscitation of brain injury and hemorrhagic shock. J Surg Res 1991;50: 284–92.
104. Qureshi AI, Suarez JI. Use of hypertonic saline solutions in treatment of cerebral edema and intracranial hypertension. Crit Care Med 2000;28:3301–13.
105. Nakayama S, Kramer GC, Carlsen RC, et al. Infusion of very hypertonic saline to bled rats: membrane potentials and fluid shifts. J Surg Res 1985;38:180–6.
106. Arjamaa O, Karlqvist K, Kanervo A, et al. Plasma ANP during hypertonic NaCl infusion in man. Acta Physiol Scand 1992;144:113–9.
107. Fisher B, Thomas D, Peterson B. Hypertonic saline lowers raised intracranial pressure in children after head trauma. J Neurosurg Anesthesiol 1992;4:4–10.
108. Peterson B, Khanna S, Fisher B, et al. Prolonged hypernatremia controls elevated intracranial pressure in head-injured pediatric patients. Crit Care Med 2000;28:1136–43.
109. Khanna S, Davis D, Peterson B, et al. Use of hypertonic saline in the treatment of severe refractory posttraumatic intracranial hypertension in pediatric traumatic brain injury. Crit Care Med 2000;28:1144–51.
110. Sterns RH, Riggs JE, Schochet SS Jr. Osmotic demyelination syndrome following correction of hyponatremia. N Engl J Med 1986;314:1535–42.
111. Qureshi AI, Suarez JI, Bhardwaj A. Malignant cerebral edema in patients with hypertensive intracerebral hemorrhage associated with hypertonic saline infu-sion: a rebound phenomenon? J Neurosurg Anesthesiol 1998;10:188–92.

112. Cordobes F, Lobato RD, Rivas JJ, et al. Post-traumatic diffuse brain swelling: isolated or associated with cerebral axonal injury. Clinical course and intracranial pressure in 18 children. Childs Nerv Syst 1987;3:235–8.
113. Kasoff SS, Lansen TA, Holder D, et al. Aggressive physiologic monitoring of pediatric head trauma patients with elevated intracranial pressure. Pediatr Neurosci 1988;14:241–9.
114. Bruce DA, Schut L, Bruno LA, et al. Outcome following severe head injuries in children. J Neurosurg 1978;48:679–88.
115. Berger MS, Pitts LH, Lovely M, et al. Outcome from severe head injury in children and adolescents. J Neurosurg 1985;62:194–9.
116. Cruz J, Nakayama P, Imamura JH, et al. Cerebral extraction of oxygen and intracranial hypertension in severe, acute pediatric brain trauma: preliminary novel management strategies. Neurosurgery 2002;50:774–9.
117. Stiefel MF, Udoetuk JD, Storm PB, et al. Brain tissue oxygen monitoring in pediatric patients with severe traumatic brain injury. J Neurosurg 2006;105:281–6.
118. Piatt JH Jr, Schiff SJ. High dose barbiturate therapy in neurosurgery and intensive care. Neurosurgery 1984;15:427–44.
119. Demopoulos HB, Flamm ES, Pietronigro DD, et al. The free radical pathology and the microcirculation in the major central nervous system disorders. Acta Physiol Scand Suppl 1980;492:91–119.
120. Kassell NF, Hitchon PW, Gerk MK, et al. Alterations in cerebral blood flow, oxygen metabolism, and electrical activity produced by high dose sodium thiopental. Neurosurgery 1980;7:598–603.
121. Taylor A, Butt W, Rosenfeld J, et al. A randomized trial of very early decompressive craniectomy in children with traumatic brain injury and sustained intracranial hypertension. Childs Nerv Syst 2001;17:154–62.
122. Hejazi N, Witzmann A, Fae P. Unilateral decompressive craniectomy for children with severe brain injury. Report of seven cases and review of the relevant literature. Eur J Pediatr 2002;161:99–104.
123. Figaji AA, Fieggen AG, Peter JC. Early decompressive craniotomy in children with severe traumatic brain injury. Childs Nerv Syst 2003;19:666–73.
124. Ruf B, Heckmann M, Schroth I, et al. Early decompressive craniectomy and duraplasty for refractory intracranial hypertension in children: results of a pilot study. Crit Care 2003;7:R133–8.
125. Jagannathan J, Okonkwo DO, Dumont AS, et al. Outcome following decompressive craniectomy in children with severe traumatic brain injury: a 10-year single-center experience with long-term follow up. J Neurosurg 2007;106:268–75.
126. Cho DY, Wang YC, Chi CS. Decompressive craniotomy for acute shaken/impact baby syndrome. Pediatr Neurosurg 1995;23:192–8.
127. Kan P, Amini A, Hansen K, et al. Outcomes after decompressive craniectomy for severe traumatic brain injury in children. J Neurosurg 2006;105:337–42.
128. Marion DW, Obrist WD, Carlier PM, et al. The use of moderate therapeutic hypothermia for patients with severe head injuries: a preliminary report. J Neurosurg 1993;79:354–62.
129. Natale JE, Joseph JG, Helfaer MA, et al. Early hyperthermia after traumatic brain injury in children: risk factors, influence on length of stay, and effect on short-term neurologic status. Crit Care Med 2000;28:2608–15.
130. Adelson PD, Ragheb J, Kanev P, et al. Phase II clinical trial of moderate hypothermia after severe traumatic brain injury in children. Neurosurgery 2005;56:740–54.

131. Biswas AK, Bruce DA, Sklar FH, et al. Treatment of acute traumatic brain injury in children with moderate hypothermia improves intracranial hypertension. Crit Care Med 2002;30:2742–51.
132. Hutchison JS, Ward RE, Lacroix J, et al. Hypothermia therapy after traumatic brain injury in children. N Engl J Med 2008;358:2447–56.
133. Young B, Rapp RP, Norton JA, et al. Failure of prophylactically administered phenytoin to prevent post-traumatic seizures in children. Childs Brain 1983; 10:185–92.
134. Lewis RJ, Yee L, Inkelis SH, et al. Clinical predictors of post-traumatic seizures in children with head trauma. Ann Emerg Med 1993;22:1114–8.
135. Abend NS, Huh JW, Helfaer MA, et al. Anticonvulsant medications in the pediatric emergency room and intensive care unit. Pediatr Emerg Care 2008;24(10): 705–18.
136. Levy DI, Rekate HL, Cherny WB, et al. Controlled lumbar drainage in pediatric head injury. J Neurosurg 1995;83:453–60.
137. Spinella PC, Dominguez T, Drott HR, et al. S-100B protein-serum levels in healthy children and its association with outcome in pediatric traumatic brain injury. Crit Care Med 2003;31:939–45.
138. Berger RP, Adelson PD, Richichi R, et al. Serum biomarkers after traumatic and hypoxemic brain injuries: insight into the biochemical response of the pediatric brain to inflicted brain injury. Dev Neurosci 2006;28:327–35.
139. Ruppel RA, Kochanek PM, Adelson PD, et al. Excitatory amino acid concentrations in ventricular cerebrospinal fluid after severe traumatic brain injury in infants and children: the role of child abuse. J Pediatr 2001;138:18–25.
140. Satchell MA, Lai Y, Kochanek PM, et al. Cytochrome c, a biomarker of apoptosis, is increased in cerebrospinal fluid from infants with inflicted brain injury from child abuse. J Cereb Blood Flow Metab 2005;25:919–27.
141. Bayir H, Kagan VE, Tyurina YY, et al. Assessment of antioxidant reserves and oxidative stress in cerebrospinal fluid after severe traumatic brain injury in infants and children. Pediatr Res 2002;51:571–8.
142. Berger RP, Kochanek PM. Urinary S100B concentrations are increased after brain injury in children: a preliminary study. Pediatr Crit Care Med 2006;7: 557–61.
143. Berger R, Richichi R. Derivation and validation of an equation for adjustment of neuron-specific enolase concentrations in hemolyzed serum. Pediatr Crit Care Med 2009;10(2):260–3.
144. Stiefel MF, Spiotta A, Gracias VH, et al. Reduced mortality rate in patients with severe traumatic brain injury treated with brain tissue oxygen monitoring. J Neurosurg 2005;103:805–11.
145. Narotam PK, Burjonrappa SC, Raynor SC, et al. Cerebral oxygenation in major pediatric trauma: its relevance to trauma severity and outcome. J Pediatr Surg 2006;41:505–13.
146. Bittigau P, Sifringer M, Genz K, et al. Antiepileptic drugs and apoptotic neurodegeneration in the developing brain. Proc Natl Acad Sci U S A 2002;99: 15089–94.
147. Young C, Jevtovic-Todorovic V, Qin YQ, et al. Potential of ketamine and midazolam, individually or in combination, to induce apoptotic neurodegeneration in the infant mouse brain. Br J Pharmacol 2005;146:189–97.
148. Olney JW, Young C, Wozniak DF, et al. Do pediatric drugs cause developing neurons to commit suicide? Trends Pharmacol Sci 2004;25:135–9.

149. Fredriksson A, Archer T, Alm H, et al. Neurofunctional deficits and potentiated apoptosis by neonatal NMDA antagonist administration. Behav Brain Res 2004;153:367–76.
150. Jevtovic-Todorovic V, Hartman RE, Izumi Y, et al. Early exposure to common anesthetic agents causes widespread neurodegeneration in the developing rat brain and persistent learning deficits. J Neurosci 2003;23:876–82.
151. Kaindl AM, Asimiadou S, Manthey D, et al. Antiepileptic drugs and the developing brain. Cell Mol Life Sci 2006;63:399–413.
152. McAuliffe JJ, Joseph B, Vorhees CV. Isoflurane-delayed preconditioning reduces immediate mortality and improves striatal function in adult mice after neonatal hypoxia-ischemia. Anesth Analg 2007;104:1066–77.
153. Zhan X, Fahlman CS, Bickler PE. Isoflurane neuroprotection in rat hippocampal slices decreases with aging: changes in intracellular Ca^{2+} regulation and N-methyl-D-aspartate receptor-mediated Ca^{2+} influx. Anesthesiology 2006;104:995–1003.
154. Zhao P, Zuo Z. Isoflurane preconditioning induces neuroprotection that is inducible nitric oxide synthase-dependent in neonatal rats. Anesthesiology 2004;101:695–703.
155. Kurth CD, Priestley M, Watzman HM, et al. Desflurane confers neurologic protection for deep hypothermic circulatory arrest in newborn pigs. Anesthesiology 2001;95:959–64.
156. Loepke AW, Priestley MA, Schultz SE, et al. Desflurane improves neurologic outcome after low-flow cardiopulmonary bypass in newborn pigs. Anesthesiology 2002;97:1521–7.
157. Bittigau P, Sifringer M, Pohl D, et al. Apoptotic neurodegeneration following trauma is markedly enhanced in the immature brain. Ann Neurol 1999;45:724–35.
158. Loepke AW, Soriano SG. An assessment of the effects of general anesthetics on developing brain structure and neurocognitive function. Anesth Analg 2008;106:1681–707.
159. Statler KD, Alexander H, Vagni V, et al. Isoflurane exerts neuroprotective actions at or near the time of severe traumatic brain injury. Brain Res 2006;1076:216–24.

Pharmacologic Management of Acute Pediatric Pain

F. Wickham Kraemer, MD[a,b,*], John B. Rose, MD[a,c]

KEYWORDS

- Pediatric pain management
- Acute • Pediatric pain pharmacology

The accurate assessment and effective treatment of acute pain in children in the hospital setting is a high priority. Evidence is growing that pediatric patients of all ages, even the most extremely premature neonates, are capable of experiencing pain as a result of tissue injuries due to medical illnesses, therapeutic and diagnostic procedures, trauma, and surgery.[1,2] If pain is not recognized and adequately treated, the resulting physiologic and behavioral responses can be potentially harmful, resulting in long-lasting negative effects on the developing nociceptive system.[3,4]

The complex processes by which noxious thermal, chemical, or mechanical stimuli are transformed, transmitted, modified, and perceived as pain by an individual are collectively referred to as nociception. Many of these processes lend themselves to pharmacologic interventions that can attenuate or block the transmission of pain. Pain treatment plans that target a single step in the nociceptive process with a single medication may be less effective than plans that target multiple steps by using a combination of analgesics.[5–9] Although opiates continue to be mainstays in the treatment of moderate to severe acute pain, by combining them with drugs and techniques that target other components of nociceptive pathways it may be possible to reduce the opiate consumption, provide equivalent or superior analgesia, and reduce the incidence and severity of opiate-related adverse drug events such as nausea, vomiting, constipation, pruritus, respiratory and central nervous system depression, and urinary retention.[7,10] In recent years regional analgesic techniques supplemented with systemic opiate or nonsteroidal anti-inflammatory drug (NSAID) therapy have emerged as invaluable methods for controlling severe acute postoperative pain in

[a] University of Pennsylvania, School of Medicine, Department of Anesthesiology and Critical Care, 3400 Spruce Street, Philadelphia, PA 19104, USA
[b] Department of Anesthesiology and Critical Care Medicine, Children's Hospital of Philadelphia, 34th and Civic Center Boulevard, Philadelphia, PA 19104, USA
[c] Pain Management Service, Department of Anesthesiology and Critical Care Medicine, Children's Hospital of Philadelphia, 34th and Civic Center Boulevard, Philadelphia, PA 19104, USA
* Corresponding author. University of Pennsylvania, School of Medicine, Philadelphia, PA 19104.
E-mail address: KRAEMER@email.chop.edu (F. W. Kraemer).

Anesthesiology Clin 27 (2009) 241–268
doi:10.1016/j.anclin.2009.07.002
1932-2275/09/$ – see front matter © 2009 Elsevier Inc. All rights reserved.

children. It should also be mentioned that especially for the treatment of moderate to severe pain in children, many hospitals now use Pediatric Acute Pain Management Services to develop individual pain treatment plans; closely monitor their implementation, safety, and efficacy; and make adjustments to the treatment plan if necessary to improve analgesia, ensure patient safety, or decrease unwanted side effects of analgesic therapy. This article provides an overview of the most common analgesic medications and techniques used to treat acute pain in children.

ANALGESIC, ANTIPYRETIC, NONSTEROIDAL ANTI-INFLAMMATORY DRUGS

NSAIDs are used for mild to moderate pain by themselves or they may used in combination with other agents and techniques for moderate to severe pain. Although they are often categorized as weak analgesics, for pain associated with tissue inflammation, they may be superior to opioids.[11] Their use is not associated with the common adverse reactions associated with opioid therapy: respiratory depression, sedation, physical dependence, nausea, vomiting, constipation, or pruritis. All NSAIDs work by inhibition of cyclooxygenase (COX), the enzyme responsible for metabolizing arachidonic acid.[12] The inflammatory response can be triggered by several mechanisms, all of which result in cell membrane damage, including thermal or mechanical trauma, infectious agents, antigen-antibody complexes, or ischemia. Once released by traumatized or damaged cell membranes, arachidonic acid is metabolized by COX to form prostaglandins and thromboxanes. Prostaglandins and thromboxanes then sensitize peripheral nerve endings and vasodilate vessels causing pain, erythema, and inflammation. Several COX isoenzymes have been identified. The constitutive form of COX (COX-1) is present throughout the body. Prostaglandins produced by COX-1 are essential for a variety of essential functions including: regulation of kidney blood flow, protection of gastric mucosa from damage secondary to gastric acid secretion, and platelet aggregation. Therefore, complications from the use of nonselective COX inhibitors such as ibuprofen, ketorolac, and naproxen include gastric ulceration, bleeding, and impaired renal function. Analgesic efficacy and the risk for bleeding was the subject of a recent review on the perioperative use of NSAIDs.[13] The investigators conclude that although NSAIDs play a valuable part in the management of postoperative pain in children, perioperative bleeding has occurred in children who received NSAIDs. Further, the investigators comment that the available evidence from the literature reviewed fails to establish definitively that NSAID administration is responsible for causing perioperative bleeding. Risk factors for NSAID-induced renal failure include preexisting renal disease, congestive heart failure, hepatic dysfunction, hypovolemia, and the concomitant use of other nephrotoxic drugs such as aminoglycosides, furosemide, or cyclosporine.[14–17] Neonates may also be at increased risk for oliguria, reduced glomerular filtration rate, and renal compromise associated with NSAID use.[18–21] NSAIDs should be used cautiously or not at all in patients with any of these risk factors. COX-2 is an inducible isoform of cyclooxygenase. COX-2 is induced by inflammatory mediators in traumatized cells. COX-2 is also a constitutive isoform because it is present in the brain and kidney in the absence of inflammation. Most NSAIDs are nonselective COX inhibitors. The theoretical advantages of using the COX-2 inhibitors relates to a reduction in the incidence of adverse drug reactions. Unfortunately, the initial enthusiasm for COX-2 inhibitors has been tempered by the observation of increased cardiovascular morbidity, myocardial infarction, and stroke due to thrombotic events in adults treated for prolonged periods with these drugs.[22] As a result, 2 COX-2 inhibitors, rofecoxib and valdecoxib, were withdrawn from the market. Celecoxib, another COX-2 inhibitor, has been approved for use in children older than 2 years of age with juvenile rheumatoid arthritis. Celecoxib was generally well tolerated, and seems to be as effective as naproxen in this patient population.[23] Although there is some variability in analgesic response to different NSAIDs among patients, initial choice of an agent depends on other factors such as cost, the desired dosing interval, underlying medical conditions, and the patient's fasting status. The variability in analgesic response to different NSAIDs may be explained in some patients by variable gene expression and polymorphisms in genes encoding enzymes involved in prostaglandin production.[24]

The oldest drug in this class, acetylsalicylic acid (aspirin), is still commonly used in adults, but use as an analgesic in pediatric patients has nearly stopped due to its association with Reye's syndrome. However, aspirin is still used for some pediatric patients suffering from rheumatologic conditions.[25] Aspirin is available in chewable 81- mg tablets as well as tablets of 81 mg and 325 mg for oral use. Aspirin is dosed 10 to 15 mg/kg orally and administered every 4 to 6 hours. Maximum daily dose should not exceed 90 mg/kg per day.

Acetaminophen, the most widely used NSAID for the treatment of fever and pain, is unique among NSAIDs. High levels of peroxides in inflammatory tissue seem to inhibit the ability of acetaminophen to block COX. Peroxide concentrations are low in the brain, thus acetaminophen is an effective COX inhibitor centrally, a potent antipyretic, and a mild analgesic. Because it is a weak COX inhibitor in the periphery, it lacks the troublesome side effects of other NSAIDs but it is a weak anti-inflammatory agent. However, it may have several other antinociceptive effects, including N-methyl-D-aspartate (NMDA) receptor inhibition and activation of descending inhibitory serotonin pathways.[26]

A recent meta-analysis revealed that acetaminophen and ibuprofen have similar safety profiles, and equivalent efficacy in treating moderate to severe pain in children, but that ibuprofen is a more effective antipyretic.[27] Others have found that rectal acetaminophen 90 to 100 mg/kg per day did not have additional analgesic effects in 0- to 2-month-old infants with severe postoperative pain receiving continuous intravenous morphine 5 to 10 μg/kg/h after major abdominal surgery.[28]

In the United States, acetaminophen is available for oral or rectal administration. Two intravenous preparations are available outside the United States, proparacetamol and paracetamol (intravenous acetaminophen). Proparecetamol is a prodrug of acetaminophen, and is rapidly metabolized to acetaminophen after administration. Though of proven analgesic efficacy perioperatively, it requires reconstitution before administration and is associated with pain during infusion at the intravenous catheter site.[29] An intravenous acetaminophen preparation may soon be available in the United States, and has also been shown to be effective for treating postoperative pain in a variety of clinical situations and is not associated with pain at the injection site.[29–33]

Of concern is that acetaminophen is frequently misused, and acetaminophen overdose can lead to hepatic necrosis and failure.[34] Under normal circumstances, acetaminophen is metabolized in the liver primarily by glucuronidation and sulfation. However, in acetaminophen overdose, an oxidation pathway predominates via cytochrome P450. This oxidation pathway results in the production of a highly hepatotoxic metabolite.

Acetaminophen is conveniently available in many preparations including drops (80 mg/0.8 mL), elixir (160 mg/5 mL), chewable tablets (80 mg and 160 mg), tablets (325 mg and 500 mg), and suppositories (80 mg, 120 mg, 325 mg, and 650 mg). Single-dose rectal acetaminophen is administered in a dose of 35 to 45 mg/kg. Repeated rectal dosing is 20 mg/kg every 6 hours in infants and children and every 12 hours in newborns. Oral acetaminophen is administered in a dose of 10 to 15 mg/kg every 4 to 6 hours. The maximum daily acetaminophen dose depends on the age of the patient: the lesser of 4 g or 100 mg/kg per day in children; 75 mg/kg per day in infants; 60 mg/kg per day in newborns longer than 32 weeks' gestation; and 40 mg/kg per day

in newborns 28 to 32 weeks' gestation. It is important to be familiar with all preparations, so that proper instructions may be given to parents of children to avoid
accidental overdose. Strict adherence to maximum daily dosing guidelines is
important because fatal hepatic necrosis may result from acetaminophen overdose.

Ibuprofen has been the subject of several investigations in children, and analgesic
efficacy in a variety of settings has been established.[11,13,27,35] Ibuprofen is another
widely used drug in this class, and is available in several formulations for pediatric
administration. Adverse events are rare when used for a short time (less than 5
days) in treating acute pain and inflammation due to injury, infection, or illness. For
analgesia, ibuprofen can be given as a single dose of 15 mg/kg orally. However, for
repeated doses in children aged 6 months to 12 years, ibuprofen should be given
as 10 mg/kg every 6 hours orally (maximum daily dose 40 mg/kg). Ibuprofen is available in drops (50 mg/1.25 mL), elixir (100 mg/5 mL), chewable tablets (50 mg and 100
mg), and tablets (200 mg, 400 mg, 600 mg, and 800 mg). Intravenous ibuprofen is not
Food and Drug Administration (FDA) approved for the treatment of pain in pediatric
patients. Of interest, an intravenous preparation of ibuprofen has been available in
North America since 2006 and has been used successfully to treat patent ductus
arteriosus in extremely premature infants.[18,36] Although the adverse events are fewer
with intravenous ibuprofen compared with indomethacin in this patient population, oliguria, renal compromise, and renal failure still occur but may be further reduced if
ibuprofen is administered orally.[37,38] The FDA has recently approved intravenous
ibuprofen for the treatment of pain and fever in adults.

Naproxen has a longer half-life than ibuprofen, allowing it to be given every 8 to 12
hours. In adults, Naproxen 400 to 500 mg administered orally is effective in treating
postoperative pain.[39] In children, naproxen 10 mg/kg orally but not acetaminophen
20 mg/kg orally, administered 30 minutes before adenoidectomy, was found to reduce
the need for opiates postoperatively.[40] Naproxen's safety in newborns and infants has
not been established. The usual dose is 5 to 10 mg/kg orally administered every 8 to 12
hours (maximum daily dose 20 mg/kg). Naproxen is available as an elixir (125 mg/
5 mL) and tablet (220 mg, 250 mg, 375 mg, and 500 mg).

The pharmacokinetics of ketorolac have now been studied in pediatric patients 0.4
to 32 weeks old, 6 to 18 months old, and 1 to 16 years old.[41–43] Doses of ketorolac
0.5 mg/kg intravenously result in plasma levels considered therapeutic in adults in
most children. In the United States, ketorolac is the only NSAID available for the treatment of pain in pediatric patients that can be given by intravenous as well as oral
administration, making it useful in the treatment of postoperative pain in patients
who are not able to take medications orally. However, caution is warranted in using
ketorolac as acute renal failure, prolongation of bleeding times, and hypersensitivity
reactions have been reported in pediatric patients.[16,44,45] Some conclude that
short-term use (less than 5 days) of ketorolac 0.5 mg/kg intravenously every 6 hours
(maximum dose 30 mg) in children 1 to 16 years old who do not have any known
contraindication to NSAID use is safe.[46] Analgesic efficacy of ketorolac in children
as a sole analgesic for minor surgery as well as an adjuvant for management of severe
postoperative pain has been demonstrated in a variety of clinical settings.[10,47–51]
Ketorolac is available for oral administration as a tablet (10 mg) or intravenous administration as an injectable (15 mg/mL and 30 mg/mL).

OPIATE ANALGESICS

Opiates are used for the treatment of moderate to severe pain.[52–55] Opiates produce
analgesia primarily by binding to pre- and postsynaptic cell membranes in the central

nervous system through specific G-protein coupled opioid receptors and acting through a second messenger (cyclic adenosine monophosphate) or K^+ channels, resulting in neuronal inhibition by decreasing excitatory neurotransmitter release from presynaptic terminals or by hyperpolarizing the postsynaptic neuron.[52] Opioid receptors are classified as μ, κ, and δ.[4] The μ receptor is further subdivided into subclasses μ_1, which mediates supraspinal analgesia and dependence, and μ_2, which mediates respiratory depression, intestinal dysmotility, sedation, and bradycardia. Most commonly used opiates work through μ_1-receptor interaction to produce analgesia. Opiates are classified as agonists, partial agonists, agonist-antagonists, and antagonists. Examples of the μ_1 agonists include morphine, hydromorphone, methadone, fentanyl, sufentanil, remifentanil, codeine, oxycodone, and hydrocodone. Agonist-antagonist opiates, which are agonists at one receptor type and antagonists at another receptor, include nalbuphine and pentazocine. Analgesia by agonist-antagonists is mainly κ-mediated, with antagonism or partial agonism at the μ receptor. A partial agonist such as buprenorphone exerts less than full response at a receptor site. Opioid antagonists include naloxone, naltrexone, and nalmefene. Alvimopan and methylnaltrexone, two peripherally acting μ-receptor antagonists, have recently been approved for use in adult patients with opioid-induced bowel dysfunction. Side effects common to opioid agonists include respiratory depression, sedation, nausea, vomiting, pruritus, urinary retention, ileus, and constipation. Less common effects are dysphoria, hallucinations, seizures, and myoclonic movements. There is significant individual variability in the side-effect profiles of the different opiate analgesics. In the presence of unacceptable side effects, switching to a different opiate may result in lessened side effects.[56]

Despite attempts to find a new opiate with equivalent or superior analgesia and a more favorable adverse event profile, morphine remains is the standard opiate with which all others are compared.[52] Morphine can be given through multiple routes (intravenous, oral, subcutaneous, aerosolized, intrathecal, epidural, and intra-articular). Morphine is metabolized in the liver to morphine-3-glucuronide (inactive) and morphine-6-glucuronide (active), which are both excreted by the kidneys. In general, the elimination half-life is longer and the clearance is decreased in newborns compared with older children and adults. This difference is especially pronounced in preterm neonates. In addition, less morphine is protein bound in neonates, allowing a greater proportion of unbound morphine to penetrate the brain, thus increasing the risk for respiratory depression. The elimination half-life and clearance reach adult values within 2 months of age. The optimal plasma concentration of morphine needed to achieve analgesia in children is variable based on the existing data. Therefore, careful titration of morphine is required to obtain the desired level of analgesia while monitoring side effects.[57–61]

Hydromorphone is a synthetic derivative of morphine with a longer duration of action (4 to 6 hours) and elimination half-life (3 to 4 hours). Hydromorphone is approximately 10 times more lipophilic than morphine and 5 times more potent. Hydromorphone is often used as a second-line opioid to morphine and is being used more increasingly as a first-line choice, and is described as often having less associated nausea and pruritus than morphine.[62]

Methadone is a synthetic opioid that is noted for its long elimination half-life and duration of action (12 to 36 hours). Traditionally used with opioid-dependent patients, methadone is being increasingly used in cases of acute pain to provide stable levels of opioid analgesia.[52,54,63] Methadone has high bioavailability (85%), making it an attractive oral analgesic. The principal metabolite is morphine, which may explain its long duration of action. In addition to being a μ agonist, methadone also is an NMDA receptor antagonist.[64] These additional qualities make methadone an excellent long-term narcotic for chronic pain. Intraoperative use of methadone has been shown to provide prolonged analgesia in children undergoing major surgery without any increase in major adverse events.[63] Methadone has the potential to increase the QTc in susceptible individuals, so an electrocardiogram is performed before starting the drug.[65]

Fentanyl is a synthetic opioid that is 100 times more potent than morphine. Fentanyl is highly lipophilic, resulting in significant brain penetration. Fentanyl has a short duration of action because of redistribution out of the plasma into body tissues. Once these sites are saturated, the elimination half-life is actually quite long (233 $\pm$ 137 minutes in infants 3 to 12 months old; 244 $\pm$ 79 minutes in children; and 129 $\pm$ 42 minutes in adults).[66] Fentanyl is highly protein bound to $\alpha 1$ acid glycoprotein in the plasma. Neonates have reduced levels of $\alpha 1$ acid glycoprotein, resulting in higher levels of free unbound fentanyl. Metabolism is through glucuronidation in the liver to inactive metabolites that are excreted by the kidney. Because of its potency, hemodynamic stability, and brief duration of action in small doses, fentanyl is an attractive analgesic for short, painful procedures in children, especially in the intensive care unit setting.[54] Fentanyl can be given in multiple routes: intravenous, epidural, nasal, transmucosal, and transdermal. Epidural fentanyl given as a bolus has its action at spinal sites with a segmental analgesic effect, whereas an epidural infusion acts supraspinally in a nonsegmental manner.[67] Given nasally in a dose of 2 μg/kg, fentanyl provides good analgesia in children who are undergoing myringotomy tube insertion.[68] Fentanyl is available in a candy matrix preparation for transmucosal administration. Transmucosal fentanyl has been used as a premedication for painful procedures, with an onset time of 20 minutes and duration of 2 hours.[69] Fentanyl is sometimes used in opioid-tolerant cancer and sickle cell patients who have frequent bouts of acute pain. Transmucosal fentanyl is more efficient than oral administration because it bypasses the hepatic first-pass metabolism of the oral route, which reduces the availability of fentanyl by 25% to 33%. Transmucosal fentanyl provides good analgesia, but the incidence of nausea with this modality is troublesome. Fentanyl is also available as a patch for transdermal administration, but is not appropriate or recommended for acute pain management in pediatric patients because of the difficulty in quickly and safely titrating an effective dose.[53,54] Transdermal fentanyl patches (12.5, 25, 50, 75, and 100 μg/h) last for 2 to 3 days.[70] The patch has a long onset time but also a long duration that persists after it is removed.

Codeine is a commonly used oral opiate analgesic often administered in combination with acetaminophen as a tablet or oral solution.[54] However, the parent compound has an extremely low affinity for opioid receptors, and most of the analgesic effect of this drug is due to about 10% of an administered dose being metabolized by the liver, using the P450 cytochrome oxidase pathway (CYP2D6) to produce morphine. Therefore it is not surprising that codeine is one-tenth as potent as morphine. Codeine has a bioavailability of 60% after oral administration, with an onset time of 20 to 30 minutes and an elimination half-life of 2.5 to 3 hours. Codeine is excreted in the urine.

Because codeine is dependent on hepatic CYP2D6 enzyme conversion to morphine to exert analgesic effects, several important pharmacogenetic implications need to be mentioned. There is a large difference in phenotypic expression of 2D6, with about 3% of Caucasians and 40% of people of North African descent being ultrarapid metabolizers, resulting in plasma levels of morphine 50% higher than normal.[71] These individuals may have profound analgesia and a high incidence of opiate-induced adverse drug reactions. In contrast, 7% to 10% of Caucasians are poor metabolizers of codeine by CYP2D6, and receive little or no analgesia after its administration.[72] One recent case report documents the serious effects of ultrarapid metabolization in a neonate who died after exposure to breast milk from his mother who was prescribed oral codeine.[73]

Oxycodone and hydrocodone are oral analgesics commonly combined with acetaminophen in tablet or liquid form. A new formulation of oxycodone combined with ibuprofen is now available. Oxycodone also is available alone in tablet or liquid form. Caution is advised when prescribing oxycodone liquid because it comes in 1 mg/mL and 20 mg/mL strengths. The usual dosing of oxycodone is 0.05 to 0.15 mg/kg every 4 to 6 hours as needed for pain relief. These analgesics are approximately 10 times more potent than oral codeine. The bioavailability is 60% after oral administration, with an onset time of 20 to 30 minutes and duration of 4 to 5 hours. Oxycodone and hydrocodone are metabolized in the liver. Oxycodone produces an active metabolite, oxymorphone, that can accumulate in renal failure.[74] Sustained-release oxycodone is available for more prolonged analgesic needs, but negative publicity over its abuse has made it less desirable to parents.[75] Hydrocodone dosing is similar to oxycodone but because it is combined with acetaminophen in an oral solution (acetaminophen 500 mg and hydrocodone 7.5 mg per 15 mL), its usefulness in smaller children is limited.

Nalbuphine is a κ agonist and a μ antagonist. Nalbuphine produces equivalent analgesia to morphine up to doses of 200 μg/kg but increasing the dose beyond this does not result in further analgesia. κ-Mediated side effects of sedation, dysphoria, or euphoria are likely at higher doses. Nalbuphine is metabolized mainly in the liver and has a half-life of approximately 5 hours. Nalbuphine is usually given intravenously. When given orally, it has a bioavailability of only 20% to 25%. Nalbuphine is often used to antagonize μ-mediated side effects from μ-agonist opioids, especially pruritus and urinary retention.[76,77] Care is needed when using nalbuphine in opioid-dependent children in order not to induce opioid withdrawal.

Naloxone is an antagonist at all opioid receptors. Naloxone is used emergently for respiratory depression at a dose of up to 10 μg/kg intravenous. Naloxone can also be used to antagonize pruritus and opioid-induced nausea and vomiting (0.25–0.5 μg/kg/h infusion).[76,78] Naloxone is metabolized in the liver and has an elimination half-life of 60 minutes.[54] Because this is a shorter half-life than the μ agonists it is meant to counteract, continued monitoring of the patient is mandatory. Severe withdrawal can occur when naloxone is given to opioid-dependent patients.

Although not yet approved for use in pediatric patients, alvimopan and methylnaltrexone are approved for use in adults with opiate-induced bowel dysfunction either due to chronic opiate therapy during palliative care (methylnaltrexone) or postoperative ileus after bowel resection surgery (alvimopan).[79,80] Both drugs bind peripheral μ receptors throughout the gastrointestinal tract, but do not reverse central analgesic effects of μ agonists or precipitate withdrawal in opiate-dependant individuals in clinically relevant doses. Methylnatrexone does not cross the blood-brain barrier due to a highly polar methyl group substitution on the structurally similar compound, naltrexone. Alvimopan is a large, highly polar compound that also does not cross the blood-brain barrier in clinically useful doses.

Tramadol is a moderately potent analgesic that is structurally related to codeine. Tramadol provides analgesia through weak μ-opioid receptor binding, and central inhibition of norepinephrine and serotonin reuptake. Tramadol has an affinity for opioid receptors about 6000 times less potent than morphine, but an active metabolite provides the main opioid analgesic effects, which are only four times less potent than morphine.[81] As an analogue to codeine, tramadol similarly undergoes metabolism by the CYP2D6 system. This metabolism puts the utility of the drug at an uncertain level because of phenotypic differences between extensive metabolizers, poor metabolizers, intermediate metabolizers, and ultrarapid metabolizers. In neonates and infants, the CYP2D6 activity increases with maturity, so even genotype extensive metabolizers at this age should be considered to have a poor phenotype response to tramadol until hepatic function improves.[82]

As an atypical analgesic with opioid receptor binding, tramadol has a decreased side-effect profile of sedation and respiratory depression, and dependence compared with other opiate receptor agonists. However, there is a high incidence of postoperative nausea and vomiting, up to 50%, which limits its usefulness.[83] Other side effects include dizziness, pruritus, and constipation. Tramadol is associated with seizures, and should be avoided in patients with a known history of seizure activity or head trauma. In general, tramadol is safe and effective, and can be used for mild to moderate pain relief in children.[84,85]

OTHER ANALGESICS
Ketamine

Ketamine is a phencyclidine derivative and a dissociative anesthetic. Ketamine is a potent analgesic in subanesthetic doses, and is often used for short, painful procedures in children in the emergency room and intensive care unit settings.[86,87] Ketamine can be administered intravenously, orally, rectally, and intramuscularly. Because of increased secretions and possible dysphoric effects, ketamine is often combined with an anticholinergic agent and a benzodiazepine. Because of elevations of cerebral blood flow and oxygen consumption, ketamine is not recommended in children who have decreased intracranial compliance. The analgesic effects of ketamine are mediated by NMDA receptor antagonism and possibly μ-receptor agonism. Oral bioavailability is 20% to 25%. Ketamine is highly lipid soluble, with rapid redistribution. Ketamine is N-demethylated in the liver by the cytochrome P450 system.[88] Intravenous doses of 0.25 to 0.5 mg/kg can produce intense analgesia for 10 to 15 minutes, although the elimination half-life is 2 to 3 hours. There is increasing literature on the intraoperative and postoperative use of ketamine as an adjunct to opioid analgesia in adults.[89] Ketamine can be especially useful in opioid-tolerant patients undergoing procedures.

α-2 Agonists

Clonidine is an α_2-adrenergic agonist with demonstrated anxiolytic and analgesic benefits in children during the perioperative period.[90] Given orally preoperatively (4 μg/kg), clonidine decreases intraoperative anesthetic requirements and postoperative opioid consumption.[91,92] Clonidine has been administered intravenously (2 μg/kg) and has been used as an adjuvant to local anesthetics to prolong analgesia or improve analgesia in caudal (1–2 μg/kg), epidural (1 μg/kg), peripheral nerve block (1 μg/kg), and spinal anesthesia (1 μg/kg).[90,93–99] When compared with opiates as adjuncts to local anesthetics in continuous epidural infusions, clonidine seems to provide equivalent analgesia and reduce the incidence of opiate-related adverse events (nausea, vomiting, and pruritus).[94,95] Clonidine 1 μg/kg as an adjunct to bupivacaine or ropivacaine during peripheral nerve block prolongs the duration of analgesia, but may also increase the incidence of motor block.[97]

Dexmedetomidine is a centrally acting α_2 receptor agonist with an affinity for the receptor that is 8 times that of clonidine.[92] Initially studied as a sedative for adults receiving mechanical ventilation, there is now literature on the use of dexmedetomidine in children.[92,100–104] In laboratory studies, α_2-agonist analgesia mediated in the spinal cord is possible even in neonates and infants.[105,106] Although dexmedetomidine is being studied primarily as a sedative, it seems to have analgesic effects in that opioid requirements are decreased with dexmedetomidine therapy. In addition to providing some analgesic benefits and excellent sedation, dexmedetomidine is associated with minimal respiratory depression.

N-methyl-ᴅ-Aspartate Receptor Antagonists

The NMDA receptor has long been known to play a key role in the development of central sensitization following tissue injuries that result in pain.[107] Ketamine, dextromethorphan, methadone, and magnesium are all known to be NMDA receptor antagonists, and there have been numerous efforts to determine if 3 of these agents (all but methadone) possess any preventative analgesic benefits in the perioperative period. A recent review of these studies determined the evidence was best for dextromethorphan (68% of dextromethorphan and 57% of ketamine studies indicated some preventative analgesic benefit could be demonstrated but none of the studies of magnesium revealed such a benefit).[108] However, even when a benefit was found, others suggested it may be of little clinical significance.[109] The evidence for analgesic benefit of dextromethorphan in pediatric patients is contradictory.[110–113] At this time the authors of this review cannot recommend the routine use of dextromethorphan in postoperative pain management protocols for children.

γ-Aminobutyric Acid Agonists

Benzodiazepines and antispasmodic medications have long been used as adjuvants in the treatment of acute pain. Medical conditions such as cerebral palsy with spastic diplegia, hemiplegia, or quadriplegia, and surgical procedures associated with painful postoperative muscle spasms such as lower extremity tendon releases are situations whereby these agents are very useful, because muscle spasm can lead to tension on surgical incisions, leading to more pain and muscle spasm. But benzodiazepines are also useful in the relief of fear and anxiety in patients without these conditions. Fear and anxiety are factors that can result in magnification of postoperative pain. Also of interest is new literature illuminating the role of γ-aminobutyric acid (GABA) in the transmission and perception of pain. GABA agonists have shown antinociceptive activity in animal models of acute, inflammatory, and neuropathic pain.[114] As the primary inhibitory neurotransmitter, GABA is widely distributed throughout the central nervous system, and has many clinical functions beyond pain control, such as anxiolysis, amnesia, muscle relaxation, and anticonvulsant activity. GABA receptors are located along pain transmission pathways from primary afferent A-δ and C fibers through the spinothalamic tract, and in supraspinal sites like the thalamus and periaqueductal gray matter that are involved with pain perception.[115] Being so ubiquitous is a detriment, as current medications such as baclofen, diazepam, midazolam, and lorazepam are not specific GABA agonists. GABA agonists have serious side effects, primarily sedation and tolerance, which can limit their clinical usefulness. More specific GABA agonists are being developed that do not cause tolerance (CGP44532) and do not cause sedation (CGP35024) at antinociceptive doses.[115]

In vitro studies have demonstrated that several benzodiazepines interact with κ receptors but not μ receptors, and this may explain the clinical observation of analgesic efficacy of benzodiazepines administered in the intrathecal and epidural spaces.[116] Caudal midazolam 50 μg/kg given alone or in combination with 0.25% bupivacaine 1 mL/kg reduced postsurgical pain in children undergoing unilateral inguinal hernia repair.[117] However, before this intervention can be advocated, more studies to determine safety as well as efficacy are needed.

Diazepam and baclofen are two common GABA agonists used in pain management. Diazepam is administered orally (0.1–0.2 mg/kg every 6 hours) or intravenously (0.05–0.1 mg/kg every 6 hours) for centrally mediated muscle relaxation. Baclofen is most often used in chronic painful conditions related to muscle spasticity. Continuous intrathecal administration of minute doses by an implantable pump is necessary for severe congenital spasms, but oral administration can be used to supplement the infusion or for acute exacerbations of pain due to muscle spasticity. Both medications can cause sedation and respiratory depression, which are increased with the concomitant administration of opiates for pain. Flumazenil (0.01–0.02 mg/kg up to maximum 0.2 mg per dose, with repeat dosing every minute up to 1 mg maximum total dose) can acutely antagonize a diazepam overdose. The acetylcholinesterase inhibitor, physostigmine, is a controversial antagonist of excessive sedation and coma caused by baclofen toxicity. Several case series report contradictory results regarding physostigmine reversal of sedation after accidental baclofen overdose.[118,119] Knowledge of GABA agonist benefits and side effects is key to their safe integration into a comprehensive acute pain management plan.

Local Anesthetics

Local anesthetics reversibly bind sodium channels. Once bound, the channels are inactive and stop the propagation of nerve signals to the brain. These drugs prevent the transmission of pain. The two classes of local anesthetics are amides and esters, which describe the central bond between the aromatic ring and amine group found in each class. Amides are metabolized by the liver, whereas esters are broken down by plasma esterases. Carl Koller, in 1884, was the first physician to use a local anesthetic for surgical anesthesia.[120] Koller applied a cocaine solution topically for ophthalmologic surgery. Today local anesthetics are administered topically, subcutaneously, transdermally, intravenously, perineurally, or administered in the intrathecal or epidural space.

The selection of local anesthetic depends on the metabolic maturity of the child as well as the delivery site. In children, tetracaine and bupivacaine are most commonly used intrathecally due to their prolonged half-lives, because neonates and infants have higher rates of cerebrospinal fluid (CSF) turnover and larger ratios of CSF volume to weight, which decrease the effectiveness of local anesthetics. Epidurally, ropivacaine, bupivacaine, and 2-chloroprocaine are commonly used. Ropivacaine has replaced bupivacaine at the authors' institution due to decreased toxicity in neonates and infants. Bosenberg and colleagues[121] showed that although ropivacaine provided effective analgesia in infants, the plasma concentration of unbound ropivacaine was not influenced by the duration of infusion for up to 48 to 72 hours. This result contrasts with bupivacaine in infants, in whom the unbound concentration of bupivacaine (considered the toxic moiety) during epidural infusion increased until the end point of 48 hours.[122] 2-Chloroprocaine avoids much of the potential toxicity of amides because plasma esterase activity, though measurably reduced in neonates, is sufficient for ester metabolism. Besides a larger therapeutic window, ropivacaine has a better side-effect profile, with less motor blockade than an equipotent analgesic dose of bupivacaine.[123]

Toxicity of local anesthetics and the technical expertise required to deliver the drugs to the site of action are the two main reasons local anesthetic use is not as ubiquitous in the pediatric population. **Table 1** lists commonly accepted maximum doses of local anesthetics. With the advent of lipid infusions for acute local anesthetic toxicity, the use of regional techniques is expanding in children. There is a case report of

Table 1
Local anesthetic maximal doses (mg/kg)

Drug	Spinal	Epidural	Infusion (h)	Peripheral	Infiltrate
2-Chloroprocaine	NR	10–30	30	8–10	8–10
Lidocaine	1–2.5	5–7	2–3	5–7	5–7
Bupivacaine	0.3–0.5	2–3	0.4	2–3	2–3
Ropivacaine	NR	2.5–4	0.4–0.5	2.5–4	2.5–4
Levobupivacaine	NR	2.5–4	0.4	2.5–4	2.5–4

Abbreviation: NR, not recommended.

a successful treatment of local anesthetic overdose with 20% lipid infusion in a child receiving a regional anesthetic for postoperative pain control.[124]

When using local anesthetics to block the transmission of pain, preventing systemic toxicity requires more vigilance with children. Most regional techniques are performed under general anesthesia or heavy sedation to allow the placement of a needle the child would not otherwise tolerate. This technique eliminates many of the signs of central nervous system toxicity such as agitation, confusion, twitching, drowsiness, apnea, and sensory disturbances (tinnitus, metallic taste, diplopia, circumoral paresthesias). Cardiovascular signs such as hypotension, bradycardia, and ventricular arrhythmias might be the only signs of acute toxicity in an anesthetized child. Measures taken to prevent toxicity include gentle aspiration on the syringe before incremental, small-volume injections, using pharmacologic markers like epinephrine when appropriate, and monitoring the patient until the peak blood concentration occurs.

TECHNIQUES FOR POSTOPERATIVE PAIN MANAGEMENT
Measuring Pain

Just as it would be inconceivable to manage hypertension without knowing the patient's blood pressure, to effectively manage pain one must have a gauge of the patient's pain intensity. Pain assessment tools are an essential prerequisite for pain treatment plans in children. Tremendous advances have been made in recent years, but assessing the perceived pain in neonates, infants, and nonverbal or developmentally delayed children is still a difficult challenge. There are dozens of pain assessment measures now available to guide clinicians in managing pain. **Table 2** lists examples of pediatric pain scales. Children of 8 years and older can reliably report pain on the visual analog scale used in adult pain management. Younger children between 3 and 7 years of age can report pain using face scales (a series of drawings depicting increasing levels of distress) after undergoing surgery.[131] The younger the child, the less likely he or she can make clear delineations between levels of pain using pain scales.[132]

For neonates and infants, pain assessment tools often rely on behavioral observations by caregivers and physiologic changes in the patient, which is often the case in cognitively impaired children as well. Problems arise in that pain is a subjective experience that cannot completely translate from patient to patient. An infant's behavioral response to a heel lance with facial grimacing, crying, and motor activity might mimic the behavior found in another infant who is experiencing hunger. Most infants with colic manifest pain facies that rate highly in infant focused pain scales, yet pain management plans are not offered to these children.[133] Another problem is that

Table 2
Pediatric pain scales

Scale	Type	Ages	Scoring Indicators
PIPP[125]	Behavioral and physiologic parameters Procedural pain	Term and preterm Infants	Gestational age Behavioral state Heart rate, SpO_2 Facial expression
CRIES[126]	Behavioral and physiologic parameters Postoperative pain	32–60 weeks	Crying, increased O_2 Increased vital signs, Expression Sleeplessness
FLACC[127]	Behavioral parameters	<3 years or unable to self-report	Face, Legs, Activity, Cry, Consolability
Faces[128]	Self-report	3–12 years	Happy face to saddest face yield numeric 0–10 score
VAS[129,130]	Self-report	Children >7 years	0 = no pain 10 = maximum pain

physiologic responses such as an increased heart rate, which could be a sign of pain or hypovolemia, are not specific or sensitive to pain alone. However, due to the lack of a reliable, validated, biologic marker, current pediatric pain scales must be used and updated as research allows.

Postoperative Pain Management Strategies

Traditionally acute pediatric pain was managed with opiate analgesics alone, but fear of severe adverse events such as central nervous system and respiratory depression related to their use often resulted in inadequate pain control. Now, successful pain management strategies target several of the complex elements of pain transduction, transmission, modulation, and perception. Balanced or multimodal analgesia plans with NSAIDs acting on the periphery, regional anesthetic blockade of peripheral nerves, nerve roots, or spinal cord, and opiates acting centrally have become increasingly popular to maximize acute pain control in pediatric patients. This balanced approach can minimize the occurrence of adverse drug reactions attributed to each component of the multimodal plan because generally lower doses of each component are required to produce equivalent or superior analgesia. Shortfalls in the opioid-only strategy such as delays in dosing, inadequate dosing, intramuscular route of delivery, and failure to recognize an individual patient's pain can all be ameliorated by long-acting regional techniques including continuous peripheral nerve catheters, scheduled dosing of NSAIDs, patient-controlled analgesia, and management of breakthrough pain with additional opiates.

Individual children have widely variable pain perceptions of similar conditions, resulting in different analgesic needs. These differences are based on past experiences, culture, and genetics. Individuals will also vary in pain control requirements depending on time, activity, and level of emotional stress. At rest, the perceived pain is usually less than when the child is changing position, taking a deep breath, receiving needed nursing care, undergoing a dressing change, or undergoing diagnostic and therapeutic procedures. Likewise, anxiety and pain can increase when the child must undergo multiple procedures, diagnostic tests, or participate in regular physical therapy or routine nursing care and physical examinations. Effective pain management plans take a proactive position in dealing with background pain, and have allowances to provide adequate analgesia for breakthrough pain experienced for any reason.

Patient-Controlled Analgesia

Patient-controlled analgesia (PCA) is an excellent delivery system for treating moderate to severe pain in children as young as 5 years old in some circumstances, with proper education and routinely in normal 7-year-old children.[134] There are reports of younger children successfully using PCA, especially in patients with chronic needs. When used with adequate monitoring, PCA is a safe, effective method of delivering opioids. PCA has a high patient, family, and staff satisfaction.[135] The high rate of success is related to meeting patient needs. PCA provides a highly reliable dispensing system that the patient can use to titrate opioids to individual needs. Patients can receive immediate relief of pain without being subjected to the inherent delays of hospital care that are out of their control, such as understaffing and other patients' need for more emergent attention. More responsibility and control for the minute to minute management of pain is given to the patient who can titrate down their demand for opiates during periods of lesser pain at rest, or increase their demand for opiates with more frequent button pushes when they are experiencing more pain associated with various activities. The patient feels the pain and self-administers medication until a satisfactory improvement is perceived.

Opioids have serious side effects that are mitigated with the appropriate use of PCA. Most institutions have monitoring requirements in place for the safe delivery of narcotics. Minimum safety measures should include continuous respiratory rate, pulse oximetry, heart rate with frequent blood pressure monitoring, pain assessment, and level of consciousness. As the blood concentration of the infused opiate increases due to increased demand from the patient, the side effects of somnolence and sedation become more clinically significant and will prevent the child from administering an opiate overdose. In this situation it is understood that the patient is the only one to activate the PCA demand button. In other situations, nurses and parents can safely deliver narcotics via PCA to children younger than 6 years or with developmental delay, but different parameters must be set to prevent accidental overdose by caregivers.[136] A recent study showed that PCA by proxy had the same prevalence of adverse events compared with PCA by the patient, but the need for rescue intervention was greater in patients on PCA by proxy.[137] By allowing the patient or proxy to control pain with frequent, small doses of medications, PCA systems maintain a narrower range of plasma concentration of opioids with lower peaks and higher troughs, resulting in less respiratory and central nervous system depression and more consistent pain control.

The infusion pump is programmed to deliver a specified (demand) dose of medication when the system is activated, typically by depressing a button. The minimum time between delivered doses is the lockout time, designed to prevent drug accumulation and to allow the effect of the drug to begin before a second dose is administered. During the lockout time, no demand doses are delivered regardless of how many times the button is pushed. Finally, a total maximum dose is set as a final precaution against overdosing. The total maximum dose is usually calculated in 1- or 4-hour limits. The pump will not administer any medication once this maximum dose is reached, until time passes to allow for the patient to eliminate the narcotic. The pump records data on the patient's drug usage including number of attempts and actual opioid injections. This information can be useful in changing the parameters on the pump to achieve better pain control.

Basal infusions are another component of PCA systems. Basal infusions allow for a continuous infusion of medication independent of the demand dosing. The goal of the basal infusion is to provide some nominal pain relief during sleep when the patient would not be activating the PCA pump, and has been advocated by some investigators for pediatric patients expected to experience severe postoperative pain, such as adolescents after posterior spinal fusion.[134] This infusion would seem to prevent acute troughs in blood levels and therefore reasonably blunt an acute exacerbation of pain. However, there is literature that shows no differences in pain scores or demand dosing between patients with or without basal infusions, and that basal infusions constitute a risk factor for increasing adverse respiratory events in children.[137–139] Opioid-naïve patients are especially at risk with basal infusions, which should most likely be avoided except in rare instances like posterior spinal fusion. Although potentially useful, basal infusions circumvent the inherent safety balance between PCA usage in an alert patient and a narcotic-induced somnolence to prevent overuse of the PCA system. **Table 3** lists the PCA dosing guidelines for several opiate analgesics.

As safe and effective as the PCA infusion is, there are problems that need to be addressed. Patients invariably will maximize the PCA and still need more opioid for pain control. Medications used for other purposes might sedate the patient, thus preventing him or her from using the PCA. Finally, the pump itself might fail. All of these situations and others require orders for the nurse to give additional pain relief, usually the same medication as found in the pump, given intravenously every 3 hours for severe, breakthrough pain. Side effects of the opioids are often encountered even with frequent, small doses so rescue orders are part of the authors' PCA treatment plan. For severe respiratory depression, naloxone 10 μg/kg intravenously will reverse the opioid effect. The half-life of the opioid antagonist is usually shorter than the offending opioid, so vigilance is necessary to prevent a recurrence of sedation. Ondansetron 100 to 150 μg/kg intravenously every 8 hours is used as first-line treatment for nausea and vomiting. For opioid-induced pruritus, nalbuphine 50 μg/kg every 4 hours can be effective, as well as naloxone infusion of 0.25 μg/kg every hour for severe pruritus, especially with neuraxial opioids. Adjunct medications for inflammation and muscle spasms are also routinely ordered with PCA.

Continuous Intravenous Opiate Infusion

In young children with moderate to severe pain who cannot use a PCA due to age, physical disability, or cognitive impairment, a continuous intravenous (CIV) infusion can provide stable pain relief. Steady plasma drug levels are one benefit compared with intermittent bolus dosing. There is a decreased reliance on often busy nursing staff. As with PCA, rescue medication must be ordered for breakthrough pain. Because of the pharmacokinetics of infusions, a bolus dose is usually given as the

Table 3
PCA dosing guidelines

Drug	Demand Dose (μg/kg)	Lockout Interval (min)	Basal Infusion (μg/kg/h)	1-h/4-h Limit (μg/kg)	As Needed IV Rescue Dose (μg/kg)
Morphine	20	8–10	0–20	100/300	50
Hydromorphone	4	8–10	0–4	20/60	10
Fentanyl	0.5	6–8	0–0.5	2.5/4	0.5–1.0
Nalbuphine	20	8–10	0–20	100/300	50

infusion is started to achieve a therapeutic drug level. Careful, slow titration is warranted in neonates and infants as the pharmacokinetics of narcotics differ widely according to age. Morphine has an elimination half-life of 9 hours in preterm infants, 6.5 hours in neonates, and 2 hours in older infants and children.[140] The CIV frequently provides a foundation for pain control at rest, but any increase in activity or nursing care necessitates intermittent administration of rescue analgesic medication for so-called breakthrough pain (**Table 4**).

Epidural Analgesia

Continuous epidural analgesia (CEA) has become an indispensible tool for managing severe postoperative pain in neonates, infants, and children after a wide variety of surgical procedures. CEA reduces the surgical stress response and hospitalization time, and may improve outcomes in specific pediatric populations.[141] Dolin and colleagues[142] collected pooled postoperative pain scores from 165 studies and found

Table 4 Opioid dosing regimens		
Opioid	Route/Age Group	Dose/Interval
Morphine	Oral, immediate release: infants and children	0.3 mg/kg every 3–4 h
	Oral, sustained release: infants and children	0.25–0.5 mg/kg every 8–12 h
	IV bolus:	
	Preterm neonate	10–25 µg/kg every 2–4 h
	Full-term neonate	25–50 µg/kg every 3–4 h
	Infants and children	50–100 µg/kg every 3–4 h
	IV Infusion:	
	Preterm neonate	2–5 µg/kg/h
	Full-term neonate	5–10 µg/kg/h
	Infants and children	15–30 µg/kg/h
Hydromorphone	Oral: infants and children	40–80 µg/kg every 4 h
	IV bolus: infants and children	10–20 µg/kg every 3–4 h
	IV infusion: infants and children	3–5 µg/kg/h
Fentanyl	Intranasal	1–2 µg/kg
	Transdermal	12.5, 25, 50, 75, 100 µg/h patches
	IV bolus	0.5–1 µg/kg every 1–2 h
	IV infusion	0.5 µg/kg/h
Methadone	Oral or IV bolus: infants and children	0.1–0.2 mg/kg every 12–36 h
Nalbuphine	IV bolus:	
	Preterm neonate	10–25 µg/kg every 2–4 h
	Full-term neonate	25–50 µg/kg every 2–4 h
	Infants and children	50–100 µg/kg every 2–4 h
	IV infusion:	
	Preterm neonate	5–10 µg/kg/h
	Full-term neonate	10–15 µg/kg/h
	Infants and children	20 µg/kg/h
Codeine	Oral	0.5–1 mg/kg every 4 h
Oxycodone	Oral	0.05–0.15 mg/kg every 4 h
Hydrocodone	Oral	0.1–0.2 mg/kg every 4 h

that the mean incidence of moderate to severe pain in patients with a PCA was 35.8% and 10.4%, whereas patients with CEA had incidences of 20.9% and 7.8%.

The placement of the tip of the epidural catheter close to the center of the surgical dermatomes to be blocked is an essential prerequisite for adequate pain relief, especially in neonates when the potential for local anesthetic toxicity greatly reduces the volume of epidural infusate that can be safely administered. In infants, a caudal insertion site for the catheter is frequently chosen because a styleted catheter can be easily advanced to thoracic levels. Another insertion point is the interspace of L5 and S1, called the modified midline Taylor approach, which also allows for a relatively easy advancement of the catheter to high lumbar and thoracic levels.[143] Whenever an epidural catheter is threaded from a caudal or lower lumbar entry site to a thoracic level, intraoperative confirmation of the correct desired position of the epidural catheter is performed by radiography after administration of a nonionic contrast medium (0.3 mL of Omnipaque 180 [iohexol], GE Health Care), or by fluoroscopy with an opaque stylet in place, or with contrast. Tsui and colleagues[144] have described a technique using nerve stimulation to confirm epidural catheter placement. Ultrasound-guided epidural catheter insertion and placement is another safe method in infants.[145]

Most, if not all epidural catheters are placed under general anesthesia. A large study in Great Britain and Ireland, consisting of 10,633 epidurals in children, did not correlate any problems to the use of general anesthesia while placing the epidurals.[146] Of course, precautions still are necessary when the child is anesthetized to ensure incorrect placement. Several anatomic differences between children and adults regarding epidural catheter placement merit discussion. The distance from skin to the epidural space or depth is the most obvious difference between adults and children. Other anatomic differences are the softer ligamentum flavum in children, making a false loss of resistance during placement of the epidural catheter more common in children. The conus medullaris ends at L3 in neonates and does not reach the adult L1 level until 1 year of age. Infants have a higher CSF volume to weight ratio, as well as a faster rate of CSF production and absorption than adults. Locating the epidural space with a loss-of-resistance technique should be conducted with saline as opposed to air to avoid air embolus, cord compression, or a patchy block.[147]

The risk of local anesthetic toxicity is one of many problems that need to be continually monitored during CEA. A dedicated team of physicians and nurses should be immediately available to manage any emergent problems with pain control or side effects in patients with CEA. The epidural insertion site should be evaluated daily by a member of the pain management team for signs of infection. Standardized protocols and order sets include patient monitoring parameters as well as neurologic assessment (mental status, motor check, and pain scores) every 4 hours. Standard safety equipment includes a working intravenous line, breathing circuit, mask, oxygen, and suction at the bedside for each patient with a CEA. Instructions for the patient's nurse on contacting members of the pain management service should be readily available. A specialized team of caregivers can anticipate medication side effects of CEA and proactively address these problems.

A common problem with CEA includes inadequate pain control. This problem is often due to incorrect dermatomal placement, catheter problems (kinking, obstruction, leaking, or breaking) pump malfunction, insufficient solution concentration/rate, or catheter migration/dislodgement from the original location. First, testing the catheter with a safe, short-acting bolus medication to ensure its continued usefulness is recommended (**Table 5**). If the epidural is functioning, then changing the rate or concentration, or adding adjuvants within the infusion may improve pain control.

Table 5 Example of bolus testing of epidural		
3% Chloroprocaine Epidural Test Dose		
Patient Weight (kg)	Bolus Volume	Total Volume
0–10	0.2 mL/kg	0.8 mL/kg
11–25	0.15 mL/kg	0.6 mL/kg
26–40	0.1 mL/kg	0.4 mL/kg
41–70	4 mL	16 mL
>70	5 mL	20 mL

Inadequate or failed CEA should be expeditiously replaced with another strategy for pain control such as CIV or PCA in appropriate children.

The medications used in CEA, specifically the opiates, are significant sources of side effects. Motor block is a late sign of compartment syndrome and also a direct effect of local anesthetics. Decreasing the concentration of the local anesthetic solution and also the rate can allow a sensory block and pain relief to remain without the disconcerting feeling of paralysis. Systemic local anesthetic toxicity is rare with infusions, but infants with immature hepatic function and decreased protein binding are at a greater risk. **Table 6** lists CEA dosing guidelines. Opioid adjuvants to CEA infusions commonly cause nausea, vomiting, pruritus, urinary retention, sedation, and respiratory depression. Reducing the amount of opiate in the epidural solution is an option, but medications to counteract the opioid-induced side effects are usually required, as if the opiates were given intravenously.

Patient-controlled epidural analgesia (PCEA) combines the benefits of CEA and PCA. Children 5 years or older have the ability to effectively use this technique.[148] As with PCA, the analgesic benefit is that the patient can adjust the pain medication to meet an increase in pain sensation due to episodes of increased activity or care. The basal infusion is administered at 0.1 to 0.2 mL/kg/h. Demand doses range form 0.05 to 0.1 mL/kg with a lockout time of 20 to 30 minutes, to accrue a total dose of 0.2 to 0.4 mL/kg/h (the total hourly dose should not exceed 20 mL).

Intrathecal Morphine

Intrathecal morphine has been used for many years to treat pain in children following a variety of surgical procedures.[149–154] An early report using relatively high doses of morphine 20 µg/kg (n = 29) and 30 µg/kg (n = 27) reported satisfactory analgesia

Table 6 CEA dosing guidelines					
Patient	Ropivacaine (mg/mL)	Fentanyl (µg/mL)	Morphine (µg/mL)	Clonidine (µg/mL)	Rate Ropivacaine (max. mg/kg/h)
Newborn 0–2 months	1 (0.5–1.0)	0.2	NR	0.04	0.2 (0.15–0.25)
Infant	1 (0.5–1.5)	2 (2–5)	25	0.4	0.25 (0.15–0.3)
Child (lumbar)	1.5 (1–2)	2 (2–5)	25–50	0.4–0.6	0.3 (0.2–0.4)
Child (thoracic)	1.5 (1–2)	2 (2–5)	NR	0.4–0.6	0.3 (0.2–0.4)

Abbreviation: NR, not recommended.

of 22 hours or more in children following open heart surgery.[149] Clinically significant respiratory depression occurred between 3.5 and 4.5 hours after intrathecal morphine administration in six patients receiving morphine 30 µg/kg versus three children who received the lower dose.[149] Since this time several reports comparing high- and low-dose intrathecal morphine for postsurgical pain in children have shown that analgesic benefit is not improved by increasing the dose of intrathecal morphine.[153,154] Intrathecal morphine 2 or 5 µg/kg administered intraoperatively provided equivalent analgesia and side-effect profiles in children after spinal fusion surgery, but the children who received morphine 5 µg/kg had lower blood loss.[150] Intrathecal morphine 4 to 5 µg/kg provided satisfactory analgesia in 187 children after a variety of surgical procedures, with minimal respiratory depression.[152] Thus it seems that the ideal dose of intrathecal morphine is 2 to 5 µg/kg.

Regional Anesthesia

Regional anesthesia in children is increasingly popular, not only as an adjunct to anesthesia but as a technique for managing postoperative pain.[155] One reason for the renewed interest in pediatric regional anesthesia is that the use of nerve stimulators and ultrasound has improved the success rate of nerve blocks and theoretically may make placement of blocks safer in anesthetized children. This differs from the standard in adults whereby blocks are placed under minimal to no sedation so that one can confirm analgesia, and so that the adult patients can communicate the occurrence of paresthesias if they occur, or symptoms indicate intravascular injection of local anesthetics. Giaufre and colleagues[156] presented data in more than 9000 peripheral nerve and regional field block techniques, and reported zero complications despite the fact that 89% of the patients were under "light general anesthesia." Moreover, studies indicate that in animals use of volatile anesthetics for general anesthesia confers some protection against cardiotoxicity in the event of an accidental overdose of local anesthetic.[157] Using ultrasound is safe and has been shown to be efficacious in pediatric regional anesthesia.[158] Ultrasound guidance of regional anesthetic blockade is reviewed in greater detail elsewhere in this issue. Whenever possible, regional anesthesia should be used as part of a comprehensive pediatric pain management program, but implementation should always focus on safety and minimizing risks.

The caudal block is one of the most commonly performed regional anesthetics in pediatrics.[159] For the majority of hernia surgery, the caudal block is the technique of choice, but it can also yield excellent analgesia for lower extremity surgery, and has been reported for patent ductus arteriosus ligation.[158–160] Typical doses include ropivacaine 0.1% to 0.2% and bupivacaine 0.125% to 0.25% with epinephrine in volumes of 0.5 to 2 mL/kg (not to exceed toxic doses measured in mg/kg). The relatively short duration of analgesia following a single-injection block can be mitigated adding clonidine, 1 to 2 µg/kg, to prolong the block.[161] Motor block with higher concentrations of bupivacaine are a major complaint in ambulatory children. One of the most frequent complications with caudals is inadvertent needle placement into the vasculature, intrathecal space, or even bone in very young children; yet, this rate remains low (overall morbidity 0.7 per 1000), due to methods of detection including ultrasound visualization, aspiration of the needle or catheter, and test dosing with epinephrine.[155,156] The caudal block is a mainstay of pediatric regional anesthesia, with a long history of safety.

All peripheral nerve blocks used in adult patients can be performed in children too.[158] **Table 7** lists examples of common peripheral nerve blocks. Pediatric regional anesthesia is incorporating single-shot and continuous (via percutaneously placed

Table 7			
Common pediatric peripheral nerve blocks			
Region	Block	Effective Analgesia	Technique
Upper extremity	Interscalene	Shoulder/arm/elbow	SS/CPNB
	Infraclavicular	Elbow/forearm	SS/CPNB
	Axillary	Forearm/hand	SS/CNPB
Lower extremity	Femoral	Thigh/knee	SS/CPNB
	Sciatic	Leg/ankle/foot	SS/CPNB
	Ankle	Foot	SS
Trunk	Ilioinguinal/iliohypogastric	Inguinal hernia/lower abdomen	SS
	Rectus sheath	Umbilicus/superficial abdomen	SS
	Intercostal/paravertebral	Thoracic	SS/CPNB
	Lumbar plexus	Hip/pelvis/leg	SS/CPNB
Miscellaneous	Penile	Penis	SS
	Supraorbital/supratrochlear	Forehead/headache	SS
	Greater/lesser occipital	Occiput/headache	SS

Abbreviations: SS, single shot; CPNB, continuous peripheral nerve block.

catheters) nerve blocks as part of a balanced pain management strategy aimed at reducing side effects and inefficiencies associated with traditional opiate-based plans. Prolonged analgesia via continuous nerve blocks or very long duration local anesthetics will allow patients to recover safely at home. This therapy will require standardized, advanced ultrasound-guided regional anesthesia training and newer pharmacologic treatments to come into routine practice.[162,163]

SUMMARY

During the past 2 to 3 decades, pediatric pain management has gained tremendous knowledge with respect to the understanding of developmental neurobiology, developmental pharmacology, the use of analgesics in children, the use of regional techniques in children, and of the psychological needs of children in pain. A wide range of opioid, NSAID, and nontraditional medications are available to treat a variety of pain types.

Teams of health care professionals specializing in managing pain in children are designing pain management plans for their patients that are proactive, and not only covering baseline pain but also anticipating breakthrough pain associated with nursing care, physical therapy, wound care, and diagnostic and therapeutic procedures, and prescribing contingent analgesics to be administered if needed during these events. Titration is an optimal way to approach opioid dosing, to maximize comfort and safety while minimizing side effects. Careful assessment and reassessment of pain and response to analgesics is required to tailor care to individual patients. Many adverse effects of opioids are idiosyncratic, so changing from one to another can resolve many problems such as itching, dysphoria, and nausea. Children are now benefiting from many techniques for effective management of pain in adult patients (PCA, CEA, PCEA, and continuous peripheral nerve blocks), as experience has shown that they are safe and effective in pediatric populations.

REFERENCES

1. Anand KJS, Hickey PR. Pain and its effects in the human neonate and fetus. N Engl J Med 1987;317:1321–9.

2. Fitgerald M, Beggs S. The neurobiology of pain: developmental aspects. Neuroscientist 2001;7:246–57.
3. Lidow MS. Long-term effects of neonatal pain on nociceptive systems. Pain 2002;99:377–83.
4. Walker SM, Franck LS, Fitzgerald M, et al. Long-term impact of neonatal intensive care and surgery on somatosensory perception in children born extremely preterm. Pain 2009;141:79–87.
5. Elia N, Lysakowski C, Tramer MR. Does multimodal analgesia with acetaminophen, nonsteroidal anti-inflammatory drugs, or selective cyclooxygenase inhibitors and patient-controlled analgesia morphine offer advantages over morphine alone? Anesthesiology 2005;103:1296–304.
6. Morton NS. Simple and systemic management of postoperative pain. In: Finley GA, McGrath PJ, editors. Progress in pain research and management, Acute and procedure pain in infants and children, vol. 20. Seattle (WA): IASP Press; 2001. p. 13–32.
7. Korpela R, Korvenoja P, Meretoja OA. Morphine-sparing effect of acetaminophen in pediatric day-case surgery. Anesthesiology 1999;91:442–7.
8. Morton NS, O'Brien K. Analgesic efficacy of paracetamol and diclofenac in children receiving PCA morphine. Br J Anaesth 1999;82:715–7.
9. Kokki H, Tuovinen K, Hendolin H. The effect of intravenous ketoprofen on postoperative epidural sufentanil analgesia in children. Anesth Analg 1999;88:1036–41.
10. Watcha MF, Jones MB, Lagueruela RG, et al. Comparison of ketorolac and morphine as adjuvants during pediatric surgery. Anesthesiology 1992;76:368–72.
11. Clark E, Plint AC, Correll R, et al. A randomized, controlled trial of acetaminophen, ibuprofen and codeine for acute pain relief in children with musculoskeletal trauma. Pediatrics 2007;119:460–7.
12. Kokki H. Nonsteroidal anti-inflammatory drugs for postoperative pain. Paediatr Drugs 2003;5:103–23.
13. Romsing J, Walther-Larsen S. Peri-operative use of nonsteroidal anti-inflammatory drugs in children: analgesic efficacy and bleeding. Anaesthesia 1997;52:673–83.
14. Moffett BS, Wann TI, Carberry KE, et al. Safety of ketorolac in neonates and infants after cardiac surgery. Paediatr Anaesth 2006;16:424–8.
15. Burd RS, Tobias JD. Ketorolac for pain management after abdominal procedures in infants. South Med J 2002;95:331–3.
16. Buck ML, Norwood VF. Ketorolac-induced acute renal failure in a previously healthy adolescent. Pediatrics 1996;98:294–6.
17. Kallanagowdar C, LeBreton A, Aviles DH. Acute renal failure. Clin Pediatr 2006;45:771–3.
18. Van Overmeire B, Smets K, Lecoutre D, et al. A comparison of ibuprofen and indomethacin for closure of patent ductus arteriosus. N Engl J Med 2000;343:674–81.
19. Allegaert K, Cossy V, Debeer A, et al. The impact of ibuprofen on renal clearance in preterm infants is independent of gestational age. Pediatr Nephrol 2005;20:740–3.
20. Jacqz-Aigrain E, Anderson BJ. Pain control: non-steroidal anti-inflammatory agents. Semin Fetal Neonatal Med 2006;11:251–9.
21. Devavaram P. Ketorolac and renal compromise in neonates. Pediatrics 2007;119:421–2.

22. Ardoin SP, Sundy JS. Update on nonsteroidal anti-inflammatory drugs. Curr Opin Rheumatol 2006;18:221–6.
23. Foeldvari I, Szer IS, Zemel LS, et al. A prospective study comparing celecoxib with naproxen in children with juvenile rheumatoid arthritis. J Rheumatol 2009; 36:174–82.
24. Lee Y, Kim H, Wu T, et al. Genetically mediated interindividual variation in analgesic response to cyclooxygenase inhibitory drugs. Clin Pharmacol Ther 2006; 79:407–18.
25. Cron RQ, Sharma S, Sherry DD. Current treatment by United States and Canadian pediatric rheumatologists. J Rheumatol 1999;26:2036–8.
26. Dugan ST, Scott LJ. Intravenous paracetamol (acetaminophen). Drugs 2009;69: 101–13.
27. Perrott DA, Piira T, Goodenough B, et al. Efficacy and safety of acetaminophen vs ibuprofen for treating children's pain or fever. Arch Pediatr Adolesc Med 2004;158:521–6.
28. Van der Marel CD, Peters JWB, Bouwmeester NJ, et al. Rectal acetaminophen does not reduce morphine consumption after major surgery in young infants. Br J Anaesth 2007;98:372–9.
29. Moller PL, Juhl GI, Payen-Champenois C, et al. Intravenous acetaminophen (paracetamol): comparable analgesic efficacy, but better local safety than its prodrug proparacetamol, for postoperative pain after third molar extraction. Anesth Analg 2005;101:90–6.
30. Goracs TS, Lambert M, Rinne T, et al. Efficacy and tolerability of ready-to-use intravenous paracetamol solution as monotherapy or as an adjunct to analgesic therapy for postoperative pain in patients undergoing elective ambulatory surgery: open, prospective study. Int J Clin Pract 2009;63:112–20.
31. Murat I, Baujard C, Foussat C, et al. Tolerance and analgesic efficacy of new i.v. paracetamol solution in children after inguinal hernia repair. Paediatr Anaesth 2005;15:663–70.
32. Capici F, Ingelmo PM, Davidson A, et al. Randomized, controlled trial of duration of analgesia following intravenous or rectal acetaminophen after adenotonsillectomy in children. 2008;100:251–5.
33. Alhashemi JA, Daghistani MF. Effects of intraoperative i.v. acetaminophen vs i.m. meperidine on post-tonsillectomy pain in children. Br J Anaesth 2006;96: 790–5.
34. Dlugosz CK, Chater RW, Engle JP. Appropriate use of nonprescription analgesics in pediatric patients. J Pediatr Health Care 2006;20:316–25.
35. Kokki H, Hendolin H, Maunuksela EL, et al. Ibuprofen in the treatment of postoperative pain in small children. A randomized, double-blind-placebo controlled parallel group study. Acta Anaesthesiol Scand 1994;38:467–72.
36. Pai VB, Sakadjian A, Puthoff TD. Ibuprofen lysine for the prevention and treatment of patent ductus arteriosus. Pharmacotherapy 2008;28:1162–82.
37. Cherif A, Jabnoun S, Khrouf N. Oral ibuprofen in early closure of patent ductus arteriosus in very premature infants. Am J Perinatol 2007;24:339–46.
38. Cherif A, Khrouf N, Jabnoun N, et al. Randomized pilot study comparing oral ibuprofen with intravenous ibuprofen in very low birth weight infants with patent ductus arteriosus. Pediatrics 2008;122:e1256–61.
39. Mason L, Edwards JE, Moore RA, et al. Single dose oral naproxen and naproxen sodium for acute post-operative pain. [update in Cochrane Database Syst Rev 2009;(1):CD004234; PMID: 19160232]. Cochrane Database Syst Rev 2004;(4):CD004234.

40. Korpela R, Silvola J, Laakso E, et al. Oral naproxen but not acetaminophen reduces the need for rescue analgesic after adenoidectomy in children. Acta Anaesthesiol Scand 2007;51:726–30.
41. Zuppa AF, Mondick JT, Davis L, et al. Population pharmacokinetics of ketorolac in neonates and infants. Am J Ther 2009;16:143–6.
42. Lynn AM, Bradford H, Kantor ED, et al. Postoperative ketorolac tromethamine in infants aged 6-18 months: the effect on morphine usage, safety assessment, and stereo-specific pharmacokinetics. Anesth Analg 2007;104: 1040–51.
43. Dsida RM, Wheeler M, Birmingham PK, et al. Age-stratified pharmacokinetics of ketorolac tromethamine in pediatric surgical patients. Anesth Analg 2002;94: 266–70.
44. Bean-Lejewski JD, Hunt RD. Effect of ketorolac on bleeding time and postoperative pain in children: a double-blind, placebo-controlled comparison with meperidine. J Clin Anesth 1996;8:25–30.
45. Castillo-Zamora C, Castillo-Peralta LA, Nava-Ocampo AA. Report of an anaphylactoid reaction to ketorolac in two pediatric surgical patients. Ther Drug Monit 2006;28:458–62.
46. Houck CS, Wilder RT, McDermott JS, et al. Safety of intravenous ketorolac therapy in children and cost savings with a unit dosing system. J Pediatr 1996;129:292–6.
47. Watcha MF, Ramirez-Ruiz M, White PF, et al. Perioperative effects of oral ketorolac and acetaminophen in children undergoing bilateral myringotomy. Can J Anaesth 1992;39:641–2.
48. Vetter TR, Heiner EJ. Intravenous ketorolac as an adjuvant to pediatric patient-controlled analgesia with morphine. J Clin Anesth 1994;6:110–3.
49. Munro HM, Walton SR, Malviya S, et al. Low dose ketorolac improves analgesia and reduces morphine requirements following posterior spinal fusion in adolescents. Can J Anaesth 2002;49:461–6.
50. Park JM, Houck CS, Sethna NF, et al. Ketorolac suppresses bladder spasms after pediatric ureteral reimplantation. Anesth Analg 2000;91:11–5.
51. Papacci P, De Francisci G, Iacobucci T, et al. Use of intravenous ketorolac in the neonate and premature babies. Paediatr Anaesth 2004;14:487–92.
52. Intrussi CE. Clinical pharmacology of opioids for pain. Clin J Pain 2002; 18(Suppl):s3–13.
53. Rose JB. Pediatric analgesic pharmacology. In: Litman RS, Hines RL, editors. Pediatric anesthesiology: the requisites in anesthesiology. Philadelphia: Elsevier Mosby; 2004. p. 196–205.
54. Yaster M, Kost-Beyerly S, Maxwell LG. Opioid agonists and antagonists. In: Schechter NL, Berde CB, Yaster M, editors. Pain in infants, children, and adolescents. 2nd edition. Philadelphia Baltimore (MD): Lippincott, Williams, Wilkins; 2003. p. 181–224.
55. Stein C, Rossow CE. Analgesia: receptor ligands and opiate narcotics. In: Evers AS, Maze M, editors. Anesthetic pharmacology: physiologic principles and clinical practice. Philadelphia: Churchill Livingstone; 2004.
56. Quigley C. Opioid switching to improve pain relief and drug tolerability. Cochrane Database Syst Rev 2004;(3):CD004847.
57. Kart T, Christup LL, Rasmussen M. Recommended use of morphine in neonates, infants, and children based on a literature review: part 1 pharmacokinetics. Paediatr Anaesth 1997;7:5–11.

58. Kart T, Christup LL, Rasmussen M. Recommended use of morphine in neonates, infants, and children based on a literature review: part 2 clinical use. Paediatr Anaesth 1997;7:93–101.
59. Bouwmeester NJ, Anderson BJ, Tibboel D, et al. Developmental pharmacokinetics of morphine and its metabolites in neonates, infants, and young children. Br J Anaesth 2004;92(2):208–17.
60. Hunt A, Joel S, Dick G, et al. Population pharmacokinetics of oral morphine and its glucuronides in children receiving morphine as immediate-release liquid or sustained-release tablets for cancer pain. J Pediatr 1999;135:47–55.
61. Lynn AM, Nespera MK, Opheim KE, et al. Respiratory effects of intravenous morphine infusions in neonates, infants, and children after cardiac surgery. Anesth Analg 1993;77:695–701.
62. Quigley C, Wiffen P. A systematic review of hydromorphone in acute and chronic pain. J Pain Symptom Manage 2003;25(2):169–78.
63. Berde CB, Beyer JE, Bournaki MC, et al. Comparison of morphine and methadone for prevention of postoperative pain in 3- to 7-year old children. J Pediatr 1991;119:136–41.
64. Weschules DJ, Bain KT. A systematic review of opioid conversion ratios used with methadone for the treatment of pain. Pain Med 2008;9:595–612.
65. Andrews CM, Krantz MJ, Wedam EF, et al. Methadone induced mortality in the treatment of chronic pain: role of QT prolongation. Cardiol J 2009;16:210–7.
66. Singleton MA, Rosen JI, Fisher DM. Plasma concentrations of fentanyl in infants, children, and adolescents. Can J Anaesth 1987;34:152–5.
67. Ginosar Y, Riley ET, Angst MS. The site of action of epidural fentanyl in humans: the difference between infusion and bolus administration. Anesth Analg 2003; 97:1428–38.
68. Galinken JL, Fazi LM, Cuy RM, et al. Use of intranasal fentanyl in children undergoing myringotomy and tube placement during halothane and sevoflurane anesthesia. Anesthesiology 2000;93(6):1378–83.
69. Schechter NL, Weisman SJ, Rosenblum M, et al. The use of oral transmucosal fentanyl citrate for painful procedures in children. Pediatrics 1995;95: 335–9.
70. Collins JJ, Dunkel IJ, Gupta SK. Transdermal fentanyl in children with cancer pain: feasibility, tolerability, and pharmacokinetic correlates. J Pediatr 1999; 134:319–23.
71. Madadi P, Koren G. Pharmacogenetic insights into codeine analgesia: implications to pediatric codeine use. Pharmacogenomics 2008;9:1267–84.
72. Gasche Y, Daali Y, Fathi M, et al. Codeine intoxication associated with ultrarapid CYP2D6 metabolism. N Engl J Med 2004;351:2827–31.
73. Koren G, Cairns J, Chtayat D, et al. Pharmacogenetics of morphine poisoning in a breastfed neonate of a codeine prescribed mother. Lancet 2006;368:704.
74. Kirvela M, Lindgren L, Seppola T. The pharmacokinetics of oxycodone in uremic patients undergoing renal transplantation. J Clin Anesth 1996;8:13–8.
75. Czarnecki ML, Jandrisevits MD, Theiler SC, et al. Controlled-release oxycodone for the management of pediatric postoperative pain. J Pain Symptom Manage 2004;27(4):379–86.
76. Kendrick WD, Woods AM, Daly MY. Naloxone versus nalbuphine infusion for epidural morphine-induced pruritus. Anesth Analg 1996;82:641–7.
77. Malinovsky JM, Lepage JY, Karam G. Nalbuphine reverses urinary effects of epidural morphine: a case report. J Clin Anesth 2002;14:535–8.

78. Maxwell LG, Kaufmann SC, Bitzer S, et al. The effects of a small-dose naloxone infusion on opioid-induced side effects and analgesia in children and adolescents treated with intravenous patient-controlled analgesia: a double-blind, prospective, randomized, controlled study. Anesth Analg 2005;100:953–8.

79. Thomas J, Karver S, Cooney GA, et al. Methylnaltrexone for opioid-induced constipation in advanced illness. N Engl J Med 2008;358:2332–43.

80. Viscussi ER, Gan TJ, Leslie JB, et al. Peripherally acting mu-opioid antagonists and postoperative ileus: mechanisms of action and clinical applicability. Anesth Analg 2009;108:1811–22.

81. Poulsen L, Arendt-Nielsen L, Brosen K, et al. The hypoalgesic effect of tramadol in relation to CYP2D6. Clin Pharmacol Ther 1996;60:636–44.

82. Van den Anker JN, Tibboel D, Van Schaik RH. Pharmacogenetics and pharmacogenomics of analgesic drugs. In: Anand KJS, Stevens BJ, McGrath PJ, editors. Pain in neonates and infants. 3rd edition. Philadelphia: Elsevier; 2007. p. 103–13.

83. Pang WW, Wu HS, Tung CC. Tramadol 2.5 mgx (kg^{-1}) appears to be the optimal intraoperative loading dose before patient-controlled analgesia. Can J Anaesth 2003;50(1):48–51.

84. Finkel JC, Rose JB, Schmitz ML, et al. Evaluation of the efficacy and tolerability of oral tramadol hydrochloride tablets for the treatment of post-surgical pain in children. Anesth Analg 2002;94:1469–73.

85. Rose JB, Finkel JF, Arguedas-Mohs A, et al. Oral tramadol for treatment of pain of 7-30 days duration in children. Anesth Analg 2003;96:78–81.

86. Zempky WT, Cravero JP. Relief of pain and anxiety in pediatric patients in emergency medical systems. AAP Committee on Pediatric Emergency Medicine and Section on Anesthesiology and Pain Medicine. Pediatrics 2004;114:1348–56.

87. Parker RI, Mahan RA, Giugliano D. Efficacy and safety of intravenous midazolam and Ketamine as sedation for therapeutic an diagnostic procedures in children. Pediatrics 1997;99:427–31.

88. Malinovsky JM, Servin F, Cozian A. Ketamine and norketamine plasma concentrations after IV, nasal, and rectal administration in children. Br J Anaesth 1996;77:203–7.

89. Himmelscher S, Durieux ME. Ketamine for perioperative pain management. Anesthesiology 2005;102(1):211–20.

90. Bergendahl H, Lonnqvist P-A, Eksborg S. Clonidine in paediatric anaesthesia: review of the literature and comparison with benzodiazepines for premedication. Acta Anaesthesiol Scand 2006;50:135–43.

91. Mikawa K, Nishina K, Maekawa N. Oral clonidine premedication reduces postoperative pain in children. Anesth Analg 1996;82:225–30.

92. Schmidt AP, Valinetti EA, Bandeira DB, et al. Effects of preanesthetic administration of midazolam, clonidine, or dexmedetomidine on postoperative pain and anxiety in children. Paediatr Anaesth 2007;17:667–74.

93. Hansen TG, Henneberg SW, Walther-Larsen S, et al. Caudal bupivacaine supplemented with caudal or intravenous clonidine in children undergoing hypospadius repair: a double-blind study. Br J Anaesth 2004;92:223–7.

94. Cucchiaro G, Adzick NS, Rose JB, et al. A comparison of epidural bupivacaine-fentanyl and bupivacaine-clonidine in children undergoing the NUSS procedure. Anesth Analg 2006;103:322–7.

95. Saudan S, Habre W, Ceroni D, et al. Safety and efficacy of patient controlled epidural analgesia following pediatric spinal surgery. Paediatr Anaesth 2008;18:132–9.

96. Kaabachi O, Zarghouni A, Ouezini R, et al. Clonidine 1 μg/kg is a safe and effective adjuvant to plain bupivacaine in spinal anesthesia in adolescents. Anesth Analg 2007;105:516–9.
97. Cucchiaro G, Ganesh A. The effects of clonidine on postoperative analgesia after peripheral nerve blockade in children. Anesth Analg 2007;104:532–7.
98. Vetter TR, Carvallo D, Johnson JL, et al. A comparison of single-dose caudal clonidine, morphine, or hydromorphone combined with ropivacaine in pediatric patients undergoing ureteral re-implantation. Anesth Analg 2007;104: 1356–63.
99. Rochette A, Raux O, Troncin R, et al. Clonidine prolongs spinal anesthesia in newborns: a prospective dose-ranging study. Anesth Analg 2004;98:56–9.
100. Hall JE, Uhrich TD, Barney JA, et al. Sedative, amnestic, and analgesic properties of small-dose dexmedetomidine infusions. Anesth Analg 2000;90: 699–705.
101. Walker J, MacCallum M, Fischer C, et al. Sedation using dexmedetomidine in pediatric burn patients. J Burn Care Res 2006;27:206–10.
102. Chrysostomou C, Di Filippo S, Manrique AM, et al. Use of dexmedetomidine in children after cardiac and thoracic surgery. Pediatr Crit Care Med 2006;7: 126–31.
103. Olutoye O, Kim T, Giannoni C, et al. Dexmedetomidine as an analgesic for pediatric tonsillectomy and adenoidectomy. (Letter). Paediatr Anaesth 2007;17: 1007–8.
104. Saadawy I, Boker A, Elshahawy MA, et al. Effect of dexmedetomidine on the characteristics of bupivacaine in a caudal block in pediatrics. Acta Anaesthesiol Scand 2009;53:251–6.
105. Yaksh TL. Neonates have a spinal alpha receptor too, as do adults. (Commentary). Br J Pharmacol 2007;151:1139–40.
106. Walker SW, Fitzgerald M. Characterization of spinal α-adrenergic modulation of nociceptive transmission and hyperalgesia throughout postnatal development in rats. Br J Pharmacol 2007;151:1334–42.
107. Woolf CJ, Thompson SW. The induction and maintenance of central sensitization is dependent on N-methyl-D-aspartic acid receptor activation: implications for the treatment of post-injury pain hypersensitivity states. Pain 1991;44:293–9.
108. McCartney CJL, Sinha A, Katz J. A Qualitative systematic review of the role of N-methyl-D-aspartate receptor antagonists in preventative analgesia. Anesth Analg 2004;98:1385–400.
109. Duedahl TH, Romsing J, Moiniche S, et al. A qualitative systematic review of peri-operative dextromethorphan in post-operative pain. Acta Anaesthesiol Scand 2006;50:1–13.
110. Rose JB, Cuy R, Cohen DE, et al. Preoperative oral dextromethorphan does not reduce pain or analgesic consumption in children after adenotonsillectomy. Anesth Analg 1999;88:749–53.
111. Dawson GS, Seidman P, Ramadan HH. Improved postoperative pain control in pediatric adenotonsillectomy with dextromethorphan. Laryngoscope 2001;111: 1223–6.
112. Hasan RA, Kartush JM, Thomas JD, et al. Oral dextromethorphan reduces perioperative analgesic administration in children undergoing tympanomastoid surgery. Otolaryngol Head Neck Surg 2004;131:711–6.
113. Ali SM, Shahrbano S, Ulhaq TS. Tramadol for pain relief in children undergoing adenotonsillectomy: a comparison with dextromethorphan. Laryngoscope 2008; 118:1547–9.

114. Patel S, Naeem S, Kesingland A, et al. The effects of GABA_B agonists and gabapentin on mechanical hyperalgesia in models of neuropathic and inflammatory pain in the rat. Pain 2001;90:217–26.
115. Enna SJ, McCarson KE. The role of GABA in the mediation and perception of pain. Adv Pharmacol 2006;54:1–27.
116. Cox RF, Collins MA. The effects of benzodiazepines on human opioid receptor binding and function. Anesth Analg 2001;93:354–8.
117. Naguib M, el Gammel M, Elhattab YS, et al. Midazolam for caudal analgesia in children: comparison with caudal bupivacaine. Can J Anaesth 1995;42: 758–64.
118. Muller-Schweffe G, Penn RD. Physostigmine in the treatment of intrathecal baclofen overdose: report of three cases. J Neurosurg 1989;71:273–5.
119. Delhaas EM, Brouwers JR. Intrathecal baclofen overdose: report of 7 events. Int J Clin Pharmacol Ther Toxicol 1991;29:274–80.
120. Ruetsch YA, Boni T, Borgeat A. From cocaine to ropivacaine: the history of local anesthetics. Curr Top Med Chem 2001;1:175–82.
121. Bosenberg AT, Thomas J, Cronje L, et al. Pharmacokinetics and efficacy of ropivacaine for continuous epidural infusion in neonates and infants. Paediatr Anaesth 2005;15:739–49.
122. Meunier JF, Goujard E, Dubousset AM, et al. Pharmacokinetics of bupivacaine after continuous epidural infusion in infants with and without biliary atresia. Anesthesiology 2001;95:87–95.
123. Zink W, Graf BM. Benefit-risk assessment of ropivacaine in the management of postoperative pain. Drug Saf 2004;27:1093–114.
124. Ludot H, Tharin JY, Belouadah M, et al. Successful resuscitation after ropivaciane and lidocaine-induced ventricular arrhythmia following posterior lumbar plexus block in a child. Anesth Analg 2008;106:1572–4.
125. Stevens B, Johnston C, Petryshen P, et al. Premature infant pain profile: development and initial validation. Clin J Pain 1996;12:13–22.
126. Krechel SW, Bildner J. CRIES: a new neonatal postoperative pain measurement score. Initial testing of validity and reliability. Paediatr Anaesth 1995;5:53–61.
127. Merkel SI, Voepel-Lewis T, Shayevitz JR, et al. The FLACC: a behavioral scale for scoring postoperative pain in young children. Pediatr Nurs 1997;23:293–7.
128. Bieri D, Reeve RA, Champion GD, et al. The faces pain scale for the self-assessment of the severity of pain experienced by children: development, initial validation, and preliminary investigation for the ratio scale properties. Pain 1990;41: 139–50.
129. McGrath PA, Seifert CE, Speechley KN, et al. A new analogue scale for assessing children's pain: an initial validation study. Pain 1996;64:435–43.
130. Johnston CC. Psychometric issues in the measurement of pain. In: Finley GA, McGrath PJ, editors. Measurement of pain in infants and children, Progress in pain research and management, vol. 10. Seattle (WA): IASP Press; 1998. p. 5–20.
131. Beyer JE, McGrath PJ, Berde CB. Discordance between self-report and behavioral pain measures in children aged 3-7 years after surgery. J Pain Symptom Manage 1990;5:350–6.
132. Decruynaere C, Thonnard JL, Plaghki L. How many response levels do children distinguish on faces scales for pain assessment? Eur J Pain 2009;13:641–8.
133. Anand KJS, Stevens BJ, McGrath PJ. Pain in neonates and infants. 3rd edition. Philadelphia: Elsevier; 2007. p. 91–101.
134. McDonald AJ, Cooper MG. Patient-controlled analgesia: an appropriate method of pain control in children. Paediatr Drugs 2001;3:273–84.

135. Lehman AK. Recent developments in patient-controlled analgesia. J Pain Symptom Manage 2005;29(5 Suppl):S72–89.
136. Monitto CL, Greenberg RS, Kost-Beyerly S, et al. The safety and efficacy of parent-nurse-controlled analgesia in patients less than six years of age. Anesth Analg 2000;91:573–9.
137. Voepel-Lewis T, Marinkovic A, Kostrzewa A, et al. The prevalence of and risk factors for adverse events in children receiving patient-controlled angalgesia by proxy or patient controlled analgesia after surgery. Anesth Analg 2008;107:70–5.
138. Dal D, Kanbak M, Caglar M, et al. A background infusion of morphine does not enhance postoperative analgesia after cardiac surgery. Can J Anaesth 2003;50:476–9.
139. Doyle E, Robinson D, Morton NS. Comparison of patient-controlled analgesia with and without a background infusion after lower abdominal surgery in children. Br J Anaesth 1993;71:670–3.
140. Berde CB, Sethna NF. Analgesics for the treatment of pain in children. N Engl J Med 2002;347:1094–103.
141. McNeely JK, Rarber NE, Rusy LM, et al. Epidural analgesia improves outcome following pediatric fundoplication: a retrospective analysis. Reg Anesth 1997;22:16–23.
142. Dolin SJ, Cashman JN, Bland JM. Effectiveness of acute postoperative pain management: I. Evidence from published data. Br J Anaesth 2002;89:409–23.
143. Gunter JB. Thoracic epidural anesthesia via the modified Taylor approach in infants. Reg Anesth Pain Med 2000;25:561–5.
144. Tsui BC, Gupta S, Finucane B. Confirmation of epidural catheter placement using nerve stimulation. Can J Anaesth 1998;45:640–4.
145. Rapp HJ, Folger A, Grau T. Ultrasound-guided epidural catheter insertion in children. Anesth Analg 2005;101:333–9.
146. Llewellyn N, Moriarty A. The national pediatric epidural audit. Paediatr Anaesth 2007;17:520–33.
147. Polaner D, Suresh S, Cote CJ. Pediatric regional anesthesia. In: Cote CJ, Todres IJ, Ryan JF, et al, editors. A practice of anesthesia for infants and children. 3rd edition. Philadelphia: WB Saunders; 2001. p. 636–74.
148. Birmingham PK, Wheeler M, Suresh S, et al. Patient-controlled epidural analgesia in children: can they do it? Anesth Analg 2003;96:686–91.
149. Jones SEF, Beasley JM, MacFarlane DWR, et al. Intrathecal morphine for postoperative pain relief in children. Br J Anaesth 1984;56:137–40.
150. Gall O, Aubineau JV, Berniere J, et al. Analgesic effect of low-dose intrathecal morphine after spinal fusion in children. Anesthesiology 2001;94:447–52.
151. Krechel SW, Helikson MA, Kittle D, et al. Intrathecal morphine (ITM) for postoperative pain control in children: a comparison with nalbuphine patient controlled analgesia (PCA). Paediatr Anaesth 1995;5:177–83.
152. Ganesh A, Kim A, Casale P, et al. Low-dose intrathecal morphine for postoperative analgesia in children. Anesth Analg 2007;104:271–6.
153. Eschertzhuber S, Hohlrieder M, Keller C, et al. Comparison of high- and low-dose intrathecal morphine for spinal fusion in children. Br J Anaesth 2008;100:538–43.
154. Harris MM, Kahana MD, Park TS. Intrathecal morphine for postoperative analgesia in children after selective dorsal root rhizotomy. Neurosurgery 1991;28:519–22.
155. Silvani P, Camporesi A, Agostino MR, et al. Caudal anesthesia in pediatrics: an update. Minerva Anestesiol 2006;72:453–9.

156. Giaufre E, Dalens B, Gombert A. Epidemiology and morbidity of regional anes-
     thesia in children: a one-year prospective survey of the French-Language
     Society of Pediatric Anesthesiologists. Anesth Analg 1996;83:904–12.
157. Copeland SE, Ladd LA, Gu XQ, et al. The effects of general anesthesia on the
     central nervous and cardiovascular system toxicity of local anesthetics. Anesth
     Analg 2008;106:1429–39.
158. Ivani G, Mossetti V. Pediatric regional anesthesia. Minerva Anestesiol 2009;75:
     1–6.
159. Henderson K, Sethna NF, Berde CB. Continuous caudal anesthesia for inguinal
     repair in former preterm infants. J Clin Anesth 1993;5:129–33.
160. Lin YC, Sentivany-Collins SK, Peterson KL, et al. Outcomes after single injection
     caudal epidural versus continuous infusion epidural via caudal approach for
     postoperative analgesia in infants and children undergoing patent ductus arte-
     riosus ligation. Paediatr Anaesth 1999;9:139–43.
161. Constant I, Gall O, Gouyert I, et al. Addition of clonidine or fentanyl to local anes-
     thetics prolongs the duration of surgical analgesia after single-shot caudal block
     in children. Br J Anaesth 1998;80:294–8.
162. Sites B, Chan VW, Neal JM, et al. American Society of Regional Anesthesia and
     Pain Medicine; European Society of Regional Anaesthesia and Pain Therapy
     Joint Committee. The American Society of Regional Anesthesia and Pain Medi-
     cine and the European Society of Regional Anaesthesia and Pain Therapy Joint
     Committee recommendations for education and training in ultrasound-guided
     regional anesthesia. Reg Anesth Pain Med 2009;34:40–6.
163. Gerner P, Binshtok AM, Wang CF, et al. Capsaicin combined with local anes-
     thetics preferentially prolongs sensory/nociceptive block in rat sciatic nerve.
     Anesthesiology 2008;109:872–8.

Is Anesthesia Bad for the Newborn Brain?

Mary Ellen McCann, MD, MPH, FAAP[a,b],*, Sulpicio G. Soriano, MD, FAAP[a,b]

KEYWORDS

- Neonate • Anesthesia • Neurotoxicity • Neuroapoptosis
- Neurocognition

Advances in surgical techniques, pediatric anesthesia, and intensive care have all contributed to improved survival rates of preterm and newborn infants receiving general anesthesia for a variety of surgical procedures and imaging studies. Recognition of functional nociceptive pathways in these patients has led to the development of general anesthetic techniques designed to ameliorate the stress response associated with painful procedures and decreased perioperative mortality and morbidity.[1,2] However, reports of anesthetic-induced neurotoxicity in immature animal models have raised questions about the overall safety of general anesthesia in human babies.

Landmark reports have linked the administration of commonly used anesthetic and sedative drugs to neurodegeneration and behavioral deficits in neonatal rats.[3,4] This phenomenon has subsequently been verified on other mammalian species. Subsequently, these studies have fueled contentious debates on the clinical relevance of these findings in the perioperative care of pediatric patients.[5-9] Because the neurotoxic potential of general anesthesia in infants is a recent controversy within the pediatric anesthesia community, there are very few clinical studies available at present to help answer this question. In this article, the authors review the relevant preclinical and clinical data that are currently available on this topic.

The developing brain begins with an excess of neurons, which must be physiologically pruned by cell death or apoptosis. This physiologic neurodegeneration is an essential part of normal development.[10] Maturation of the central nervous system is influenced by external cues. As the immature central nervous system is extremely sensitive to its environment, various exposures and physiologic insults have the potential to amplify this neurodegenerative process. Establishment of synaptic connections between neurons is an essential process in the formation of neuronal

This work was supported by the CHMC Anesthesia Foundation.
[a] Department of Anesthesia (Pediatrics), Harvard Medical School, 25 Shattuck Street, Boston, MA, USA
[b] Department of Anesthesiology, Perioperative and Pain Medicine, Children's Hospital Boston, 300 Longwood Avenue, Boston, MA 02115, USA
* Corresponding author. Department of Anesthesiology, Perioperative and Pain Medicine, Children's Hospital Boston, 300 Longwood Avenue, Boston, MA 02115.
E-mail address: mary.mccann@childrens.harvard.edu (M.E. McCann).

Anesthesiology Clin 27 (2009) 269–284
doi:10.1016/j.anclin.2009.05.007
1932-2275/09/$ – see front matter © 2009 Elsevier Inc. All rights reserved.

circuitry and survival. The neurologic development of all mammalian species is similar, although the duration of this development is different and loosely correlates with the lifespan of the organism. In humans, rapid brain growth begins in the intrauterine period and continues for the first 2 to 3 years of life. Disruption of this process leads to central nervous system (CNS) developmental abnormalities and, in many cases, fetal death.[11] General anesthetics given to immature animals have been found to increase the level of apoptosis leading to "overpruning" and abnormally small number of neurons remaining. Many different types of general anesthetics, sedatives, and anticonvulsants have been implicated in animal models, but all are believed to be related to alterations of synaptic transmissions involving the γ-amino butyric acid (GABA) or N-methyl-D-aspartate (NMDA) receptors.

Programmed cell death or apoptosis differs from other forms of neuronal cell death in that it is mediated by the caspase enzyme system within the cytosol. Several pathways have been discovered that activate the effector caspase system. The intrinsic pathway is a mitochondrial-dependent pathway, in which anesthetic drugs cause an increase in mitochondrial membrane permeability and release in cytochrome c into the cytosol, which then recruits the caspase system. The intrinsic system is activated quickly (within 2 hours of exposure to anesthetic drugs), and in rat studies, melatonin has been found to decrease the release of cytochrome c into the cytosol and therefore decrease the degree of apoptosis.[12,13]

An extrinsic pathway has also been described that involves activation of a protein called Fas, a tumor necrosing factor, which also activates the caspase system. This pathway takes longer to get activated by anesthetics than the intrinsic pathway.[12]

Although neurotrophins such as nerve growth factor, brain-derived neurotrophic factor (BDNF), and neurotrophic factor are necessary for neuronal survival, they have also been implicated in causing increased neuroapoptosis.[14] One recent study in rats suggested that a triple agent cocktail frequently used in pediatric anesthesia (midazolam, isoflurane, and nitrous oxide) significantly enhanced the BDNF-activated neuroapoptotic cascades in the cerebral cortex and thalamus.[15] Prolonged exposure to ketamine also increases BDNF levels in the developing rat brain.[16] The "triple agent cocktail" has also been found to negatively affect levels of synaptic proteins important in activity-induced synaptic plasticity (eg, synaptophysin, synaptobrevin, amphiphysin, SNAP-25, and CaM kinase H).[17] This might explain the consistent finding that anesthetic agents appear to have the greatest neurodegenerative impact when exposure occurs during the period of rapid synaptogenesis. Experimental studies in animals have found that β-estradiol may provide some protection against anesthetic-induced neurotoxicity by this pathway.[18]

PRECLINICAL DATA
Type of Exposures

NMDA antagonists: dose and duration
The neurotoxic effect of ketamine has been extensively investigated in mice, rats, and rhesus monkeys. Rat pups, given doses of 20 to 25 mg/kg every 90 minutes for at least seven doses on postnatal day seven, show evidence of neurotoxicity, whereas juvenile rats given the same doses for four or less times show no neurotoxicity.[19–21] In mice, single doses of greater than 10 mg/kg intraperitoneally are associated with neuroapoptosis and impaired learning once the mice reach adulthood.[22,23] Newer investigations on rhesus monkeys have revealed that there is increased neurodegeneration in monkeys that were exposed prenatally to roughly twice the standard ketamine concentrations (20–50 mg/kg/h for 24 hours) used in humans.[24] Neonatal

monkeys exposed to the same doses of ketamine on the fifth day of life also developed increased neurodegeneration of the frontal cortex. However, older monkeys exposed on the 35th day of life did not exhibit any neurodegeneration, even though the plasma ketamine levels of these monkeys was 10 times that found in anesthetized humans.[24] This same study also demonstrated that when the exposure time was reduced from 24 hours to 3 hours, there was no neurodegeneration found even in the postnatal day 5 monkeys.[24]

Primary cell cultures derived from neonatal rat and rhesus monkey frontal cortex exhibited increased DNA fragmentation and apoptosis when incubated in 10 to 20 μM ketamine solution for 6 to 48 hours.[25,26] Primary neuronal cell culture preparations show decrease in dendritic branches and length of dendrites in 2 μg/mL ketamine for 8 hours or 5 μg/mL for 4 hours.[27]

Mice given a single dose of ketamine 25 mg/kg subcutaneously on day 10 did not demonstrate any neurodegeneration, but when the ketamine was combined with either thiopental 5 mg/kg or propofol 10 mg/kg, there was increased neurodegeneration and impaired learning in adult mice.[28] Juvenile mice develop accelerated neuro-apoptosis after a single dose of ketamine (20–40 mg/kg) subcutaneously.[22,23] The administration of nitrous oxide, a mild NMDA receptor antagonist, for 6 hours is associated with increased caspase 3 expression in the infant mouse but not in the infant rat.[4,12,29] Nitrous oxide was also found to significantly increase the degree of neuro-apoptosis in neonatal rat pups and neonatal mouse hippocampal cultures exposed to isoflurane.[29] These data demonstrate that neurodegeneration increases with increasing doses and duration of exposure to NMDA antagonists. These changes are amplified when ketamine is given in combination with other anesthetic agents.

GABAnergic agonists: dose and duration

The anesthetics and sedatives that are implicated in causing increased apoptosis in immature mammals by way of being GABA agonists include benzodiazepines, barbiturates, ethanol, propofol, and volatile anesthetics. GABA is the principal fast-acting excitatory transmitter in the neonatal brain. In contrast to mature neurons, excessive stimulation of this receptor causes excitotoxicity of the neurons and results in cell death in these immature neuronal populations.[30]

The preclinical data on benzodiazepine administration seems to be species specific, with neonatal mice being more susceptible to the effects of benzodiazepines than neonatal rats. Young mice given a dose of diazepam 5 mg/kg developed increased neurodegeneration, although these mice later did not develop neurocognitive behavioral deficits.[31] However, neonatal rats required higher doses of diazepam (10–30 mg/kg) before they demonstrated increased neurodegeneration.[32] In addition, neonatal mice were susceptible to the neurotoxic effects of midazolam at doses of 9 mg/kg but neonatal rats were not.[4,23] The benzodiazepines, clonazepam (0.5–4 mg/kg intraperitoneally) and diazepam (10–30 mg/kg), but not midazolam, are associated with increased neurotoxicity after a single dose given intraperitoneally or subcutaneously to neonatal rats.[31,32] So a variety of different benzodiazepines in single doses can induce neuroapoptosis in both rats and mice.

There is evidence in neonatal rats that both pentobarbital 5 to 10 mg/kg and phenobarbital 40 to 100 mg/kg lead to increased apoptosis, but simultaneous administration of estradiol prevented this neurotoxicity.[32,33] Estradiol has been found to increase the levels of prosurvival proteins, such as extracellular signal-regulated kinase and protein kinase B, rather than to alter GABA or NMDA currents in hippocampal neuronal cultures.[33] In addition, thiopental given to neonatal mice in a dose of 5 to 25 mg/kg did not lead to apoptosis.[28]

Although etomidate has been shown to be a potent GABAnergic transmitter inhibitor, there are no preclinical studies in juvenile animals that demonstrate increased apoptosis.[34] Propofol has shown to have a dose-dependent neurotoxicity in neonatal mice. Doses of 200 mg/kg intraperitoneally are needed to induce a surgical plane of anesthesia in a neonatal mouse.[35] Exposure to a single subclinical dose of 10 mg/kg did not lead to either increased neurologic degeneration or functional neurologic impairments, but exposure to a higher dose of 50 to 60 mg/kg in neonatal mice did lead to neurodegeneration and long-term functional impairments,[28,35] even though this dose is only one-fourth the total dose needed for surgical anesthesia in a mouse. Similar findings were also found in rats with a single high dose of propofol (60 mg/kg subcutaneously) but not with a small dose (10 mg/kg subcutaneously).[28]

Exposure to halothane or enflurane for as little as 0.5 hour prenatally is associated with learning impairments in mice, and exposure to 2 hours prenatally of halothane 2.5% leads to learning disabilities in rats.[36] Prolonged exposure to halothane in subclinical doses of 25 to 200 ppm in young rats leads to decrease in cerebral synaptic density and dendritic numbers.[37–39]

Isoflurane exposure in young rats and mice has been studied extensively and has been found to lead to increased apoptosis in a manner dependent on the dose duration of exposure. Studies of isoflurane exposure in young rats or mice demonstrate that the rats need to be exposed for at least 4 hours of 0.75% isoflurane for evidence of neurotoxicity[4,12,29,40] to induce increased caspase 3 and 9 activation. The effects of isoflurane on neonatal rodent neurons are potentiated by midazolam and nitrous oxide and ameliorated by xenon and dexmedetomidine.[4,12,15,29,41] Isoflurane in combination with midazolam and nitrous oxide has also been shown to increase neuroapoptosis in guinea pigs.[42]

Sevoflurane has also been shown to increase neuroapoptosis in neonatal mice. Exposure to a subanesthetic concentration of sevoflurane (1.7%) for 2 hours resulted in caspase 3 activation and neurodegeneration in 7-day-old mouse pups.[31,43] Another group examined the effect of exposure to sevoflurane for 6 hours in 6-day-old mice and reported increased neuroapoptosis and abnormal social and learning behaviors.[44]

Timing of Exposure

All animals studied thus far have shown that the timing of exposure is critical in inducing neurotoxicity. It is generally believed that the exposure needs to occur when the CNS is developing, especially during the period of rapid synaptogenesis. Early studies in rats with a potent NMDA receptor antagonist, MK-801, showed that rats were most vulnerable to neurodegeneration from birth to day 14 of life, with peak sensitivity occurring on day seven of life. Fetal rats had a minimal increase in MK-801–induced neurodegeneration during the late fetal period (days 19–21) but none before this period.[19] The period of sensitivity in the rat appears to be correlated to some extent with the peak expression of the NR1 subunit of the NMDA receptor in the developing rat brain. These data suggest that the rat is most sensitive to NMDA receptor–mediated neurotoxicity during early neuronal pathway development, referred to as the "brain-growth spurt period" or period of synaptogenesis.[45] Mice have been shown to have the same period of vulnerability. Other potential neurotoxic agents, such as isoflurane and ketamine, have also shown peak effects on rodent brains during this period of synaptogenesis. Rats exposed to 0.75% to 1.5% isoflurane for 6 hours demonstrate evidence of neurotoxicity if the exposure occurs on postnatal day seven but do not exhibit any evidence of neurotoxicity if exposed on days 10 to 14 and only exhibit neurotoxicity on postnatal days 1 to 3 when exposed to

1.5% isoflurane.[4,12,29] In rhesus monkeys, the period of most susceptibility is from postconception day 122 to postnatal day five. At postnatal day 35, there was no neuroapoptosis seen in monkeys exposed to ketamine infusions. In humans, the brain growth spurt begins in the third trimester of gestation and extends through the third year of life.[46] So it would appear that the period of susceptibility to neuroapoptosis for humans would extend through this time period. However, the period of maximal susceptibility to neuron-apoptotic injury in humans is controversial. Efforts to determine the point of maximum vulnerability for humans have also been addressed using neuroinformatics, an analysis that combines neuroscience, evolutionary science, statistical modeling, and computer science, and this analysis reveals that the maximal point of vulnerability for humans may be at 17 to 20 weeks postconception, which is before the third trimester of pregnancy.[47,48] This analysis is bolstered by additional work examining the most ethanol-sensitive times for the human conceptus using data from seasonal alcohol consumption and determining lag times, which suggests that the human fetus is most sensitive to fetal alcohol syndrome during the 18th to 20th week postconception.[49] Ethanol is a potent neurotoxin that has NMDA antagonist and GABA mimetic properties, which are believed to be responsible for its apoptotic action. Single doses of ethanol intoxication given to rodents can activate a massive wave of apoptotic neurodegeneration.[5] So, although the period of maximal vulnerability has been determined for several mammalian species, there are still great uncertainties about this period in humans.

Exposure Effects or Outcomes

The histopathologic brain findings in exposed animals include increased apoptotic neurodegeneration of the laterodorsal thalamus, hippocampus, cortex, and caudate putamen.[23,31,50] A few studies have demonstrated neurodegeneration with pre- or postnatal exposure initially but then no functional neurocognitive deficits later when the animals reached maturity, perhaps indicating neurologic plasticity.[22,31,51,52] Most of the studies that revealed widespread neurodegeneration on histopathology also revealed neurocognitive behavioral issues later in the life of the exposed animals. The functional deficits described include disruption of spontaneous activity, learning acquisition, and impaired memory retention in adult mice that were exposed to propofol, or a combination of propofol with thiopental, or ketamine during the neonatal period.[31] There were also more errors in maze tasks and learning tasks found in adult rats exposed to halothane or a combination of isoflurane, midazolam, and nitrous oxide, exposed either prenatally or postnatally.[4,53,54]

CLINICAL HUMAN DATA

There are several difficulties in extrapolating the results from rat and small mammal studies to the human population. There are uncertainties about the determination of the timing of potential vulnerability during human development. Other possible confounders exist. Human infants are very carefully monitored during anesthesia, with great care taken to ensure that they are hemodynamically and electrophysiologically stable throughout the perioperative period, with additional attention paid to their ongoing nutritional needs. It is impossible to care for newborn infant rats with the same attention because of the limitations imposed on researchers by the extreme small size of these research subjects. In addition, there may be some genetic factors within humans that allow for greater brain plasticity after general anesthesia.

Although not much data have been published yet specifically examining the possible effects of anesthesia, there are several published reports on the neurodevelopmental outcomes of children who were born prematurely or who have had surgery at a young age. Because of the multiple confounders in most of these studies, it is difficult to conclusively determine whether general anesthetics are safe for young children. There are many known predictors of poor neurodevelopmental outcomes, such as low birth weight, prematurity, morbidity at birth, and low maternal socioeconomic status, which are not controlled for in some of these studies. In addition, it is probable that the perioperative events surrounding surgery independent of the general anesthesia may impact on neurologic development of young children, such as perioperative fasting, transport, hypothermia, hemodynamic instability, and stress response secondary to surgical stimulus.

Prenatal Human Exposure to General Anesthesia

In a study of Japanese full-term infants who were exposed to nitrous oxide during the last stages of delivery, there was statistically significant increase in neurologic sequelae at postnatal day five compared with infants who were not exposed to anesthesia.[55] These sequelae included weaker habituation to sound, stronger muscular tension, fewer smiles, and resistance to cuddling. Exposure to either short duration of general anesthesia or a small amount of local anesthesia for maternal dental procedures during pregnancy was found to be associated with a prolongation of visual pattern preference in the neonates and lower scores at age 4 on the Peabody Picture Vocabulary Test but no differences between cases and controls at age 4 on the Wechsler Preschool Primary Scales of Intelligence (WPPI) or the Stanford-Binet Intelligence Test. This study was limited by the small number of participants (39 total patients with nine patients prenatally exposed to anesthesia) and possibility of confounding by indication (maternal stress and morbidity).[56,57]

Neonatal or Early Infantile Human Exposure to General Anesthesia

Several studies have reported the neurodevelopmental outcomes of neonates who have had surgery at a very young age. Most of the studies have been cohort or case-control studies, and the primary exposure examined has not been anesthesia but surgery. The Victorian Infant Collaborative Study Group did a case-control study of infants born less than 27 weeks postconception who had patent ductus arteriosus (PDA) ligation, inguinal hernia repair, gastrointestinal surgery, neurosurgery, and tracheotomy, and compared them with age-matched controls who did not require surgery, for a total of 221 infants. They found that there was an increased incidence of cerebral palsy, blindness, deafness, and WPPI <3 standard deviation below the mean.[58] In another study involving almost 4000 extremely low-birth-weight infants, there was a higher incidence of cerebral palsy and lower Bayley Scales of Infant Development 2 scores in patients who had been treated surgically for necrotizing enterocolitis (NEC) compared with those treated with peritoneal drainage.[59] Five other smaller studies corroborated the findings that premature infants treated for NEC surgically have more neurocognitive deficits compared with those treated medically.[60–64] However, infants with isolated tracheoesophageal fistula repair, when tested in late childhood, did not have statistically different intelligence quotient (IQ) measurements compared with the general population.[65,66] These children were exposed to general anesthesia at a later postconceptual age than the age of the children in the NEC studies. A study that compared PDA ligation with indomethacin treatment revealed that there was an increase in cerebral palsy, cognitive delay, hearing loss, and blindness in the surgically treated group. Multiple outcome studies in children who have had cardiac surgeries as neonates have demonstrated increased incidence of cerebral palsy, lower IQs, speech and language impairment, and motor dysfunction.[67–75]

A prospective randomized trial that compared surgery for transposition of the great vessels followed 155 patients and did neurologic assessments at ages 1, 2.5, 4, and 8 years found that although the mean scores for most outcomes were within normal limits, the neurodevelopmental status of the cohort as a whole was below expectation, including academic achievement, fine motor function, visual spatial skills, working memory, hypothesis generating and testing, sustained attention, and higher-order language skills.[67–69]

There have also been some studies examining the neurocognitive outcomes of infants exposed to prolonged sedation in the neonatal intensive care unit. In the Neonatal Outcome and Prolonged Analgesia in Neonates (NOPAIN) trial, Anand and colleagues[76] noted that there was a poorer neurologic outcome and increased mortality in premature infants sedated for prolonged periods of time with midazolam compared with placebo or morphine. Poor neurologic outcomes (grade 3–4 intraventricular hemorrhages, periventricular malacia, and death) occurred in 24% of neonates in the placebo group, 32% in the midazolam group, and 4% in the morphine group, leading a Cochrane review to find that there was no evidence to support the use of midazolam in the neonatal intensive care unit (NICU).[77]

With the exception of the NOPAIN trial, the exposure of interest in these studies was not general anesthesia or sedatives; therefore, it is difficult to draw conclusions about the poorer neurologic outcomes found in most studies of infants who had surgical treatment rather than medical treatment. Most of the studies done in these infants were case-control or cohort studies rather than randomized control trials. Thus, there were many possible confounding variables that may have affected the neurologic outcome measures. The degree of presurgical morbidity may be one of the reasons that some infants had surgery for PDA and NEC rather than medical therapy. In children undergoing inguinal herniorrhaphies, a possible confounder might be a complicated respiratory neonatal course, which has been linked to both a higher incidence of inguinal hernias and to poorer neurologic outcomes.[78] The effects of surgery in these studies cannot be separated from the effects of general anesthesia. Neonates often receive increased inspired oxygen during transport to the operating rooms and during surgical procedures, which can be another source of neurotoxicity.[79] In the elderly, the inflammatory response activated by the trauma of surgery can accelerate neurodegenerative disease.[80,81] It is not known if the surgical inflammatory response leads to long-term neurologic development issues in children.

Early Childhood Human Exposure to General Anesthesia

Many of the agents suspected of causing neurotoxicity have been administered for prolonged periods to children in intensive care for the purposes of sedation. There are several very small case series that report short-term neurologic abnormalities in children exposed to these agents.[82–86] These findings are difficult to interpret because there are many reasons, in addition to the actions of the sedatives, that may be causative of the neurologic sequelae, including concomitant hypoxia, hypotension, infection, and antecedent neurologic trauma.

Midazolam, when given in conjunction with opioids, is associated with agitation, muscle twitching, myoclonus, chorea, facial grimacing, hallucinations, and disorientation in 11% to 50% of patients when it is discontinued after an infusion in children.[82–86] Symptoms usually resolve completely within 7 days. In two small case series (total number of patients, 48), when pentobarbital was given as a sedation agent for at least 1 day in conjunction with benzodiazepines, it was associated with agitation, anxiety, sweating, and muscle twitching in up to 35% of patients on cessation.[83,87] However, there were no short-term neurologic sequelae found in a very small series of six patients who were sedated with pentobarbital from 4 to 28 days.[88]

No neurologic sequelae other than immediate sedation were found in a case series of 18 children aged 1 month to 7 years given an inadvertent overdose of ketamine (13–56 mg/kg).[89] In a pilot study of children sedated with repetitive doses of ketamine or propofol for radiation therapy for retinoblastoma, a trend toward learning deficits and seizure disorders was noted in the sedated group compared with the nonsedated group.[90]

In 3 case series involving a total of 25 patients aged 1 month to 19 years who received isoflurane in conjunction with benzodiazepines for 1 to 497 minimum alveolar concentration (MAC)-hours, temporary neurologic sequelae included agitation, non-purposeful movement, myoclonus, hallucinations, and confusion on cessation of the volatile gas.[91–93] All symptoms resolved within a few days, and normal neurologic follow-up 4 to 6 weeks later was reported for all 12 patients in one of the case series.

Several studies have attempted to quantify the psychologic changes that may occur after an anesthetic and surgery in young children. In a large meta-analysis at a medical center, more maladaptive behaviors postoperatively were noted in children who were younger and whose parents were more anxious on induction.[94] Several studies have noted that the maladaptive behaviors determined by parental report occur more frequently in children less than 3 years of age compared with older children.[95–97] The maladaptive behaviors most often reported are night terrors, oppositional behavior, bedwetting, and changes in feeding routines. Young children given a mida-zolam premedication in addition to their general anesthetic exhibit less maladaptive behaviors compared with those who do not get a premedication, although by 6 months, 20% of children will still exhibit some behavioral problems that parents attri-bute to the surgical experience.[98]

There has been interest in doing epidemiologic studies to determine whether general anesthesia is associated with learning disabilities. In a large retrospective cohort study of 5357 children, 593 patients were identified as having one or more general anesthetics before age 4 years.[99] This study found that there were significantly more reading, written language, and math learning disabilities in children who had been exposed to two or more general anesthetics but no increase in disabilities in those children who had been exposed to a single anesthetic. The risk for learning disabilities also increased with the cumulative duration of the general anesthesia. In another epidemiologic study, a birth cohort of 5000 patients was identified from the New York State Medicaid billing codes.[100] Of this group, 625 patients underwent inguinal herniorraphy at a young age. After controlling for gender and low birth weight, the authors found nearly a twofold increase in developmental and behavioral issues. In a pilot study to test the feasibility of using a validated child behavior checklist in 314 children who had urologic surgery, it was determined that there was more disturbed neurobehavioral development in children who underwent surgery before age 24 months compared with those who underwent surgery after age 24 months, although the differences between the two groups were not statistically significant.[101] These studies are provocative, but the data do not reveal whether anesthesia itself may contribute to developmental issues or whether the need for anesthesia is a marker for other unidentified factors that contribute to these.

Beneficial Effects of Anesthesia for Newborns

Isoflurane and other NMDA antagonists, such as ketamine, in preclinical studies in the setting of hypoxia decrease the total amount of neuronal loss. At least in in vivo exper-iments, this protection is greater in hippocampal slides derived from 5-day-old rats compared with 23-month-old rats.[102] Although only hypothermic protection has been shown to improve clinical outcome in perinatal hypoxic-ischemic encephalopathy, additional benefit may require adjunctive agents.[103] The entry of calcium into the neuron appears to be the key element in cell death, and it is known that during asphyxia, excessive glutamate is released, which stimulates the voltage-dependent NMDA receptor to open with an accumulation of excess intracellular calcium.[104] MK-801, a potent NMDA receptor antagonist, has been shown to limit the extent of cortical neuronal infarction after asphyxia in 7-day-old rat pups.[105] The picture of the role of NMDA antagonist in cerebral protection is further clouded by the fact that perinatal hypoxic-ischemic injury is associated with more concomitant apoptotic cell death in infants than similar injury to the adult CNS.[106]

There is accumulating evidence that pain systems develop and function very early in the gestational period.[107] It is believed that the nociceptive nervous system is mostly mature by 23 to 25 weeks postconceptual age in humans but that the antinociceptive system develops later in infancy leaving premature and term infants more sensitive to pain than adults.[108] Animal models have shown that sensory nerve fibers involved in nociception grow out of the dorsal root ganglia during the prenatal period and eventually innervate the skin starting with the trunk and ending with the limbs.[109] The larger-diameter A fibers migrate first from the dorsal root to the periphery to form a cutaneous nerve plexus, which is followed by migration of C fibers. The last elements to appear are descending fibers from the brainstem, which modulate excitation and inhibition.[107,108]

Several short-term and long-term consequences of tissue damage during this developmental period have been reported.[108,109] In immature animal models, chronic painful stimuli can provoke cell death in the cortical, thalamic, hypothalamic, amydaloid, and hippocampal areas of the neonatal rat brain.[110]

Although many nervous system responses may resolve after an injury has healed, tissue damage during certain critical periods of development may have a more lasting effect even into adulthood.[108,109] There are several clinical correlates in which exposure to painful stimulation has altered human behavior. In a cohort study of 87 infants who had undergone circumcision, circumcision with EMLA (eutectic mixture of local anesthetics) pretreatment, and no circumcision, those infants who underwent circumcision without pretreatment had the highest pain scores on vaccination at age 4 to 6 months.[111] There are changes in pain thresholds in children who are graduates of NICUs, which can persist until the children reach their teenage years.[112] Several possible mechanisms exist to account for this, including alterations in synaptic connectivity and signaling, changes in the balance of inhibition versus excitation, and increased terminal density in the injured area resulting from increased concentration of nerve growth factor.[108,109] Early postnatal pain may also affect neurodevelopment through stress responses. In a study designed to evaluate the relationship between early pain and stress, repeated painful experiences seemed to affect subsequent responses to open field habituation, an index of emotionality.[113]

SUMMARY

Although certain emerging data suggest that common general anesthetics may be neurotoxic to immature animals, there are also data suggesting that these same anesthetics may be neuroprotective against hypoxic-ischemic injury, and that inadequate analgesia during painful procedures may lead to increased neuronal cell death in animals and long-term behavioral changes in humans. The challenge for the pediatric anesthesia community is to design and implement studies in human infants to ascertain the safety of general anesthesia. It is likely that the answer to whether general anesthetics are neurotoxic to young babies will require many different study approaches, including epidemiologic, case-control, and randomized control trials.[114–116] The permanent neurocognitive damage caused by general anesthetics is likely to be subtle in nature, if it exists, and thus may be difficult to measure. It may take many years of following cohorts of youngsters until maturity before some of these possible neurocognitive abnormalities are manifest. In the meantime, it is important to continue the preclinical studies to elucidate the general anesthetics least likely to be neurotoxic in the setting of painful stimulation.

REFERENCES

1. Hickey PR, Hansen DD. High-dose fentanyl reduces intraoperative ventricular fibrillation in neonates with hypoplastic left heart syndrome. J Clin Anesth 1991;3:295–300.
2. Anand KJ, Hansen DD, Hickey PR. Hormonal-metabolic stress responses in neonates undergoing cardiac surgery. Anesthesiology 1990;73:661–70.
3. Ikonomidou C, Bittigau P, Koch C, et al. Neurotransmitters and apoptosis in the developing brain. Biochem Pharmacol 2001;62:401–5.
4. Jevtovic-Todorovic V, Hartman RE, Izumi Y, et al. Early exposure to common anesthetic agents causes widespread neurodegeneration in the developing rat brain and persistent learning deficits. J Neurosci 2003;23:876–82.
5. Olney JW, Wozniak DF, Farber NB, et al. The enigma of fetal alcohol neurotoxicity. Ann Med 2002;34:109–19.
6. Soriano SG, Anand KJ, Rovnaghi CR, et al. Of mice and men: should we extrapolate rodent experimental data to the care of human neonates? Anesthesiology 2005;102:866–8, author reply 8–9.
7. Todd MM. Anesthetic neurotoxicity: the collision between laboratory neuroscience and clinical medicine. Anesthesiology 2004;101:272–3.
8. Anand KJ. Anesthetic neurotoxicity in newborns: should we change clinical practice? Anesthesiology 2007;107:2–4.
9. Olney JW. New insights and new issues in developmental neurotoxicology. Neurotoxicology 2002;23:659–68.
10. Buss RR, Oppenheim RW. Role of programmed cell death in normal neuronal development and function. Anat Sci Int 2004;79:191–7.
11. Kuida K, Zheng TS, Na S, et al. Decreased apoptosis in the brain and premature lethality in CPP32-deficient mice. Nature 1996;384:368–72.
12. Yon JH, Daniel-Johnson J, Carter LB, et al. Anesthesia induces neuronal cell death in the developing rat brain via the intrinsic and extrinsic apoptotic pathways. Neuroscience 2005;135:815–27.
13. Yon JH, Carter LB, Reiter RJ, et al. Melatonin reduces the severity of anesthesia-induced apoptotic neurodegeneration in the developing rat brain. Neurobiol Dis 2006;21:522–30.
14. Head BP, Patel HH, Niesman IR, et al. Inhibition of p75 neurotrophin receptor attenuates isoflurane-mediated neuronal apoptosis in the neonatal central nervous system. Anesthesiology 2009;110:813–25.
15. Lu LX, Yon JH, Carter LB, et al. General anesthesia activates BDNF-dependent neuroapoptosis in the developing rat brain. Apoptosis 2006;11:1603–15.
16. Ibla JC, Hayashi H, Bajic D, et al. Prolonged exposure to ketamine increases brain derived neurotrophic factor levels in developing rat brains. Curr Drug Saf 2009;4:11–6.

17. Nikizad H, Yon JH, Carter LB, et al. Early exposure to general anesthesia causes significant neuronal deletion in the developing rat brain. Ann N Y Acad Sci 2007; 1122:69–82.

18. MacLusky NJ, Chalmers-Redman R, Kay G, et al. Ovarian steroids reduce apoptosis induced by trophic insufficiency in nerve growth factor-differentiated PC12 cells and axotomized rat facial motoneurons. Neuroscience 2003;118: 741–54.

19. Ikonomidou C, Bosch F, Miksa M, et al. Blockade of NMDA receptors and apoptotic neurodegeneration in the developing brain. Science 1999;283: 70–4.

20. Hayashi H, Dikkes P, Soriano SG. Repeated administration of ketamine may lead to neuronal degeneration in the developing rat brain. Paediatr Anaesth 2002;12: 770–4.

21. Scallet AC, Schmued LC, Slikker W Jr, et al. Developmental neurotoxicity of ketamine: morphometric confirmation, exposure parameters, and multiple fluorescent labeling of apoptotic neurons. Toxicol Sci 2004;81:364–70.

22. Rudin M, Ben-Abraham R, Gazit V, et al. Single-dose ketamine administration induces apoptosis in neonatal mouse brain. J Basic Clin Physiol Pharmacol 2005;16:231–43.

23. Young C, Jevtovic-Todorovic V, Qin YQ, et al. Potential of ketamine and midazolam, individually or in combination, to induce apoptotic neurodegeneration in the infant mouse brain. Br J Pharmacol 2005;146:189–97.

24. Slikker W Jr, Zou X, Hotchkiss CE, et al. Ketamine-induced neuronal cell death in the perinatal rhesus monkey. Toxicol Sci 2007;98:145–58.

25. Wang C, Sadovova N, Fu X, et al. The role of the N-methyl-D-aspartate receptor in ketamine-induced apoptosis in rat forebrain culture. Neuroscience 2005;132: 967–77.

26. Wang C, Sadovova N, Hotchkiss C, et al. Blockade of N-methyl-D-aspartate receptors by ketamine produces loss of postnatal day 3 monkey frontal cortical neurons in culture. Toxicol Sci 2006;91:192–201.

27. Vutskits L, Gascon E, Potter G, Tassonyi E, Kiss JZ. Low concentrations of ketamine initiate dendritic atrophy of differentiated GABAergic neurons in culture. Toxicology 2007;234:216–26.

28. Fredriksson A, Pontén E, Gordh T, et al. Neonatal exposure to a combination of N-methyl-D-aspartate and gamma-aminobutyric acid type A receptor anesthetic agents potentiates apoptotic neurodegeneration and persistent behavioral deficits. Anesthesiology 2007;107:427–36.

29. Ma D, Williamson P, Januszewski A, et al. Xenon mitigates isoflurane-induced neuronal apoptosis in the developing rodent brain. Anesthesiology 2007;106: 746–53.

30. Nunez JL, Alt JJ, McCarthy MM. A new model for prenatal brain damage. I. GABAA receptor activation induces cell death in developing rat hippocampus. Exp Neurol 2003;181:258–69.

31. Fredriksson A, Archer T, Alm H, et al. Neurofunctional deficits and potentiated apoptosis by neonatal NMDA antagonist administration. Behav Brain Res 2004;153:367–76.

32. Bittigau P, Sifringer M, Genz K, et al. Antiepileptic drugs and apoptotic neurodegeneration in the developing brain. Proc Natl Acad Sci U S A 2002;99:15089–94.

33. Asimiadou S, Bittigau P, Felderhoff-Mueser U, et al. Protection with estradiol in developmental models of apoptotic neurodegeneration. Ann Neurol 2005;58: 266–76.

34. Cheng VY, Martin LJ, Elliott EM, et al. Alpha5GABAA receptors mediate the amnestic but not sedative-hypnotic effects of the general anesthetic etomidate. J Neurosci 2006;26:3713–20.
35. Cattano D, Young C, Straiko MM, et al. Subanesthetic doses of propofol induce neuroapoptosis in the infant mouse brain. Anesth Analg 2008;106:1712–4.
36. Chalon J, Tang CK, Ramanathan S, et al. Exposure to halothane and enflurane affects learning function of murine progeny. Anesth Analg 1981;60:794–7.
37. Uemura E, Bowman RE. Effects of halothane on cerebral synaptic density. Exp Neurol 1980;69:135–42.
38. Uemura E, Ireland WP, Levin ED, et al. Effects of halothane on the development of rat brain: a golgi study of dendritic growth. Exp Neurol 1985;89:503–19.
39. Uemura E, Levin ED, Bowman RE. Effects of halothane on synaptogenesis and learning behavior in rats. Exp Neurol 1985;89:520–9.
40. Stratmann G, Sall JW, May LD, et al. Isoflurane differentially affects neurogenesis and long-term neurocognitive function in 60-day-old and 7-day-old rats. Anesthesiology 2009;110:834–48.
41. Sanders RD, Xu J, Shu Y, et al. Dexmedetomidine attenuates isoflurane-induced neurocognitive impairment in neonatal rats. Anesthesiology 2009; 110:1077–85.
42. Rizzi S, Carter LB, Ori C, et al. Clinical anesthesia causes permanent damage to the fetal guinea pig brain. Brain Pathol 2008;18:198–210.
43. Zhang X, Xue Z, Sun A. Subclinical concentration of sevoflurane potentiates neuronal apoptosis in the developing C57BL/6 mouse brain. Neurosci Lett 2008;447:109–14.
44. Satomoto M, Satoh Y, Terui K, et al. Neonatal exposure to sevoflurane induces abnormal social behaviors and deficits in fear conditioning in mice. Anesthesiology 2009;110:628–37.
45. Mellon RD, Simone AF, Rappaport BA. Use of anesthetic agents in neonates and young children. Anesth Analg 2007;104:509–20.
46. Dobbing J, Sands J. Comparative aspects of the brain growth spurt. Early Hum Dev 1979;3:79–83.
47. Clancy B, Finlay BL, Darlington RB, et al. Extrapolating brain development from experimental species to humans. Neurotoxicology 2007;28:931–7.
48. Clancy B, Kersh B, Hyde J, et al. Web-based method for translating neurodevelopment from laboratory species to humans. Neuroinformatics 2007;5:79–94.
49. Renwick JH, Asker RL. Ethanol-sensitive times for the human conceptus. Early Hum Dev 1983;8:99–111.
50. Olney JW, Wang H, Qin Y, et al. Pilocarpine pretreatment reduces neuroapoptosis induced by midazolam or isoflurane in infant mouse brain. Program No 286.15, Neuroscience Meeting Planner, Society for Neuroscience. Atlanta (GA), 2006.
51. Loepke AW, Istaphanous GK, McAuliffe JJ 3rd, et al. The effects of neonatal isoflurane exposure in mice on brain cell viability, adult behavior, learning, and memory. Anesth Analg 2009;108:90–104.
52. Li Y, Liang G, Wang S, et al. Effects of fetal exposure to isoflurane on postnatal memory and learning in rats. Neuropharmacology 2007;53:942–50.
53. Smith RF, Bowman RE, Katz J. Behavioral effects of exposure to halothane during early development in the rat: sensitive period during pregnancy. Anesthesiology 1978;49:319–23.
54. Quimby KL, Aschkenase LJ, Bowman RE, et al. Enduring learning deficits and cerebral synaptic malformation from exposure to 10 parts of halothane per million. Science 1974;185:625–7.

55. Eishima K. The effects of obstetric conditions on neonatal behaviour in Japanese infants. Early Hum Dev 1992;28:253–63.
56. Blair VW, Hollenbeck AR, Smith RF, et al. Neonatal preference for visual patterns: modification by prenatal anesthetic exposure? Dev Med Child Neurol 1984;26: 476–83.
57. Hollenbeck AR, Grout LA, Smith RF, et al. Neonates prenatally exposed to anesthetics: four-year follow-up. Child Psychiatry Hum Dev 1986;17:66–70.
58. Surgery and the tiny baby: sensorineural outcome at 5 years of age. The Victorian Infant Collaborative Study Group. J Paediatr Child Health 1996;32: 167–72.
59. Hintz SR, Kendrick DE, Stoll BJ, et al. Neurodevelopmental and growth outcomes of extremely low birth weight infants after necrotizing enterocolitis. Pediatrics 2005;115:696–703.
60. Blakely ML, Tyson JE, Lally KP, et al. Laparotomy versus peritoneal drainage for necrotizing enterocolitis or isolated intestinal perforation in extremely low birth weight infants: outcomes through 18 months adjusted age. Pediatrics 2006; 117:e680–7.
61. Walsh MC, Kliegman RM, Hack M. Severity of necrotizing enterocolitis: influence on outcome at 2 years of age. Pediatrics 1989;84:808–14.
62. Tobiansky R, Lui K, Roberts S, et al. Neurodevelopmental outcome in very low birthweight infants with necrotizing enterocolitis requiring surgery. J Paediatr Child Health 1995;31:233–6.
63. Chacko J, Ford WD, Haslam R. Growth and neurodevelopmental outcome in extremely-low-birth-weight infants after laparotomy. Pediatr Surg Int 1999;15: 496–9.
64. Simon NP, Brady NR, Stafford RL, et al. The effect of abdominal incisions on early motor development of infants with necrotizing enterocolitis. Dev Med Child Neurol 1993;35:49–53.
65. Lindahl H. Long-term prognosis of successfully operated oesophageal atresia-with aspects on physical and psychological development. Z Kinderchir 1984;39: 6–10.
66. Bouman NH, Koot HM, Hazebroek FW. Long-term physical, psychological, and social functioning of children with esophageal atresia. J Pediatr Surg 1999;34: 399–404.
67. Bellinger DC, Rappaport LA, Wypij D, et al. Patterns of developmental dysfunction after surgery during infancy to correct transposition of the great arteries. J Dev Behav Pediatr 1997;18:75–83.
68. Bellinger DC, Wypij D, duPlessis AJ, et al. Neurodevelopmental status at eight years in children with dextro-transposition of the great arteries: the Boston Circulatory Arrest Trial. J Thorac Cardiovasc Surg 2003;126:1385–96.
69. Bellinger DC, Wypij D, Kuban KC, et al. Developmental and neurological status of children at 4 years of age after heart surgery with hypothermic circulatory arrest or low-flow cardiopulmonary bypass. Circulation 1999;100:526–32.
70. Miller G, Tesman JR, Ramer JC, et al. Outcome after open-heart surgery in infants and children. J Child Neurol 1996;11:49–53.
71. Hovels-Gurich HH, Seghaye MC, Dabritz S, et al. Cognitive and motor development in preschool and school-aged children after neonatal arterial switch operation. J Thorac Cardiovasc Surg 1997;114:578–85.
72. Hovels-Gurich HH, Seghaye MC, Schnitker R, et al. Long-term neurodevelopmental outcomes in school-aged children after neonatal arterial switch operation. J Thorac Cardiovasc Surg 2002;124:448–58.

73. Karl TR, Hall S, Ford G, et al. Arterial switch with full-flow cardiopulmonary bypass and limited circulatory arrest: neurodevelopmental outcome. J Thorac Cardiovasc Surg 2004;127:213–22.
74. Limperopoulos C, Majnemer A, Shevell MI, et al. Neurodevelopmental status of newborns and infants with congenital heart defects before and after open heart surgery. J Pediatr 2000;137:638–45.
75. Mahle WT, Clancy RR, Moss EM, et al. Neurodevelopmental outcome and life-style assessment in school-aged and adolescent children with hypoplastic left heart syndrome. Pediatrics 2000;105:1082–9.
76. Anand KJ, Barton BA, McIntosh N, et al. Analgesia and sedation in preterm neonates who require ventilatory support: results from the NOPAIN trial. Neonatal outcome and prolonged analgesia in neonates. Arch Pediatr Adolesc Med 1999;153:331–8.
77. Ng E, Taddio A, Ohlsson A. Intravenous midazolam infusion for sedation of infants in the neonatal intensive care unit. Cochrane Database Syst Rev 2000; 1:CD002052.
78. Brooker RW, Keenan WJ. Inguinal hernia: relationship to respiratory disease in prematurity. J Pediatr Surg 2006;41:1818–21.
79. van der Walt J. Oxygen–elixir of life or Trojan horse? Part 2: oxygen and neonatal anesthesia. Paediatr Anaesth 2006;16:1205–12.
80. Cunningham C, Campion S, Lunnon K, et al. Systemic inflammation induces acute behavioral and cognitive changes and accelerates neurodegenerative disease. Biol Psychiatry 2009;65:304–12.
81. Palin K, Cunningham C, Forse P, et al. Systemic inflammation switches the inflammatory cytokine profile in CNS Wallerian degeneration. Neurobiol Dis 2008;30:19–29.
82. Bergman I, Steeves M, Burckart G, et al. Reversible neurologic abnormalities associated with prolonged intravenous midazolam and fentanyl administration. J Pediatr 1991;119:644–9.
83. Fonsmark L, Rasmussen YH, Carl P. Occurrence of withdrawal in critically ill sedated children. Crit Care Med 1999;27:196–9.
84. Khan RB, Schmidt JE, Tamburro RF. A reversible generalized movement disorder in critically ill children with cancer. Neurocrit Care 2005;3:146–9.
85. Hughes J, Gill A, Leach HJ, et al. A prospective study of the adverse effects of midazolam on withdrawal in critically ill children. Acta Paediatr 1994;83: 1194–9.
86. Franck LS, Naughton I, Winter I. Opioid and benzodiazepine withdrawal symp-toms in paediatric intensive care patients. Intensive Crit Care Nurs 2004;20: 344–51.
87. Yanay O, Brogan TV, Martin LD. Continuous pentobarbital infusion in children is associated with high rates of complications. J Crit Care 2004;19:174–8.
88. Tobias JD, Deshpande JK, Pietsch JB, et al. Pentobarbital sedation for patients in the pediatric intensive care unit. South Med J 1995;88:290–4.
89. Green SM, Clark R, Hostetler MA, et al. Inadvertent ketamine overdose in chil-dren: clinical manifestations and outcome. Ann Emerg Med 1999;34:492–7.
90. McCann ME, Petersen RA, Marcus K, et al. Does repeated exposure to anesthetic drugs lead to neurodevelopmental disabilities? Anesthesiology 2006;105:A966.
91. Arnold JH, Truog RD, Rice SA. Prolonged administration of isoflurane to pedi-atric patients during mechanical ventilation. Anesth Analg 1993;76:520–6.

92. Kelsall AW, Ross-Russell R, Herrick MJ. Reversible neurologic dysfunction following isoflurane sedation in pediatric intensive care. Crit Care Med 1994; 22:1032–4.
93. Sackey PV, Martling CR, Radell PJ. Three cases of PICU sedation with isoflurane delivered by the 'AnaConDa'. Paediatr Anaesth 2005;15:879–85.
94. Kain ZN, Caldwell-Andrews AA, Maranets I, et al. Preoperative anxiety and emergence delirium and postoperative maladaptive behaviors. Anesth Analg 2004;99:1648–54.
95. Kain ZN, Caldwell-Andrews AA, Weinberg ME, et al. Sevoflurane versus halothane: postoperative maladaptive behavioral changes: a randomized, controlled trial. Anesthesiology 2005;102:720–6.
96. Eckenhoff JE. Relationship of anesthesia to postoperative personality changes in children. AMA Am J Dis Child 1953;86:587–91.
97. Keaney A, Diviney D, Harte S, et al. Postoperative behavioral changes following anesthesia with sevoflurane. Paediatr Anaesth 2004;14:866–70.
98. Kain ZN, Mayes LC, Wang SM, et al. Postoperative behavioral outcomes in children: effects of sedative premedication. Anesthesiology 1999;90:758–65.
99. Wilder RT, Flick RP, Sprung J, et al. Early exposure to anesthesia and learning disabilities in a population-based birth cohort. Anesthesiology 2009;110: 796–804.
100. DiMaggio CJ, Sun L, Kakavouli A, et al. Exposure to anesthesia and the risk of developmental and behavioral disorders in young children. Anesthesiology 2008;109:A1415.
101. Kalkman CJ, Peelen L, Moons KG, et al. Behavior and development in children and age at the time of first anesthetic exposure. Anesthesiology 2009;110: 805–12.
102. Zhan X, Fahlman CS, Bickler PE. Isoflurane neuroprotection in rat hippocampal slices decreases with aging: changes in intracellular Ca2+ regulation and N-methyl-D-aspartate receptor-mediated Ca2+ influx. Anesthesiology 2006; 104:995–1003.
103. Sanders RD, Ma D, Brooks P, et al. Balancing paediatric anaesthesia: preclinical insights into analgesia, hypnosis, neuroprotection, and neurotoxicity. Br J Anaesth 2008;101:597–609.
104. Levene M. Role of excitatory amino acid antagonists in the management of birth asphyxia. Biol Neonate 1992;62:248–51.
105. Ford LM, Sanberg PR, Norman AB, et al. MK-801 prevents hippocampal neurodegeneration in neonatal hypoxic-ischemic rats. Arch Neurol 1989;46:1090–6.
106. Nakajima W, Ishida A, Lange MS, et al. Apoptosis has a prolonged role in the neurodegeneration after hypoxic ischemia in the newborn rat. J Neurosci 2000;20:7994–8004.
107. Walco GA. Needle pain in children: contextual factors. Pediatrics 2008; 122(Suppl 3):S125–9.
108. Fitzgerald M. The development of nociceptive circuits. Nat Rev Neurosci 2005; 6:507–20.
109. Fitzgerald M, Howard F. The neurologic basis of pediatric pain. In: Schecter NL, Berde CB, Yaster M, editors. Pain in infants, children and adolescents. Philadelphia: Lippincott, Williams and Wilkins; 2003. p. 19–42.
110. Anand KJ, Garg S, Rovnaghi CR, et al. Ketamine reduces the cell death following inflammatory pain in newborn rat brain. Pediatr Res 2007;62: 283–90.

111. Taddio A, Katz J, Ilersich AL, et al. Effect of neonatal circumcision on pain response during subsequent routine vaccination. Lancet 1997;349: 599–603.
112. Hermann C, Hohmeister J, Demirakca S, et al. Long-term alteration of pain sensitivity in school-aged children with early pain experiences. Pain 2006;125: 278–85.
113. Page GG, Blakely WP, Kim M. The impact of early repeated pain experiences on stress responsiveness and emotionality at maturity in rats. Brain Behav Immun 2005;19:78–87.
114. Sun LS, Li G, Dimaggio C, et al. Anesthesia and neurodevelopment in children: time for an answer? Anesthesiology 2008;109:757–61.
115. Davidson AJ, McCann ME, Morton NS, et al. Anesthesia and outcome after neonatal surgery: the role for randomized trials. Anesthesiology 2008;109: 941–4.
116. Hansen TG, Flick R. Anesthetic effects on the developing brain: insights from epidemiology. Anesthesiology 2009;110:1–3.

The Fontan Patient

Philip D. Bailey, Jr, DO*, David R. Jobes, MD

KEYWORDS

- Fontan • Cavopulmonary anastomosis • Single ventricle
- Noncardiac surgery • Anesthetic considerations

SINGLE VENTRICLE/FONTAN PHYSIOLOGY: ANATOMIC FEATURES AND STAGED RECONSTRUCTION

In the early 1970s, Fontan[1] and Kreutzer[2] independently introduced a technique to surgically repair tricuspid atresia that resulted in routing systemic venous return to the pulmonary arteries by way of a complete cavopulmonary anastomosis without the benefit of an interposed subpulmonic ventricle. This procedure was designed anatomically to separate the pulmonary and systemic circulations, and aimed physiologically at creating nearly normal arterial saturations while reducing the pressure and volume load of the heart to that of a normal systemic ventricle.

Univentricular congenital heart anomalies include a wide spectrum of defects that result in one of the ventricular chambers either being absent or severely hypoplastic making a biventricular repair impossible (**Fig. 1**). Hypoplastic left heart syndrome (HLHS), tricuspid atresia, and unbalanced atrioventricular canal are examples of anatomic defects that produce univentricular anatomy or functionally a single ventricle. Regardless of the specific defect, a series of 3-staged surgical procedures are usually required to achieve separation of the pulmonary and systemic circulation.

In the neonatal period, the first stage of the univentricular pathway involves creating a shunt to provide an arterial source of pulmonary blood flow, ensuring unobstructed systemic outflow, and providing adequate mixing of blood at the atrial level with an unrestricted atrial defect (**Fig. 2**). The second stage, typically performed between 6 and 9 months of age, involves the creation of a superior cavopulmonary anastomosis (bidirectional Glenn or hemi-Fontan) and the removal of the existing systemic to pulmonary artery shunt (**Fig. 3**). The third stage, Fontan completion, typically occurs between 15 and 24 months of age and involves inclusion of the inferior vena cava blood flow into the pulmonary artery by way of a lateral tunnel or extracardiac conduit, with or without fenestration of the conduit (**Fig. 4**).

A fenestration is often created to limit pressure in the Fontan circuit with the intention of reducing the systemic residua and sequelae of increased venous pressure

Division of Cardiothoracic Anesthesiology, Department of Anesthesiology and Critical Care Medicine, The Children's Hospital of Philadelphia, 34th and Civic Center Boulevard, Philadelphia, PA 19104, USA
* Corresponding author.
E-mail address: baileyp@email.chop.edu (P.D. Bailey).

Anesthesiology Clin 27 (2009) 285–300
doi:10.1016/j.anclin.2009.05.004
1932-2275/09/$ – see front matter © 2009 Elsevier Inc. All rights reserved.

anesthesiology.theclinics.com

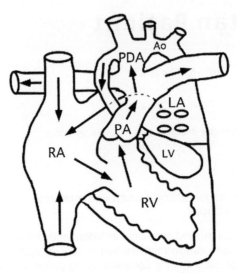

Fig. 1. Pre-Norwood anatomy. Direction of blood flow indicated by the *arrows*. Ao, aorta; LA, left atrium; LV, left ventricle; PA, pulmonary artery; PDA, patent ductus arteriosus; RA, right atrium; RV, right ventricle. (*Reprinted from* Walker SG, Stuth EA. Single-ventricle physiology: perioperative implications. Semin Pediatr Surg 2004;13(3):191; with permission from Elsevier.)

(eg, effusions). The fenestration may also help preserve preload of the systemic ventricle and cardiac output to a varying degree when pulmonary blood flow is decreased, albeit at the expense of systemic desaturation. Systemic oxygen saturation should be greater than 85% to 90%. Systemic saturation less than 85% to 90% may suggest excessive flow across the fenestration, extremely low mixed venous oxygen saturation, pulmonary arteriovenous malformations, or an additional venous channel diverting blood around the pulmonary circulation.[3]

Following completion of the Fontan, cardiac output is completely dependent on pulmonary blood flow and is not entirely determined by the heart, but by transpulmonary blood flow, which itself is determined by the pulmonary vascular resistance (PVR). Unlike the second stage, whereby reduced pulmonary blood flow will result in decreased systemic oxygenation, reduced pulmonary blood flow after completion of the Fontan results in reduced cardiac output in addition to systemic deoxygenation. Children tend to tolerate decreased systemic oxygenation far better than diminished cardiac output. Other disadvantages of the Fontan circulation include chronic venous hypertension, systemic venous congestion, and decreased cardiac output at rest and during exercise.[4] Therefore, when caring for the Fontan patient it is paramount that these physiologic principles are understood and appropriate measures are taken to preserve pulmonary blood flow.

Improved surgical and medical management has led to an increase in survival after staged univentricular palliative procedures. Subsequently, improved survival has led to a progressive increase in the number of patients who will present for noncardiac surgical interventions with Fontan physiology. Indeed, over a recent 3-year period, 247 patients with univentricular heart defects underwent noncardiac surgery at the Children's Hospital of Philadelphia.[3] Although most of these procedures occurred between stage II and the Fontan operation, surgery was performed at every stage and age along the univentricular pathway. Procedures ranged in complexity and

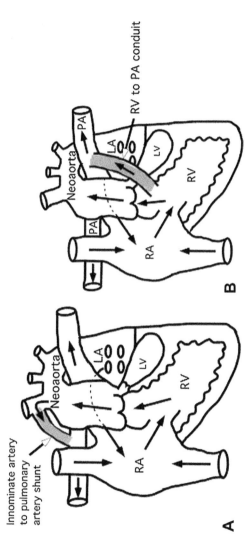

Fig. 2. HLHS status post stage I (Norwood) palliation. (*A*) The current standard for providing pulmonary blood flow is the systemic artery to pulmonary artery (Blalock-Taussig) shunt. (*B*) A recent innovation is a modification in which a systemic ventricle to pulmonary artery conduit is used. Direction of blood flow indicated by the *arrows*. LA, left atrium; LV, left ventricle; PA, pulmonary artery; RA, right atrium; RV, right ventricle. (*Reprinted from* Walker SG, Stuth EA. Single-ventricle physiology: perioperative implications. Semin Pediatr Surg 2004;13(3):192; with permission from Elsevier.)

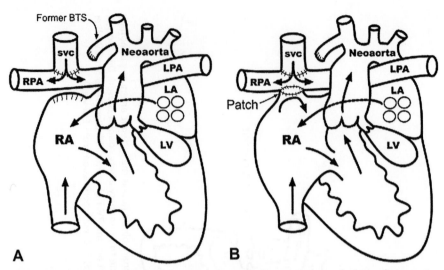

Fig. 3. Technical variants of stage II partial cavapulmonary anastomosis, immediate postoperative period. Note the ventricular dilation and hypertrophy caused by volume overload during the preceding stage. (*A*) The bidirectional Glenn. (*B*) The hemi-Fontan. This procedure is physiologically identical to the Glenn, but with an additional anastomosis from the proximal SVC to the RPA. This anastomosis is then occluded with a patch, which is removed during subsequent Fontan completion. Direction of blood flow indicated by the *arrows.* BTS, Blalock-Taussig shunt; LA, left atrium; LPA, left pulmonary artery; LV, left ventricle; RA, right atrium; RPA, right pulmonary artery; RV, right ventricle; SVC, superior vena cava. (*Reprinted from* Walker SG, Stuth EA. Single-ventricle physiology: perioperative implications. Semin Pediatr Surg 2004;13(3):195; with permission from Elsevier.)

urgency from emergent to elective, and from simple superficial to highly complex (eg, major intracavitary, craniofacial, and so forth).

Although the urgency and complexity of the proposed procedure may vary, the general concepts that serve as a framework for the perioperative management of the Fontan patient does not. A comprehensive multidisciplinary (cardiologist, surgeon, anesthesiologist) understanding is necessary to construct the perioperative plan. The patient's cardiologist is usually in a unique position to succinctly address the patient's anatomy, physiology, and the preexisting level of cardiac impairment (ventricular dysfunction, AV valve regurgitation, outflow tract obstruction, and so forth) and therefore should be engaged throughout the entire perioperative process. Before agreeing to care for patients with Fontan physiology, consideration needs to be given to the proposed venue for the surgery and whether the infrastructure is capable of safely and comprehensively caring for the patient.[5]

PREOPERATIVE ASSESSMENT: FORMULATING THE PERIOPERATIVE PLAN
History and Physical Examination

In addition to obtaining a compete history, information from old medical records, and information from parents regarding the functional state of the patient, a letter from the child's cardiologist describing any recent changes in the patient's exercise tolerance or level of cardiac impairment as well as the details of the patient's physiology, anatomy, and any residua and sequelae of previous surgeries should be available for review. Recent illnesses should be addressed, especially respiratory tract infections because changes in airway resistance and PVR are detrimental and may pose

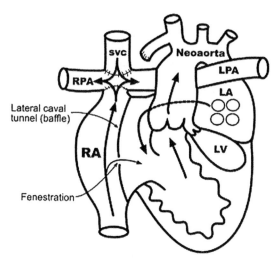

Fig. 4. The lateral caval tunnel Fontan procedure (with baffle fenestration), immediate post-operative period. Note the return to more normal ventricular size that occurs during stage II. LA, left atrium; LPA, left pulmonary artery; LV, left ventricle; RA, right atrium; RPA, right pulmonary artery; RV, right ventricle; SVC, superior vena cava. Direction of blood flow indicated by the *arrows*. (*Reprinted from* Walker SG, Stuth EA. Single-ventricle physiology: perioperative implications. Semin Pediatr Surg 2004;13(3):197; with permission from Elsevier.)

an unacceptable risk for elective surgery in the Fontan patient as pulmonary blood flow and cardiac output will decrease if respiratory complications such as laryngospasm or bronchospasm occur.[6] Determining the length of time to delay an elective procedure presents a conundrum; however, waiting 4 weeks after the symptoms resolve may be prudent to err on the side of caution rather than anesthetize the Fontan patient with suboptimal respiratory mechanics.

The physical examination, in addition to focusing on the airway, heart, and lungs, should include an examination of the extremities. The extremities should be inspected for cyanosis, edema, and vascular access sites. Vascular access may prove to be a challenge in this patient population because a minimum of three open cardiac procedures and several cardiac catheterizations have been performed before Fontan completion and many patients have had additional procedures and catheterizations after their Fontan, potentially further compromising vascular integrity/access.

Some Fontan patients may have a history of prolonged intervals of mechanical ventilation or a prior tracheostomy. A careful and detailed airway evaluation and management is therefore necessary because there is a risk of laryngeal anomalies: subglottic stenosis, laryngeal webbing, as well as vocal cord and hemi-diaphragm paralysis.[7,8] Some of these issues, such as subglottic stenosis, tend to become less problematic as the child grows. Previous anesthetic records should be reviewed and plans should be made for securing the potentially difficult airway by alternate means. This procedure is especially important in the Fontan patient because hypercarbia, hypoxia, and atelectasis will increase PVR and subsequently decrease pulmonary blood flow and cardiac output if the patient cannot be adequately ventilated.

Associated Defects

Patients with univentricular heart defects may have other congenital anomalies and genetic disorders that need to be considered when formulating an anesthetic plan.

Awareness of these associations enables the anesthesiologist to investigate and anticipate potential perioperative issues such as airway difficulties, cervical spine instability, and neurologic deficits. For example, trisomy 21 is associated with atrioventricular canal defects and heterotaxy has an association with chromosome 22q11 deletions (ie, DiGeorge syndrome). Two recently published texts are excellent sources of the anesthetic and perioperative implications of genetic syndromes.[9,10]

Current Medications

Patients may be on a spectrum of medications including, but not limited to, diuretics, digoxin, anticoagulants, antihypertensive, and antiarrhythmic agents. One needs to inquire if there have been any recent changes to the patient's medication regimen; this may indicate worsening ventricular function and a decreased ability of the heart to respond to the increased demands placed on it during the perioperative period. Communication with the patient's cardiologist is helpful to determine why changes to their medication regimen were made. It is our practice to continue the patient's medication regimen throughout the perioperative period with few exceptions although diuretics are usually withheld the day of surgery because of concern over the potential for dehydration.

Nothing by Mouth Status

Minimizing the nothing by mouth (NPO) interval, adequate preoperative hydration, and maintenance of intravascular volume are critical in patients with Fontan physiology. Avoiding dehydration is paramount because decreased preload can result in decreased pulmonary blood flow and cardiac output because the Fontan circulation is preload dependent. Scheduling patients as the first case as well as encouraging intake of clear liquid until 2 hours before the start of surgery may reduce the risks of dehydration. Verifying NPO times before surgery is important because unforeseen delays may occur despite best efforts. In this situation, if surgery is significantly delayed by more than 2 hours, patients should be allowed intake of clear liquids or an intravenous catheter should be placed and intravenous fluids started to avoid dehydration.

Laboratory Evaluation

Preoperative laboratory testing is guided by the proposed surgical procedure and the health status of the patient; however, a basic metabolic panel, complete blood count, type, and screen should be routine for most procedures regardless of the magnitude of the planned procedure. A recent ECG, an echocardiogram to assess ventricular function and Fontan pathway patency, and a chest radiograph may be indicated depending on the surgical procedure or clinical scenario. Information less than 6 months old is usually sufficient for patients who remain physiologically sound. However, if the patient is symptomatic suggesting a decrease in cardiac output and ventricular dysfunction, then the cardiologist should evaluate the patient before performing elective surgery. The cardiologist should assess the overall status of the patient, recommend, and evaluate tests as well as medical interventions to better optimize the patient. Cardiac catheterization may be indicated in patients whose ventricular function has decreased not only to help determine the cause, but to potentially intervene if appropriate before elective procedures. For most procedures, the availability of cross-matched blood will be required secondary to the increased bleeding potential in these patients. The bleeding propensity is due to elevated systemic venous pressure, the presences of collateral vessels, coagulation factor abnormalities, and antithrombotic therapy. In addition, Fontan patients typically have higher hemoglobin concentrations

bstantially reduced in Fontan patients. A progressive
rt Association class and maximal aerobic capacity has
eserve capacity is usually less than 50% of age-matched
on in exercise capacity is due to several factors: limited
o increase heart rate secondary to sinus node dysfunc-
ormalities, and an inability to increase preload

often present in Fontan patients, which may complicate
Arrhythmias, such as sinus node dysfunction and atrial
dings after the Fontan operation.[21,22] This is especially
der at the time of the Fontan completion and in patients
eration (extensive suture lines, damaged sinoatrial [SA]
pertension).[20] This finding necessitates the close moni-
arrhythmias in the perioperative period; some patients
rs and recommendations for the perioperative manage-
gement devices should be followed.[23] Effusions, pleural
atic and their significance must be established before
associated complication of the Fontan physiology that
norbidity is protein-losing enteropathy (PLE); a condition
ous congestion resulting in impaired lymphatic drainage
may lead to severe hypoalbuminemia and consideration
n in action and duration of anesthetic drugs.[27,28] Ascites
sent. It has been previously mentioned that thrombotic
s are coagulation factor abnormalities, after the Fontan
are on prophylactic anticoagulation (aspirin, Couma-
a rare complication of the Fontan physiology that is char-
of thick, tenacious rubbery cast of the tracheobronchial
tilatory management difficult.[32]
be classified as failing when these chronic complications
tment with ionotropes, diuretics, and vasodilators do not
ement and a more aggressive approach is often neces-
with a maze procedure or cardiac transplantation.[33]

everal operative techniques and issues merit specific
with Fontan physiology may be extremely sensitive to
aneuvers.

orts describing laparoscopic surgery in the Fontan
aparoscopic surgery include less postoperative pain,
a shorter hospital stay compared with open surgery.
y in patients with Fontan physiology has the increase
n and hypoxemia. Increased intraabdominal pressur
ng as well as elevated arterial carbon dioxide tensi
se PVR and decrease cardiac output to varyi
ng pressure to 10 to 12 mmHg may reduce the adve
delenburg positioning, which is commonly emplo
ay decrease preload resulting in decreased pulmo

---

due to chronic hypoxia. Therefore, a lower transfusion threshold is necessary to ensure adequate oxygen carrying capacity and delivery.

Psychosocial Issues: Premedication

Psychosocial issues are often overlooked. Depression, anxiety, and posttraumatic stress disorder are common.[11] Preoperative anxiety is common in children, and in the parents of children with a history of congenital heart disease and prior surgery. The importance of developing a rapport with the parents and the patient before the procedure should not be overlooked. Discussing the proposed plan as well as alterna- tive options for premedication, induction, and postoperative pain management is important. Children who have experienced multiple interventions often have strong preferences with regard to the choice of anesthetic premedication and method of induction; these wishes should be respected and honored whenever feasible.
Premedication should be considered depending on the physical status of the patient, the urgency, and the nature of the surgical procedure. Although oral midazo- lam (0.5 mg/kg) is appropriate, our preference is pentobarbital 4 mg/kg by mouth up to a maximum dose of 120 mg in patients without intravenous access because of its dose-related sedative properties, duration of action, and its preservation of ventilation and cardiac output; a high proportion of patients will be sleeping when administered 60 minutes before the start of the surgical procedure. Intravenous midazolam (0.05– 0.1 mg/kg), administered at the bedside by the anesthesia care-team is appropriate if the patient has intravenous access.

INTRAOPERATIVE MANAGEMENT
Monitoring

The level of monitoring will vary depending on the physiologic status of the patient and the proposed surgical procedure. The degree of invasiveness should be dictated by the patient's clinical condition and by the proposed procedure, giving one the ability to track ventilatory, hemodynamic, and metabolic parameters. There should be a low threshold for placing an arterial catheter because the risk/benefit ratio usually favors having, rather than not having, arterial access. Attention to the placement of the monitors is important to yield the most accurate information. Specifically, blood pres- sure measurements in all four extremities may be necessary to determine if there are any discrepancies secondary to prior surgical procedures or previous cut down attempts, especially if prior aortic surgery was undertaken and the possibility of an aortic coarctation exists, or if a classic Blalock-Taussig shunt has been performed and has compromised upper extremity blood flow.
Vascular access often presents a formidable challenge, especially if multiple oper- ative and interventional procedures have been preformed in the past. Evaluation of previous anesthetic records and catheterization reports may be useful to ascertain previous access sites and to determine vascular occlusion sites. Arterial and vascular access using a cut down approach may be necessary and is a useful skill to develop if one is planning on caring for patients with congenital cardiac lesions. Ultrasound may be useful in determining vessel patency and in obtaining vascular access. Central venous catheters may be useful to facilitate venous filling pressure and mixed venous oxygen saturation. However, it is our practice to forgo the routine placement of central venous catheters secondary to the need to preserve the patency of the venous archi- tecture for future interventions, prevent infection, decrease the risk of thrombosis, and concern about impaired venous return, all potentially catastrophic complications, especially in the Fontan patient.

Systemic oxygen saturation will be less than 100%. When the patient has a patent fenestration, systemic oxygen saturation typically ranges from the high 80s to the mid 90s. In addition, consideration needs to be given to the site at which temperature will be monitored. Ideally, temperature should be monitored at the core and peripheral sites; an increased gradient with elevated core temperature may be an indication of poor systemic perfusion.[12]

Induction and Maintenance

No specific anesthetic agent or regimen can be recommended. However, several general principles, including maintaining adequate preload, preserving low PVR and pulmonary blood flow, preserving sinus rhythm, preserving ventricular contractility and filling, blunting the stress response to surgery, and afterload reduction, are appropriate goals. Induction is typically accomplished by mask in the child with well-compensated Fontan physiology without intravenous access and for short, superficial procedures, assisted spontaneous ventilation by mask may be appropriate. However, the advantages of spontaneous mask ventilation and enhanced venous return must be weighed against the risk of hypercarbia, reduced oxygenation, and atelectasis, which can produce increased PVR and subsequently decrease pulmonary blood flow.[12] In the Fontan patient who has ventricular dysfunction and reduced cardiac output, induction is accomplished intravenously with agents known to have minimal myocardial depressant effects such as ketamine or etomidate.

Maintenance with volatile anesthetic agents and opioids are the mainstay of most anesthetic regimens for the Fontan patient undergoing noncardiac surgery. These agents are generally well tolerated. Nitrous oxide may be used, but the benefits need to be balanced with the potential for increasing PVR, atelectasis, and the potential for paradoxic emboli in patients with fenestration of the Fontan conduit. Neuromuscular blocking agents are usually chosen based on the length of the surgical procedure as well as the cardiodynamic profile of the agent; reversal agents are administered at the completion of the procedure unless the patient is going to remain intubated. Ensuring adequate reversal of neuromuscular blockade is important in this patient population because residual weakness postoperatively may lead to hypoventilation, hypoxemia, and hypercarbia, which are poorly tolerated in the Fontan patient. One must be cognizant of the reduced capacity of the single ventricle to respond to physiologic stress; myocardial dysfunction must always be considered, and emergency cardiac resuscitation drugs and ionotropic support readily available.[13] The authors routinely have milrinone, dopamine, and epinephrine prepared by the pharmacy anf available for all procedures. Maintenance of sinus rhythm is essential in the Fontan patient because rhythms other than sinus tend to be poorly tolerated. Atrial contribution to ventricular filling is extremely important because adequate cardiac output in the univentricular patient is dependent on it. The limited contractile and preload reserves increase the dependency on heart rate to increase cardiac output.[12]

Regional anesthesia has been described in patients with Fontan physiology.[14,15] If one decides to incorporate regional techniques to manage the patient perioperatively, then the coagulation status should be ascertained before undertaking this procedure because patients may have preexisting abnormalities of coagulation and may be taking medications that alter platelet function and coagulation to reduce the increased risk of thrombosis in the Fontan circuit. Another consideration is that neuraxial regional anesthetics induce a sympathectomy, which may result in a decrease in preload and afterload, and may be detrimental in the Fontan patient whose pulmonary blood flow and cardiac output are dependent on adequate preload; hypotension is usually more pronounced with spinal than epidural anesthesia. Therefore, epidural is usually

preferable to s[...]
controlled. Intra[...]
the effects of th[...]
a sympathecto[...]
issue as it is wi[...]

Mechanical Ve[...]

PVR plays a c[...]
cardiac output[...]
return and atria[...]
ventilation has[...]
long as hyperc[...]
tive-pressure v[...]
atelectasis, wh[...]
and cardiac o[...]
optimizes oxy[...]
low respirator[...]
positive end-e[...]
(10–15 mL/kg[...]

Fluid Manage[...]

Meticulous at[...]
ment of the Fo[...]
nary blood flo[...]
before the sta[...]
venous cathe[...]
intravascular[...]
tial length of[...]
more fluid m[...]
to calculate f[...]
tachycardia[...]
treated.

Transfusio[...]
patient is uni[...]
Venous con[...]
surgical tec[...]
depending[...]
Baseline co[...]
VIII, decrea[...]
medications[...]
the approp[...]
routinely st[...]
bleeding.

Subacute B[...]

The need[...]
nature of t[...]
Fontan co[...]
Associatio[...]
org).[18] Mo[...]
preventive[...]

Special Patient Consideratio[...]

Exercise performance is su[...]
decline in the New York Hea[...]
been described.[19] Exercise r[...]
control subjects. This reduct[...]
ventricular reserve, inability t[...]
tion and conduction abr[...]
augmentation.[20]

Chronic complications are[...]
perioperative management.[...]
tachycardia, are common fir[...]
true for patients who were ol[...]
with older versions of the op[...]
node artery, chronic atrial hy[...]
toring of Fontan patients for[...]
will have epicardial pacemak[...]
ment of cardiac rhythm mana[...]
and pericardial, are problem[...]
elective surgery.[24–26] Anothe[...]
contributes to perioperative n[...]
related to gastrointestinal ven[...]
and reduced absorption. PLE[...]
must be given to the alteratio[...]
and edema may also be pres[...]
complications are common, a[...]
operation and many patients[...]
din).[29–31] Plastic bronchitis is a[...]
acterized by the development[...]
tree making perioperative ven[...]

The Fontan circulation may[...]
are severe. Unfortunately, trea[...]
typically lead to much improv[...]
sary, such as Fontan revision[...]

Special Surgical Consideratio[...]

The physiologic impact of s[...]
discussion because patients[...]
the consequences of these m[...]

Laparoscopy

There are multiple case rep[...]
patient.[34–36] The benefits of[...]
pulmonary dysfunction, and[...]
However, laparoscopic surge[...]
potential to cause hypotensio[...]
from insufflation and position[...]
from insufflation will increa[...]
degrees.[35,36] Limiting insufflat[...]
effects of laparoscopy. Tren[...]
during laparoscopic surgery, r[...]

due to chronic hypoxia. Therefore, a lower transfusion threshold is necessary to ensure adequate oxygen carrying capacity and delivery.

Psychosocial Issues: Premedication

Psychosocial issues are often overlooked. Depression, anxiety, and posttraumatic stress disorder are common.[11] Preoperative anxiety is common in children, and in the parents of children with a history of congenital heart disease and prior surgery. The importance of developing a rapport with the parents and the patient before the procedure should not be overlooked. Discussing the proposed plan as well as alternative options for premedication, induction, and postoperative pain management is important. Children who have experienced multiple interventions often have strong preferences with regard to the choice of anesthetic premedication and method of induction; these wishes should be respected and honored whenever feasible.

Premedication should be considered depending on the physical status of the patient, the urgency, and the nature of the surgical procedure. Although oral midazolam (0.5 mg/kg) is appropriate, our preference is pentobarbital 4 mg/kg by mouth up to a maximum dose of 120 mg in patients without intravenous access because of its dose-related sedative properties, duration of action, and its preservation of ventilation and cardiac output; a high proportion of patients will be sleeping when administered 60 minutes before the start of the surgical procedure. Intravenous midazolam (0.05–0.1 mg/kg), administered at the bedside by the anesthesia care-team is appropriate if the patient has intravenous access.

INTRAOPERATIVE MANAGEMENT
Monitoring

The level of monitoring will vary depending on the physiologic status of the patient and the proposed surgical procedure. The degree of invasiveness should be dictated by the patient's clinical condition and by the proposed procedure, giving one the ability to track ventilatory, hemodynamic, and metabolic parameters. There should be a low threshold for placing an arterial catheter because the risk/benefit ratio usually favors having, rather than not having, arterial access. Attention to the placement of the monitors is important to yield the most accurate information. Specifically, blood pressure measurements in all four extremities may be necessary to determine if there are any discrepancies secondary to prior surgical procedures or previous cut down attempts, especially if prior aortic surgery was undertaken and the possibility of an aortic coarctation exists, or if a classic Blalock-Taussig shunt has been performed and has compromised upper extremity blood flow.

Vascular access often presents a formidable challenge, especially if multiple operative and interventional procedures have been preformed in the past. Evaluation of previous anesthetic records and catheterization reports may be useful to ascertain previous access sites and to determine vascular occlusion sites. Arterial and vascular access using a cut down approach may be necessary and is a useful skill to develop if one is planning on caring for patients with congenital cardiac lesions. Ultrasound may be useful in determining vessel patency and in obtaining vascular access. Central venous catheters may be useful to facilitate venous filling pressure and mixed venous oxygen saturation. However, it is our practice to forgo the routine placement of central venous catheters secondary to the need to preserve the patency of the venous architecture for future interventions, prevent infection, decrease the risk of thrombosis, and concern about impaired venous return, all potentially catastrophic complications, especially in the Fontan patient.

Systemic oxygen saturation will be less than 100%. When the patient has a patent fenestration, systemic oxygen saturation typically ranges from the high 80s to the mid 90s. In addition, consideration needs to be given to the site at which temperature will be monitored. Ideally, temperature should be monitored at the core and peripheral sites; an increased gradient with elevated core temperature may be an indication of poor systemic perfusion.[12]

Induction and Maintenance

No specific anesthetic agent or regimen can be recommended. However, several general principles, including maintaining adequate preload, preserving low PVR and pulmonary blood flow, preserving sinus rhythm, preserving ventricular contractility and filling, blunting the stress response to surgery, and afterload reduction, are appropriate goals. Induction is typically accomplished by mask in the child with well-compensated Fontan physiology without intravenous access and for short, superficial procedures, assisted spontaneous ventilation by mask may be appropriate. However, the advantages of spontaneous mask ventilation and enhanced venous return must be weighed against the risk of hypercarbia, reduced oxygenation, and atelectasis, which can produce increased PVR and subsequently decrease pulmonary blood flow.[12] In the Fontan patient who has ventricular dysfunction and reduced cardiac output, induction is accomplished intravenously with agents known to have minimal myocardial depressant effects such as ketamine or etomidate.

Maintenance with volatile anesthetic agents and opioids are the mainstay of most anesthetic regimens for the Fontan patient undergoing noncardiac surgery. These agents are generally well tolerated. Nitrous oxide may be used, but the benefits need to be balanced with the potential for increasing PVR, atelectasis, and the potential for paradoxic emboli in patients with fenestration of the Fontan conduit. Neuromuscular blocking agents are usually chosen based on the length of the surgical procedure as well as the cardiodynamic profile of the agent; reversal agents are administered at the completion of the procedure unless the patient is going to remain intubated. Ensuring adequate reversal of neuromuscular blockade is important in this patient population because residual weakness postoperatively may lead to hypoventilation, hypoxemia, and hypercarbia, which are poorly tolerated in the Fontan patient. One must be cognizant of the reduced capacity of the single ventricle to respond to physiologic stress; myocardial dysfunction must always be considered, and emergency cardiac resuscitation drugs and ionotropic support readily available.[13] The authors routinely have milrinone, dopamine, and epinephrine prepared by the pharmacy anf available for all procedures. Maintenance of sinus rhythm is essential in the Fontan patient because rhythms other than sinus tend to be poorly tolerated. Atrial contribution to ventricular filling is extremely important because adequate cardiac output in the univentricular patient is dependent on it. The limited contractile and preload reserves increase the dependency on heart rate to increase cardiac output.[12]

Regional anesthesia has been described in patients with Fontan physiology.[14,15] If one decides to incorporate regional techniques to manage the patient perioperatively, then the coagulation status should be ascertained before undertaking this procedure because patients may have preexisting abnormalities of coagulation and may be taking medications that alter platelet function and coagulation to reduce the increased risk of thrombosis in the Fontan circuit. Another consideration is that neuraxial regional anesthetics induce a sympathectomy, which may result in a decrease in preload and afterload, and may be detrimental in the Fontan patient whose pulmonary blood flow and cardiac output are dependent on adequate preload; hypotension is usually more pronounced with spinal than epidural anesthesia. Therefore, epidural is usually preferable to spinal anesthesia because the level and onset of the block is more controlled. Intravenous hydration before the onset of the block is useful to ameliorate the effects of the sympathectomy. Most peripheral nerve blocks do not usually cause a sympathectomy and therefore hypotension after placement is not as much of an issue as it is with neuraxial regional anesthetics.

Mechanical Ventilation

PVR plays a critical role in the Fontan patient because pulmonary blood flow and cardiac output are the result of the pressure difference between the systemic venous return and atrial pressure. Compared with positive-pressure ventilation, spontaneous ventilation has the advantage of enhanced venous return and pulmonary blood flow so long as hypercarbia, hypoxia, atelectasis, and acidosis are avoided.[16] However, positive-pressure ventilation will usually be required to prevent hypercarbia, hypoxia, and atelectasis, which will increase PVR and subsequently decrease pulmonary blood flow and cardiac output. A ventilatory strategy that preserves pulmonary blood flow and optimizes oxygen delivery by limiting peak inspiratory pressure (<20 cmH$_2$O), using low respiratory rates (<20 bpm), employing short inspiratory times, avoiding excessive positive end-expiratory pressure, and incorporating moderately elevated tidal volumes (10–15 mL/kg) in addition to ensuring adequate intravascular volume will be required.

Fluid Management/Transfusion

Meticulous attention to volume status is absolutely critical to the successful management of the Fontan patient because decreased preload will result in decreased pulmonary blood flow and cardiac output. Encouraging intake of clear liquid until 2 hours before the start of surgery may reduce the risks of dehydration. Placement of an intravenous catheter and hydration preoperatively may be necessary to ensure adequate intravascular volume if fasting has been prolonged or surgery is delayed any substantial length of time. Vascular capacitance is increased in the Fontan patient so even more fluid may be required than anticipated based on the formula commonly used to calculate fluid requirements. Hypovolemia should be suspected when unexplained tachycardia is present; the cause should be promptly determined and aggressively treated.

Transfusion may become necessary during the operative procedure. The Fontan patient is unique because they have venous collaterals and elevated venous pressure. Venous congestion often leads to increased perioperative bleeding despite adequate surgical technique often necessitating transfusion of packed red blood cells, and depending on the nature of the blood loss, platelets and other coagulation factors. Baseline coagulation defects exist in patients with Fontan physiology: increased factor VIII, decreased protein C and S.[17] In addition, many patients will be on outpatient medications, such as aspirin and Coumadin, that may not have been stopped for the appropriate length of time, intentionally or unintentionally; aspirin is often not routinely stopped because the risk of thrombosis is often outweighed by the risk of bleeding.

Subacute Bacterial Endocarditis Prophylaxis

The need for antibiotic prophylaxis against bacterial endocarditis is based on the nature of the surgical procedure and the proximity of the proposed procedure to the Fontan completion. The current guidelines published in 2007 by the American Heart Association (AHA) are available at the AHA Web site (http://www.americanheart.org).[18] Most patients will have a recent letter from their cardiologist with specific preventive endocarditis recommendations.

Special Patient Considerations

Exercise performance is substantially reduced in Fontan patients. A progressive decline in the New York Heart Association class and maximal aerobic capacity has been described.[19] Exercise reserve capacity is usually less than 50% of age-matched control subjects. This reduction in exercise capacity is due to several factors: limited ventricular reserve, inability to increase heart rate secondary to sinus node dysfunction and conduction abnormalities, and an inability to increase preload augmentation.[20]

Chronic complications are often present in Fontan patients, which may complicate perioperative management. Arrhythmias, such as sinus node dysfunction and atrial tachycardia, are common findings after the Fontan operation.[21,22] This is especially true for patients who were older at the time of the Fontan completion and in patients with older versions of the operation (extensive suture lines, damaged sinoatrial [SA] node artery, chronic atrial hypertension).[20] This finding necessitates the close monitoring of Fontan patients for arrhythmias in the perioperative period; some patients will have epicardial pacemakers and recommendations for the perioperative management of cardiac rhythm management devices should be followed.[23] Effusions, pleural and pericardial, are problematic and their significance must be established before elective surgery.[24-26] Another associated complication of the Fontan physiology that contributes to perioperative morbidity is protein-losing enteropathy (PLE); a condition related to gastrointestinal venous congestion resulting in impaired lymphatic drainage and reduced absorption. PLE may lead to severe hypoalbuminemia and consideration must be given to the alteration in action and duration of anesthetic drugs.[27,28] Ascites and edema may also be present. It has been previously mentioned that thrombotic complications are common, as are coagulation factor abnormalities, after the Fontan operation and many patients are on prophylactic anticoagulation (aspirin, Coumadin).[29-31] Plastic bronchitis is a rare complication of the Fontan physiology that is characterized by the development of thick, tenacious rubbery cast of the tracheobronchial tree making perioperative ventilatory management difficult.[32]

The Fontan circulation may be classified as failing when these chronic complications are severe. Unfortunately, treatment with ionotropes, diuretics, and vasodilators do not typically lead to much improvement and a more aggressive approach is often necessary, such as Fontan revision with a maze procedure or cardiac transplantation.[33]

Special Surgical Considerations

The physiologic impact of several operative techniques and issues merit specific discussion because patients with Fontan physiology may be extremely sensitive to the consequences of these maneuvers.

Laparoscopy

There are multiple case reports describing laparoscopic surgery in the Fontan patient.[34-36] The benefits of laparoscopic surgery include less postoperative pain, pulmonary dysfunction, and a shorter hospital stay compared with open surgery. However, laparoscopic surgery in patients with Fontan physiology has the increased potential to cause hypotension and hypoxemia. Increased intraabdominal pressure from insufflation and positioning as well as elevated arterial carbon dioxide tension from insufflation will increase PVR and decrease cardiac output to varying degrees.[35,36] Limiting insufflating pressure to 10 to 12 mmHg may reduce the adverse effects of laparoscopy. Trendelenburg positioning, which is commonly employed during laparoscopic surgery, may decrease preload resulting in decreased pulmonary blood flow and cardiac output. Gas embolism is possible and the risk of paradoxic embolism is increased in a patient who has a fenestration. Adequate hydration, attention to the signs of decreasing pulmonary blood flow, communication with the surgeon as well as a low threshold to convert to an open procedure is essential when performing laparoscopic surgery in patients with Fontan physiology.

One-lung Ventilation

During one-lung ventilation the nondependent lung is not ventilated and right-to-left shunting increases. Increasing ventilation in the dependent lung may be able to compensate to eliminate carbon dioxide; however, the alveolar arterial oxygen gradient will likely increase and subsequently, PVR will increase. Thoracoscopy incurs concerns similar to laparoscopy whereby the lung is partially collapsed, and in addition to a mechanical increase in PVR, the arterial carbon dioxide tension is elevated from carbon dioxide insufflation.[37–40] Limiting insufflating pressure may reduce the adverse effects of thoracoscopy. Optimizing oxygenation involves optimizing intravascular volume. Invasive use of arterial pressure monitoring will help guide ventilation and fluid management.

Positioning

Positions other than supine are often required to optimize exposure of the surgical site and special consideration is needed in the patient with Fontan physiology. In the lateral position, a mismatch between ventilation and perfusion increases PVR and decreases pulmonary blood flow. The prone position results in decreased venous return from direct compression of the abdomen and venous pooling in the lower extremities resulting in a decreased preload reduced pulmonary blood flow, and cardiac output. Bolsters and compression stockings make help attenuate these changes. Trendelenburg positioning has the potential to compromise mechanical ventilation from the abdominal contents compressing the diaphragm, which will increase PVR. In addition, reverse Trendelenburg positioning may dramatically reduce preload, pulmonary blood flow, and cardiac output.[41,42] Adequate hydration may help to reduce the severity of these changes.

Pregnancy

As the number of patients with Fontan physiology of childbearing age increases, the likelihood of having to care for a pregnant Fontan patient increases. In addition to the physiologic changes during pregnancy that must be considered, the Fontan physiology must be integrated into the clinical scenario; notably the effect of the growing uterus on venous return and pulmonary blood flow and the increase in cardiac output, blood volume, and the decrease in systemic vascular resistance that occurs during pregnancy. The ability to compensate for the increased volume load on the ventricle may be severely compromised secondary to decreased function of the systemic ventricle, especially if the systemic ventricle is the right ventricle, and when valve regurgitation is present; these changes are most pronounced after delivery when cardiac output increases substantially.[43] Left uterine displacement is absolutely essential when caring for the pregnant Fontan patient to ensure venous return. Regional anesthesia with epidural may be considered so long as one is mindful of the considerations of regional anesthesia in the Fontan patient discussed earlier.[44,45]

Emergency Surgery

Patients with Fontan physiology are not exempt from needing emergency surgical procedures. Emergency surgical procedures often add additional risk to the Fontan patient because there is often little time to optimize the patient's status. Obtaining cardiology and surgical records may be difficult and further delay may jeopardize the patient so the preoperative evaluation may need to be truncated into the most pertinent information: the nature and duration of the present illness, baseline ventricular function, and current medications.[46] The patient will most likely need a period of expeditious intravenous hydration and resuscitation before induction. Maintenance of adequate preload, judicious use of inotropes, and correcting acidosis are important to ensure an optimal outcome.

POSTOPERATIVE CONCERNS

The recovery location should be chosen with the patient's physiology and the nature of the surgical procedure in mind. Ideally, the proposed recovery venue should be discussed with the patient's cardiologist and surgeon before the procedure so that appropriate recovery arrangements may be made (ie, reserve a bed in the intensive care unit) ahead of time. Patients with well-compensated Fontan physiology may be

---

Box 1
Key points

Fontan physiology

- Cardiac output is essentially completely dependent on pulmonary blood flow.

Preoperative preparation

- Review information from patient's cardiologist; changes in patient's exercise tolerance, level of cardiac impairment, details of the patient's physiology, anatomy, and any residua and sequelae of previous surgeries.

- Minimize NPO interval, maintain intravascular volume: decreased preload results in decreased pulmonary blood flow and cardiac output.

Intraoperative management

- Vascular access often presents a challenge.

- General principles: maintain adequate preload; preserve low PVR, pulmonary blood flow, sinus rhythm, ventricular contractility and filling; blunt stress response of surgery; avoid increases in afterload.

- Ventilatory strategy: limit peak inspiratory pressure (<20 cmH$_2$O), use low respiratory rates (<20 bpm), short inspiratory times, avoid excessive positive end-expiratory pressure, moderately elevated tidal volumes (10–15 mL/kg), ensure adequate intravascular volume.

- Vascular capacitance is increased in the Fontan patient; more fluid may be required than anticipated based on the formula commonly used to calculate fluid requirements.

- Increased bleeding potential: coagulation factor deficiencies, antithrombotic therapy, venous collaterals, and venous hypertension.

Postoperative concerns

- Maintaining volume status, acid-base balance, and cardiac output are essential in the postoperative period: ensure adequate hydration and aggressively manage low cardiac output with intravenous hydration and ionotropes.

- Adequate analgesia improves pulmonary mechanics and oxygenation; enhanced vigilance is required to avoid the effects of hypercapnia secondary to opioids.

- Treat postoperative nausea and vomiting to permit adequate hydration, prevent dehydration and electrolyte loss, and allow the patient to resume their medication regimen.

considered for outpatient surgery if the procedure and postoperative course permit, and appropriate support systems are in place at home. However, hospital admission would be prudent if any aspect of the patient's condition would render them vulnerable to the routine consequences of anesthesia and surgery (nausea, vomiting, pain, inability to take fluids or medications orally, and so forth).[47]

The same concerns regarding the maintenance of volume status, acid-base balance, and cardiac output are just as applicable in the postoperative period. Low cardiac output should be aggressively managed with intravenous hydration and if necessary ionotropic support to avoid hypotension. If left untreated, hypotension will result in decreased organ perfusion and metabolic acidosis, increased PVR, decreased pulmonary blood flow, hypoxemia, and decreased cardiac output. End-organ dysfunction, especially in the older Fontan patient, can be a major problem postoperatively and is best avoided by optimizing ventricular performance and Fontan pressure.

Adequate analgesia is important in the Fontan patient because pulmonary mechanics and oxygenation are usually improved. However, enhanced vigilance is required to avoid the effects of hypercapnia secondary to opioids. Hypoventilation resulting in hypercarbia and atelectasis should be avoided in patients with Fontan physiology because elevations in arterial carbon dioxide tensions increase PVR and limit pulmonary blood flow thereby worsening hypoxemia and cardiac output. Neuraxial analgesia may be of benefit; however the benefits of neuraxial analgesia need to be balanced with the potential risk of hypotension.[48] Consideration needs to be given to the increased risk of thrombotic events; patients may receive unfractionated heparin or low molecular weight heparin as prophylaxis. In addition, postoperative nausea and vomiting should be aggressively treated to permit adequate hydration, prevent dehydration and electrolyte loss, and allow the patient to resume their medication regimen.

SUMMARY

Improved surgical and medical management has led to an increase in survival after staged univentricular palliative procedures. Subsequently, this improved survival has led to an increase in the number of patients who will present for noncardiac surgical interventions with Fontan physiology. A comprehensive understanding of normal Fontan physiology and the perturbations that the proposed surgical procedure will likely have is necessary to care for and design a comprehensive anesthetic plan that takes into account the effects of anesthetic agents, ventilation strategies, cardiovascular drugs, and various other perioperative factors. In addition, when constructing a perioperative plan, a carefully orchestrated, comprehensive, multidisciplinary (anesthesiologist, cardiologist, surgeon) care-team approach must be employed to help ensure optimal outcomes. Although no formula exists that will guarantee a particular outcome, applying the knowledge presented in this article should enable the anesthesiologist with the necessary principles to care for the Fontan patient (**Box 1**).

REFERENCES

1. Fontan F, Baudet E. Surgical repair of tricuspid atresia. Thorax 1971;26(3):240–8.
2. Kreutzer G, Galindez E, Bono H, et al. An operation for the correction of tricuspid atresia. J Thorac Cardiovasc Surg 1973;66(4):613–21.
3. Nicolson SC, Steven JM. Anesthesia for the patient with a single ventricle. In: Andropoulos DB, Stayer SA, Russell IA, editors. Anesthesia for congenital heart disease. Oxford: Blackwell Futura; 2005. p. 356–72.

4. Gewillig M. The Fontan circulation. Heart 2005;91:839–46.
5. Nicolson SC, Steven JM. Anesthetic management for HLHS. In: Rychik J, Wernovsky G, editors. Hypoplastic left heart syndrome. The Netherlands: Kluwer Academic Publishers; 2003. p. 167–91.
6. Tait AR, Malviya S, Voepel-Lewis T, et al. Risk factors for perioperative adverse events in children with upper respiratory tract infections. Anesthesiology 2001; 95:299–306.
7. Pfammatter JP, Casaulta C, Pavlovic M, et al. Important excess morbidity due to upper airway anomalies in the perioperative course in infant cardiac surgery. Ann Thorac Surg 2006;81(3):1008–12.
8. Khariwala SS, Lee WT, Koltai PJ. Laryngotracheal consequences of pediatric cardiac surgery. Arch Otolaryngol Head Neck Surg 2005;131(4):336–9.
9. Baum VC, O'Flaherty JE. Anesthesia for genetic, metabolic & dysmorphic syndromes of childhood. 2nd edition. Philadelphia: Lippincott Williams & Wilkins; 2007.
10. Bissonnette B, Luginbuehl I, Marciniak B, et al, editors Syndromes: rapid recognition and perioperative implications. New York: McGraw-Hill; 2006. p. 1–852.
11. Galli KK, Myers LB, Nicolson SC. Anesthesia for adult patients with congenital heart disease undergoing noncardiac surgery. Int Anesthesiol Clin 2001;39(4):43–71.
12. Walker SG, Eckehard SA. Single-ventricle physiology: perioperative physiology. Semin Pediatr Surg 2004;13(3):188–202.
13. Hosking MP, Beynen FM. The modified Fontan procedure: physiology and anesthetic implications. J Cardiothorac Vasc Anesth 1992;6(4):465–75.
14. Sumpelmann R, Osthaus WA. The pediatric cardiac patient presenting for noncardiac surgery. Curr Opin Anaesthesiol 2007;20:216–20.
15. Ioscovich A, Briskin A, Fadeev A, et al. Emergency cesarean section in a patient with Fontan circulation and indwelling epidural catheter. J Clin Anesth 2006;18(8): 631–4.
16. Baum VC. The adult patient with congenital heart disease. J Cardiothorac Vasc Anesth 1996;10(2):261–82.
17. Ravn HB, Hjortdal VE, Stenbog EV, et al. Increased platelet reactivity and significant changes in coagulation markers after cavopulmonary connection. Heart 2001;85:61–5.
18. American Heart Association. Endocarditis prophylaxis information. Available at: www.americanheart.org/presenter.jhtml. Accessed December 26th, 2008.
19. Fredriksen PM, Therrien J, Veldtman G, et al. Lung function and aerobic capacity in adults following modified Fontan procedure. Heart 2001;85:295–9.
20. McGowan FX. Perioperative issues in patients with congenital heart disease. Presented at: Society for Pediatric Anesthesia Annual Meeting; March 5, 2004; Phoenix, AZ.
21. Cohen MI, Bridges ND, Gaynor JW, et al. Modifications to the cavopulmonary anastomosis do not eliminate early sinus node dysfunction. J Thorac Cardiovasc Surg 2000;120(5):891–900.
22. Blaufox AD, Sleeper LA, Bradley DJ, et al. Functional status, heart rate, and rhythm abnormalities in 521 Fontan patients 6 to 18 years of age. J Thorac Cardiovasc Surg 2008;136(1):100–7.
23. Zaidan JR, Atlee JL, Belott P, et al. Practice advisory for the perioperative management of patients with cardiac rhythm management devices: pacemakers and implantable cardioverter-defibrillators: a report by the American society of anesthesiologists task force on perioperative management of patients with cardiac rhythm management devices. Anesthesiology 2005;103(1):186–98.

24. Chan SY, Lu W, Wong W, et al. Chylothorax in children after congenital heart surgery. Ann Thorac Surg 2006;82(5):1650–6.
25. Gupta A, Daggett C, Behera S, et al. Risk factors for persistent pleural effusions after extracardiac Fontan procedure. J Thorac Cardiovasc Surg 2004;127(6):1664–9.
26. Cheung EWY, Ho SA, Tang KKY, et al. Pericardial effusion after open heart surgery for congenital heart disease. Heart 2003;89(7):780–3.
27. Therrien J, Webb GD. Gatzoulis. Reversal of protein losing enteropathy with prednisone in adults with modified Fontan operations: long term palliation or bridge to cardiac transplantation? Heart 1999;82(2):241–3.
28. Vyas H, Driscoll DJ, Cetta F. Gastrointestinal bleeding and protein-losing enteropathy after the Fontan operation. Am J Cardiol 2006;98(5):666–7.
29. Odegard KC, McGowan FX Jr, Dinardo JA, et al. Coagulation abnormalities in patients with single-ventricle physiology precede the Fontan procedure. J Thorac Cardiovasc Surg 2002;123(3):459–65.
30. Odegard KC, McGowan FX Jr, Zurakowski D, et al. Coagulation factor abnormalities in patients with single-ventricle physiology immediately prior to the Fontan procedure. Ann Thorac Surg 2002;73(6):1770–7.
31. Odegard KC, McGowan FX Jr, Zurakowski D, et al. Procoagulant and anticoagulant factor abnormalities following the Fontan procedure: increased factor VIII may predispose to thrombosis. J Thorac Cardiovasc Surg 2003;125(6):1260–7.
32. Costello JM, Steinhorn D, McColley S, et al. Treatment of plastic bronchitis in a Fontan patient with tissue plasminogen activator: a case report and review of the literature. Pediatrics 2002;109(4):1–3.
33. Huddleston CB. The failing Fontan: options for surgical therapy. Pediatr Cardiol 2007;28:472–6.
34. McClain CD, McGowan FX, Kovatsis PG. Laparoscopic surgery in a patient with Fontan physiology. Anesth Analg 2006;103(4):856–8.
35. Mariano ER, Boltz MG, Albanese CT, et al. Anesthetic management of infants with palliated hypoplastic left heart syndrome undergoing laparoscopic Nissen fundoplication. Anesth Analg 2005;100(6):1631–3.
36. Taylor KL, Holtby H, Macpherson B. Laparoscopic surgery in the pediatric patient post Fontan procedure. Paediatr Anaesth 2006;16(5):591–5.
37. Diaz LK, Akpek EA, Dinavahi R, et al. Tracheoesophageal fistula and associated congenital heart disease: implications for anesthetic management and survival. Paediatr Anaesth 2005;15(10):862–9.
38. Mariano ER, Chu LF, Albanese CT, et al. Successful thoracoscopic repair of esophageal atresia with tracheoesophageal fistula in a newborn with single ventricle physiology. Anesth Analg 2005;101(4):1000–2.
39. Heggie J, Karski J. The anesthesiologist's role in adults with congenital heart disease. Cardiol Clin 2006;24:571–85.
40. Vischoff D, Fortier LP, Villeneuve E, et al. Anaesthetic management of an adolescent for scoliosis surgery with a Fontan circulation. Paediatr Anaesth 2001;11(5):607–10.
41. Rafique MB, Stuth EA, Tassone JC. Increased blood loss during posterior spinal fusion for idiopathic scoliosis in an adolescent with Fontan physiology. Paediatr Anaesth 2006;16(2):206–12.
42. van Mook WN, Peeters L. Severe cardiac disease in pregnancy, part II: impact of congenital and acquired cardiac disease during pregnancy. Curr Opin Crit Care 2005;11:435–48.
43. Buckland R, Pickett JA. Pregnancy and the univentricular heart: case report and literature review. Int J Obstet Anesth 2000;9(1):55–63.
44. Siu S, Coleman J. Heart disease and pregnancy. Heart 2001;85(6):710–5.

45. Khairy P, Ouyang DW, Fernandes SM, et al. Pregnancy outcomes in women with congenital heart disease. Circulation 2006;113(4):266–70.
46. Frankville D. Anesthesia for noncardiac surgery in children and adults with congenital heart disease. In: Lake CL, Booker PD, editors. Pediatric cardiac anesthesia. 4th edition. Philadelphia: Lippincott Williams & Wilkins; 2005. p. 601–32.
47. Diaz LK, Hall S. Anesthesia for non-cardiac surgery and magnetic resonance imaging. In: Andropoulos DB, Stayer SA, Russell IA, editors. Anesthesia for congenital heart disease. Oxford: Blackwell Futura; 2005. p. 427–52.
48. Ahmad S, Lichtenthal P. Anesthetic management of a patient with a single ventricle and modified Fontan procedure. J Cardiothorac Vasc Anesth 1993; 7(6):727–9.

Sedating the Child with Congenital Heart Disease

Laura K. Diaz, MD[a],*, Lisa Jones, CRNA[a,b]

KEYWORDS

• Sedation • Infant • Child • Congenital heart disease

In the past 2 decades the number of infants, children, and adults surviving with congenital heart disease (CHD) has continued to grow substantially.[1] This increase in the number of CHD survivors has resulted in a sharp escalation in the number of procedures requiring analgesia, sedation, or anxiolysis that these patients undergo outside the cardiac operating room. Frequently used nonoperating room venues for this group of patients include the cardiac catheterization laboratory, interventional radiology, magnetic resonance imaging (MRI), procedure rooms, or the emergency department. Frequently encountered challenges include the urgent or emergent scheduling of procedures, the physical challenges of working in remote locations, and transporting critically ill children from one venue to another.

Current cardiac catheterization procedures performed with sedation may be either diagnostic, interventional, or both. Defibrillator checks in patients with internal cardioverter-defibrillators frequently necessitate the use of sedation as well. In addition to the cardiac catheterization laboratory, other diagnostic imaging modalities such as cardiac magnetic resonance imaging (CMRI), transthoracic or transesophageal echocardiography, computed tomography (CT) with angiography, and ventilation-perfusion scans are often requested for complete evaluation of these patients. In particular, the length of CMRI scans (generally an hour or more) mandates the use of sedation for pediatric patients to provide satisfactory scanning conditions. Procedures such as placement of peripherally inserted central catheters (PICC) lines, renal dialysis catheters, or drainage of loculated pleural or pericardial effusions are frequently performed in interventional radiology with the aid of ultrasound and fluoroscopy. Procedure rooms are used for cardioversions, removal of sutures or staples, dressing changes, placement of chest tubes or pleural catheters, and performance

[a] Division of Cardiothoracic Anesthesiology, Department of Anesthesiology and Critical Care Medicine, The Children's Hospital of Philadelphia, University of Pennsylvania School of Medicine, 34th Street, Civic Center Boulevard, Philadelphia, PA 19104, USA
[b] University of Pennsylvania School of Nursing Science, Claire M. Fagan Hall, 418 Curie Boulevard, Philadelphia, PA 19104, USA
* Corresponding author.
E-mail address: diazl@email.chop.edu (L.K. Diaz).

Anesthesiology Clin 27 (2009) 301–319
doi:10.1016/j.anclin.2009.05.003
1932-2275/09/$ – see front matter © 2009 Elsevier Inc. All rights reserved.
anesthesiology.theclinics.com

of sedated echocardiograms. Cardiac patients who have additional coexisting diseases may require sedation or analgesia for other ancillary procedures such as lumbar punctures, bone marrow aspiration, radiation therapy, or gastrointestinal endoscopy.

The American Academy of Pediatrics (AAP) published the first guidelines for pediatric sedation in 1985 in response to several sedation-related deaths in a dental office.[2] In an effort to disseminate information among practitioners, standardize care, and further the safe practice of pediatric sedation, guidelines for the monitoring and management of pediatric sedation have been published by several entities in the past 5 years, including the AAP, the American Society of Anesthesiologists (ASA), the American College of Emergency Physicians (ACEP), the American Academy of Pediatric Dentists (AAPD) and the US Joint Commission on Accreditation of Healthcare Organization (JCAHO).[3–6] Efforts have been made to standardize language and sedation categories to facilitate use of these guidelines, as the initial definition of "conscious sedation" proved confusing to many practitioners. Current ASA definitions incorporate the terminology of "minimal," "moderate" or "deep" sedation, followed by general anesthesia (**Table 1**). Minimal sedation implies that the child remains normally responsive to verbal stimulation alone and that respiratory and cardiovascular functions remain at baseline; with moderate sedation the patient maintains purposeful responses to either verbal or light tactile stimulation while continuing to maintain adequate respiratory and normal cardiovascular status. Either repeated or painful stimulation is required to achieve a response from patients under deep sedation, and interventions may be necessary to appropriately maintain either or both their airway and ventilation. Cardiovascular function generally, but not always, remains at baseline in this subset of patients. General anesthesia implies a lack of response to painful stimulation, with frequent airway and ventilatory manipulations required and potential for impairment of cardiovascular status. Current ASA guidelines recommend that only personnel with training in the delivery of general anesthesia should administer deep sedation,[7] as sedation is a continuum and it is likely or even expected that children may move either between levels or to a deeper sedation level than originally intended. Children 6 years of age and younger nearly always require deep sedation to

Table 1 Levels of sedation	
Minimal sedation	Drug-induced state during which patients respond normally to verbal commands; ventilatory and cardiovascular functions are unaffected
Moderate sedation	Drug-induced depression of consciousness during which patients respond purposefully to verbal commands: older patients are interactive whereas younger patients exhibit age-appropriate behaviors. No intervention is needed to maintain a patent airway and cardiovascular function is usually maintained
Deep sedation	Drug-induced depression of consciousness during which patients are not easily aroused but respond purposefully after repeated painful or verbal stimulation. May require assistance maintaining patent airway; spontaneous ventilation may be inadequate. Partial or complete loss of protective airway reflexes may occur. Cardiovascular function is usually maintained
General anesthesia	Medically controlled state of unconsciousness with loss of protective reflexes, including the inability to maintain a patent airway independently and respond purposefully to physical stimulation or verbal command

successfully accomplish invasive procedures and it should be assumed that this level of sedation will occur in this age group.[8]

Many hospitals have developed pediatric sedation services using pediatric intensivists, hospitalists, and anesthesiologists to implement these guidelines, standardize care, and provide care to children in a variety of locations. To better delineate the frequency and nature of adverse occurrences in these patients, Cravero and colleagues recently reviewed adverse events reported from a database including 37 institutions with pediatric sedation services and a total of 49,836 pediatric propofol sedation encounters. Although serious adverse events were rare, it is sobering that nearly 1 in 65 children receiving propofol sedation experienced airway complications of stridor, laryngospasm, airway obstruction, wheezing, or apnea, while 1 in 70 required airway interventions such as placement of oral or nasal airways, bag-mask ventilation or endotracheal intubation. Children with higher ASA physical status, young patients, and those who received opiates had a higher rate of adverse events and pulmonary complications.[9]

GOALS OF SEDATION AND ANALGESIA

The desired goals of each pediatric sedation encounter should be identified and carefully considered by the practitioner before initiation of any drug therapy. Nonpharmacologic-based methods may be used to initially allay anxiety in the child and parents before the procedure, including the involvement of child-life practitioners followed by a discussion of the planned procedure, duration, and plan for provision of sedation and analgesia. Careful attention to patient and parental preferences is important, and prior adverse experiences with certain drugs or methods of drug administration should be discussed and clarified, along with any drug allergies. Most patients with CHD have had multiple hospital experiences and, as a result, not infrequently have definitive preferences in these areas.

Successful completion of most imaging studies requires anxiolysis and sedation rather than analgesia, whereas more invasive procedures will require sedation and analgesia. Likewise, minimal motion may be tolerable for certain procedures but not acceptable for imaging procedures such as CMRI. Recognition of the primary goals will allow selection of the optimal drug or drugs required to achieve satisfactory completion of the procedure with minimal patient risk, as the association between adverse patient outcome and drug overdosage or administration of multiple sedating medications has been recognized in several studies.[10,11]

PRESEDATION ASSESSMENT

Evaluation of the patient with CHD can be challenging given the wide spectrum of diagnostic categories within CHD and the variability within these subgroups. Children with unrepaired or palliated heart disease, particularly infants and cyanotic patients, are often more fragile and require comprehensive assessment before even simple procedures. An understanding of the child's underlying lesion, along with a history of previous surgical or catheter-based interventions, and knowledge regarding his or her current functional status is essential. Based on this information the need for cardiology consultation, including repeat echocardiographic evaluation or laboratory studies, can be determined.

In addition to a comprehensive cardiac medical history, details of the child's general health should be elicited along with details of any changes from his or her baseline condition, feeding and growth, activity level, and information regarding other medical issues such as gastroesophageal reflux disease (GERD), reactive airway disease, upper airway obstruction or ongoing neurologic issues. Recent illnesses, particularly upper respiratory tract infections (URIs) should be noted, as changes in airway reactivity and pulmonary vascular resistance (PVR) can be poorly tolerated in children with single ventricle physiology, decreased pulmonary compliance, or pulmonary hypertension. Careful note should be taken of current medications and the time of last administration as well as any drug allergies or adverse reactions. With the possible exception of anticoagulant medications, our practice is to continue medications throughout the periprocedural period with as little interruption as possible. For patients undergoing invasive procedures the recent American Heart Association (AHA) guidelines for bacterial endocarditis prophylaxis or the cardiologist's recommendations should also be reviewed before the procedure and appropriate prophylaxis administered.[12]

Physical examination should encompass a detailed evaluation of the child's airway, chest, and heart, with any changes from baseline status noted. Airway abnormalities such as micrognathia, macroglossia, abnormal dentition, facial dysmorphism, and tonsillar hypertrophy should be recorded. Increased tachypnea, work of breathing, or changes in oxygen saturation may require further investigation and a new chest radiograph before administration of sedative drugs. Current and potential sites of vascular access should also be evaluated, as it is frequently difficult to obtain access in this patient population. Current weight and vital signs including oxygen saturation should be recorded. Although preoperative laboratory work may not always be necessary, a recent hematocrit may yield useful information regarding the degree of secondary erythrocytosis due to chronic hypoxemia in certain patients. Following complete assessment of the patient an ASA physical status (PS) classification can be assigned. Patients with a PS classification of three or greater are at increased risk for sedation-related adverse events, and many, if not most, patients with CHD will receive such a classification. The proposed plans, along with risks, benefits, and alternatives, should then be discussed with the family and informed consent obtained.

Currently accepted nil per os (NPO) guidelines recommend a 6- to 8-hour (or longer) fast from solid foods but clear liquids may be ingested until 2 hours before receiving sedation for the procedure.[13,14] Avoidance of prolonged periods of fasting is important particularly for cyanotic and shunt-dependent patients. Procedural delays for certain imaging studies can occasionally result in extended periods of fasting; these patients are best served by offering them clear liquids if time permits, or by starting an intravenous infusion if needed. Despite adherence to these guidelines, Cravero and colleagues[9] noted four episodes of suspected aspiration accompanied by changes in respiratory status and new oxygen requirement during their evaluation of more than 49,000 propofol sedation encounters. Thus, although the necessity of fasting before sedation has been questioned by some practitioners,[15,16] the authors mandate adherence to these guidelines in practice.

THE SEDATION ENVIRONMENT
Equipment and Resuscitation Drugs

Provision of sedation or anesthesia outside the operating room for children with CHD requires a high level of skill, teamwork, organization, and the flexibility and experience to enable rapid changes in plans if necessary. Sedation of patients with CHD should only take place in a location where appropriate personnel, equipment, monitoring, and backup support mechanisms exist; preparation, equipment, and personnel should be no different than in an operating-room environment. Not only should the practitioner managing the child's sedation/analgesia possess full information regarding the patient's underlying cardiac disease, he or she must also be qualified to manage all potential ensuing complications, which requires the assistance of additional personnel such as anesthesia residents, fellows, technicians, or assistants. Available equipment should include appropriately sized pediatric monitors, resuscitative equipment including a defibrillator, and necessary medications for cardiopulmonary resuscitation (**Box 1, Table 2**). It is essential that all equipment be checked and documented to be functioning correctly, as Robbertze and colleagues[11] noted in a closed claims review of anesthesia procedures performed outside the operating room that equipment-related events accounted for a significant number of claims (21%), second only to respiratory events (38%).

Monitoring

Standard noninvasive monitoring should be used in all patients: ECG, noninvasive blood pressure, respiratory rate, pulse oximetry, and, whenever possible, capnography. Temperature monitoring is advocated as mechanisms for keeping small infants and children warm may be substandard in remote locations. Continuous visualization,

---

Box 1
Equipment/monitoring guidelines for nonoperating room anesthesia (NORA) locations

- Standard monitoring

  Electrocardiogram

  Noninvasive blood pressure

  Pulse oximetry

  Capnography

  Temperature

  Capability for invasive pressure monitoring if needed

- Anesthesia machine, fully checked AND/OR

  Source of compressed oxygen

  Self-inflating breathing-bag valve set AND/OR Mapleson circuit

- Appropriately sized neonatal and pediatric equipment

- Anesthesia cart, stocked to operating room (OR) standard

  Airway management equipment

  >   Laryngoscope blades and handles

  >   Laryngeal mask airways (LMAs)

  >   Endotracheal tubes, stylets

  >   Oral and nasal airways

  >   Nasal cannulae

  >   Face masks

  Intravenous access equipment

  Invasive monitoring equipment

  Intravenous fluids and tubing sets

- Suction device, Yankauer, and appropriate soft-tip catheters

- Defibrillator (pediatric pads/paddles) and emergency crash cart.

Table 2
Cardiac tray medications

Medication	Concentration	Dosage (Intravenous Unless Noted)
Adenosine	3 mg/mL	Bolus: 50 µg/kg; may double if necessary. Max dose: 0.25 mg/kg
Albuterol inhalation aerosol		
Amiodarone	50 mg/mL	5 mg/kg IV push for refractory VT/VF; over 20–60 minutes for perfusing tachycardia, up to 15 mg/kg
Atropine	0.4 mg/mL	0.02 mg/kg. Max dose: 1 mg
Bupivacaine 0.25%	2.5 mg/mL	1 cm³/kg
Bupivacaine 0.5%	5 mg/mL	0.5 cm³/kg
Calcium gluconate 10%	100 mg/mL	30 mg/kg
Cefazolin	1 g (for dilution)	25 mg/kg
Dexamethasone	4 mg/mL	0.1 – 0.5 mg/kg. Max dose 8 mg.
Digoxin	100 µg/mL	—
Diphenhydramine	50 mg/mL	0.25–1 mg/kg
Dobutamine	12.5 mg/mL	3–15 µg/kg/min
Dopamine	40 mg/mL	3–15 µg/kg/min
Ephedrine	50 mg/mL	0.1 mg/kg
Epinephrine 1:1000	1 mg/mL	Bolus: 1–10 µg/kg. Infusion: 0.02–0.5 µg/kg/min
Epinephrine 1:10,000	0.1 mg/mL	—
Esmolol	20 mg/mL	Bolus: 100–500 µg/kg over 1 min. Infusion: 50–300 µg/kg/min
Flumazenil	0.5 mg/mL	0.01 mg/kg, may repeat every minute. Max dose: 1 mg
Furosemide	10 mg/mL	0.5–1 mg/kg
Glycopyrrolate	0.2 mg/mL	0.01 mg/kg
Heparin	1000 units/mL	—
Hydrocortisone	100 mg/2 mL	1–2 mg/kg for adrenal insufficiency; 100 mg/m² for stress dosing
Isoproterenol	0.2 mg/mL	0.03–2 µg/kg/min
Labetalol	5 mg/mL	0.25–1 mg/kg
Lidocaine 2%	20 mg/mL	Bolus: 1–2 mg/kg. Infusion: 30–50 µg/kg/min
Magnesium sulfate	80 mg/mL (0.65 mEq/mL)	25–50 mg/kg over 1 h
Milrinone	1 mg/mL	Loading dose: 25–75 µg/kg/min. Infusion: 0.2–1 µg/kg/min
Methylprednisolone	125 mg/2 mL	30 mg/kg
Naloxone	1 mg/mL	0.01 mg/kg.
Neostigmine	0.5 mg/mL	0.07 mg/kg
Nitroglycerin	5 mg/mL	0.5–5 µg/kg/min
Nitroprusside	50 mg/2 mL	0.3 – 8 mcg/kg/min
Oxymetazoline spray		
Phenylephrine	10 mg/mL	Bolus: 1–10 µg/kg. Infusion: 0.05–0.5 µg/kg/min

(continued on next page)

Table 2 (continued)		
Medication	Concentration	Dosage (Intravenous Unless Noted)
Propofol	10 mg/mL	1–3 mg/kg
Protamine	10 mg/mL	—
Scopolamine	0.4 mg/mL	0.005–0.01 mg/kg
Sodium bicarbonate	50 mL vial	1–2 mEq/mg
Sodium chloride 0.9%	10 mL vials	—
Sterile water	10 mL vials	—
Vancomycin hydrochloride	500 mg (for dilution)	10–20 mg/kg/dose
Vecuronium	100 mg (for dilution)	0.1 mg/kg
Dextrose 50%	25 g vial	0.5–1 mL/kg

although difficult in certain environments such as MRI, is also important for assessment of airway obstruction, respiratory pattern, and secretions.

The use of continuous capnography is advocated in all patients as it can assist in identifying airway obstruction or apnea before changes in pulse oximetry or even patient visualization. Appropriately sized nasal cannulas may be taped in place through the nares or mouth to obtain readings. In a prospective study of ASA PS 1 and two patients undergoing fracture reduction in the emergency department Anderson and colleagues found that 11% of children undergoing sedation with propofol experienced airway issues requiring an intervention (jaw thrust, supplemental oxygen, or brief bag-mask ventilation). Eleven of the 14 airway issues were identified by capnography before recognition by either pulse oximetry or clinical examination.[17] Similarly, in a prospective, randomized, double-blind evaluation of 163 ASA PS 1 and two children undergoing gastrointestinal (GI) endoscopy procedures under fentanyl/midazolam sedation, the use of capnography indicated alveolar hypoventilation in 56% of procedures and apnea during 24%.[18] Cote and colleagues compared end-tidal carbon dioxide (CO_2) with blood gas CO_2 values in a population of 59 sedated children undergoing cardiac catheterization. End-tidal monitoring was accomplished using a sampling line designed to sample simultaneously from over the mouth and nares. Although end-tidal CO_2 values are not always reflective of arterial values in patients with significant intracardiac or intrapulmonary shunting, in this population a reasonable correlation between the two values was noted even in patients with intracardiac shunting. During the course of the study capnography also revealed some degree of airway obstruction requiring intervention in 13 of the 59 children (22%).[19]

Bispectral analysis and processing of the adult electroencephalogram (EEG) has been used to derive a neurophysiologic variable known as the bispectral (BIS) index. This index, a number ranging between 0 (isoelectric electroencephalogram) and 100 (awake), has been used as a guide to depth of sedation or anesthesia, and successfully correlated with reduced probabilities of awareness in adults undergoing inhalational anesthesia.[20] An index of 70 to 90 is associated with light to moderate sedation, 60 to 70 with deep sedation and 40 to 60 with general anesthesia.[21] An analysis of the BIS monitor in children 0 to 12 years of age undergoing cardiothoracic surgery showed that although the BIS number is not consistent across all children, it does remain relative during steady state anesthesia and wake-up for an individual patient.[22]

Ketamine does not follow the basic EEG pattern seen in general anesthesia, as an increase in β range activity occurs, resulting in a paradoxic increase in BIS index after ketamine administration.[23] In a sample of 47 children aged 2 to 17 years sedated with nonketamine drugs in the emergency department, a highly significant association between BIS scores and the Observer's Assessment and Alertness/Sedation Scale (OAA/S) was observed; no such association was noted for patients who were sedated with ketamine.[24] In a prospective study of 126 patients ranging in age from 4 months to 15 years undergoing cardiac catheterization under midazolam/ketamine sedation, Baysal and colleagues found that BIS monitoring allowed the use of lower doses of midazolam and ketamine in children between 1 and 6 years. Using the index as a guide to titration of sedation, fewer respiratory complications and a decreased need for oxygen supplementation were observed in the group of patients receiving BIS monitoring.[25] Other limitations to BIS monitoring include interference from certain electrical devices and the presence of preexisting abnormalities in EEG patterns.[26] Although BIS monitoring can potentially serve as a guide to administration and titration of certain sedative drugs, the lack of a validated scale for pediatric patients, particularly those less than 1 year of age, limits its usefulness in children at present. It is also important to note that performance of a certain BIS model does not necessarily apply to other models.[26]

MEDICATIONS

Although many medications may be administered by oral, nasal, inhalational, or rectal routes (**Table 3**), in caring for children with CHD the authors advocate obtaining intravenous access in most patients before administration of any medications. On rare occasions when the lack of vascular access necessitates placement of a PICC line in interventional radiology and the child currently possesses no intravenous access, the interventional radiologist will often assist in placing an intravenous line before beginning the PICC placement. Not only does intravenous administration of medications allow for greater flexibility in titrating to appropriate effect, it also ensures a route for delivery of resuscitative medications should those become necessary.

Analgesic Medications

With the exception of imaging studies, procedures outside of the OR frequently involve some level of discomfort and pain. It falls to the discretion of the anesthesia provider to determine the appropriate type and amount of analgesic medication to administer as well as delineating the appropriate time for administration of such medications; many children may receive sedation before transport to the procedural location, but it is often more prudent in critically ill children to withhold medication until the precise start of the procedure when all monitoring is in place. Along with acting as an adjunct to other purely sedative drugs such as midazolam, small doses of analgesics can also give comfort without necessitating the use of a full-fledged general anesthetic. As with any cardiac case, consideration should always be given to the patient's cardiac function and reserve before administration of any type of medication.

Dissociative: ketamine

Ketamine, an N-methyl-D-aspartate glutamate (NMDA) receptor antagonist and phencyclidine derivative, fills a unique niche in the anesthesiologist's arsenal as it is able to provide sedation and profound analgesia with a minimum of negative side effects. Upper airway tone, airway reflexes, and spontaneous ventilation are generally preserved, and ketamine's hemodynamic effects of increased systemic vascular resistance, cardiac output, and heart rate prove favorable for most patients.[27] Although ketamine can act as a direct myocardial depressant, this effect is clinically manifest only in the catecholamine-depleted patient.[28]

Table 3
Sedative and analgesic medications

Medications	Dosing	Onset	Duration	Comments
Analgesics				
Ketamine	IV: 0.5–1 mg/kg over 1 min IM: 3–7 mg/kg Infusion: 0.1 mg/kg/h	IV: 1–2 min IM: 3–5 min	IV: 10–15 min IM: 15–30 min	Antisialogogue may be necessary with higher doses; hallucinations or dysphoric dreams more likely in older patients
Fentanyl	IV: 0.5–1 µg/kg; max 50 µg/dose	IV: 2–3 min	IV: 30–60 min	Rigid chest may occur with rapid dosing; respiratory depression, facial itching, nausea may occur
Sedative-hypnotics				
Pentobarbital	IV: 1–2 mg/kg every 3–5 min; max dose 6 mg/kg or 200 mg IM: 2–6 mg/kg; max dose 200 mg	IV: 3–5 min IM: 10–20 min	IV: 30–45 min IM: 45–90 min	Contraindication: porphyria
Midazolam	PO: 0.2–0.75 mg/kg; max dose 20 mg IV: 0.05–0.1 mg/kg; max dose 10 mg	PO: 15–30 min IV: 1–2 min	PO: 60–90 min IV: 45–60 min	Paradoxic reactions possible; may be reversed with flumazenil
Propofol	IV bolus: 0.5–1 mg/kg Infusion: 50–200 µg/kg/min	1–2 min	Bolus: 5–10 min	Frequent respiratory depression; no reversal agent available. Antiemetic effect at low infusion rate
Etomidate	IV: 0.1–0.3 mg/kg	1 min	5–15 min	Myoclonus, burning on injection frequently observed
Alpha-2 agonist				
Dexmedetomidine	Bolus: 0.5–1 µg/kg Infusion: 0.2–2 µg/kg/h	IV: 3–5 min	IV: 15–30 min	May see decrease in heart rate and blood pressure; minimal respiratory effects
Reversal agents				
Naloxone	IV: 0.01 mg/kg; max dose 2 mg	1–2 min	20–40 min	Repeat dosing may be necessary; observe in recovery for 2 h after last dose. May cause catecholamine release and systemic/pulmonary hypertension
Flumazenil	IV: 0.01–0.02 mg/kg; max dose 1 mg	1–2 min	30–60 min	Repeat dosing may be necessary; observe in recovery for 2 h after last dose. Lowers seizure threshold

Ketamine produces a unique and characteristic state of cortical dissociation, clinically apparent by a nystagmic gaze and a cataleptic appearance, and accompanied by profound analgesia, sedation, and amnesia.[29] Ketamine is also singular in that it may be administered by a variety of routes (oral, rectal, nasal, intravenous, and intramuscular), although intravenous or intramuscular routes are most commonly chosen for sedation. Given intravenously in low doses (1–2 mg/kg), ketamine results in analgesia and sedation; in higher doses (4–6 mg/kg) it produces general anesthesia.[30] Ketamine induces an analgesic and dissociative state within 15 to 60 seconds after a single intravenous (IV) dose and within 3 to 5 minutes following an intramuscular (IM) dose, with unconsciousness/dissociation lasting approximately 10 to 15 minutes for IV doses and 20 to 30 minutes for IM doses. Analgesia generally persists for approximately 40 minutes with amnesia lasting for 1 to 2 hours.[31] In our practice, for short procedures such as placement of a chest tube or PICC line, particularly in children with marginal cardiac reserve, ketamine is frequently the drug of choice as it allows maintenance of cardiac stability, the flexibility to modulate sedation length as necessary, and provides excellent sedation and analgesia without requiring the use of multiple drugs.

Hallucinations or dysphoric emergence phenomena seem to occur more frequently in older patients, with a reported incidence of 10% to 20% in adult patients.[32] Although the concurrent use of midazolam in small doses with ketamine offers the advantage of decreasing the likelihood of emergence reactions, there can be considerable consequences with polypharmacy and ketamine administration. In a meta-analysis by Green and colleagues evaluating the combination of these two medications, overall airway and respiratory adverse events, particularly apnea, are significantly more frequent when benzodiazepines are coadministered. Risk factors for these adverse effects are high intravenous doses, administration to children younger than 2 years or greater than 13 years, and the coadministration of benzodiazepines. Green also found, unequivocally, that the concurrent use of anticholinergics increased adverse respiratory events overall, even though this seems like a paradoxic finding.[33] Although once routinely advocated, use of an anticholinergic medication for antisialogogue effect is only occasionally necessary with higher dosages of ketamine when oversecretion of saliva can act as an irritant to the airway.[34]

The use of ketamine in patients with pulmonary hypertension (PHTN) has been a controversial issue. A recent study by Williams and colleagues in children with severe PHTN who continued to breathe spontaneously while receiving sevoflurane 0.5 minimum alveolar concentration (MAC) showed that ketamine did not increase PVR. This study differs from most because induction and maintenance of anesthesia were accomplished with sevoflurane. Ketamine was introduced after initial catheterization measurements were obtained, and a ketamine infusion was then started. No change in mean pulmonary artery pressure or PVR index was observed after administration of a 2 mg/kg ketamine bolus followed by a 10 μg/kg/min infusion, leading to the conclusion that ketamine can be safely used in children with PHTN.[35] This is particularly useful information as children with PHTN are a challenging patient population to care for safely.

Opioids: fentanyl

Fentanyl is a short-acting synthetic opioid, and a frequently used analgesic medication in pediatric patients outside the operating room environment. Fentanyl acts primarily as a μ-agonist and is approximately 80 times as potent as morphine.[36] It offers a rapid onset of action (less than 30 seconds) and a short duration of action (20–40 minutes), which makes it an advantageous choice for sedation. Like other opioids, fentanyl provides only analgesia, without anxiolysis or amnesia, and thus it is frequently administered in conjunction with benzodiazepines to provide these elements. When given in concert with benzodiazepines it is recommended that both medications be given in reduced doses to minimize the chance of hemodynamic or respiratory compromise.[37]

Side effects from fentanyl are few but can include nasal pruritis and nausea, whereas the most significant adverse effects of fentanyl are respiratory depression and chest rigidity. Both these effects are reversible with naloxone, an opioid antagonist, although it is important to remember that the half-life of fentanyl is longer than that of naloxone and re-dosage may be necessary. In addition, naloxone administration is not innocuous, as it can result in adverse hemodynamic changes including increases in heart rate, blood pressure, and myocardial oxygen consumption. Chest wall rigidity can be life threatening, and, if not reversed by naloxone, it may be necessary to use neuromuscular blocking drugs to effectively ventilate the patient. Chest rigidity has most often been related to administration of larger fentanyl doses and a more rapid rate of infusion, but has also been reported with smaller doses or the use of infusions in the intensive care unit.[38–40] Fentanyl is generally devoid of adverse hemodynamic effects and thus can be administered even to hemodynamically fragile infants and children. The use of fentanyl infusions is frequently seen in pediatric intensive or cardiac intensive care patients and may be continued throughout the sedative encounter if desired.

Local Anesthetics

For procedures such as pleural catheter insertion, PICC line insertion, or suturing of a laceration the infiltration of local anesthetic (bupivacaine 0.25%: allowable dose 1 cm^3/kg with a maximum of 20 cm^3) around the procedural site can decrease the amount of sedation and analgesia required by most children. Topical analgesics such as EMLA (lidocaine 2.5% and prilocaine 2.5%) may also be useful before insertion of intravenous catheters, lumbar puncture, or bone marrow biopsy. For lacerated skin, a mixture of lidocaine, epinephrine, and tetracaine (LET) can be used and has an onset time of approximately 20 to 30 minutes.[41]

Sedative/Hypnotic Medications

Barbiturates

A variety of barbiturates have been used for pediatric sedation and may be differentiated clinically on the basis of their duration of action. Shorter-acting agents (duration of action 5–10 minutes) include methohexital, thiopental, and thiamylal; pentobarbital has an intermediate duration of action. Barbiturates are useful only for inducing sedation, hypnosis, and amnesia as they lack intrinsic analgesic properties. With the exception of methohexital they also possess anticonvulsant properties produced by way of dose-dependent central nervous system depression. Extravasation of barbiturates into subcutaneous tissue can result in severe irritation and local erythema due to their extremely alkaline pH, thus the patency of an intravenous line should always be ascertained before drug administration. Barbiturates should not be given in conjunction with certain neuromuscular blocking agents (pancuronium, vecuronium, atracurium), opioids (sufentanil or alfentanil) or midazolam, as decreasing the alkalinity of the drug will result in precipitation in the intravenous line and likely occlusion, particularly in small lines.[42]

Pentobarbital is frequently chosen for sedation for shorter imaging procedures such as CT. Titrated in intravenous doses of 1 to 2 mg/kg, its sedative effects become apparent in 3 to 5 minutes and last approximately 30 minutes. Although respiratory depression, apnea, and hypotension have been described with pentobarbital, in our experience these side effects are rare if the drug is judiciously titrated to effect. In a study of 195 patients ranging in age from 4 to 240 months and receiving pentobarbital for noninvasive procedural sedation, a decrease in dosage requirement was noted with increasing age. Children less than 1 year of age required a mean dose of 3.68 ± 1.68 mg/kg for sedation, whereas the mean dosage requirement for the oldest patients was 2.86 ± 1.04 mg/kg. Recovery times were not affected by age.[43] Mason and colleagues[44] compared the use of oral versus intravenous pentobarbital in infants less than 12 months of age undergoing either MR or CT imaging. The time to achieve a desired sedation level was longer with oral administration, but no difference between the two groups was observed with respect to time to discharge. The group of infants receiving IV pentobarbital demonstrated a slightly higher incidence of oxygen desaturation than those receiving the drug orally, and the sedation effectiveness was similar in both groups. The use of oral pentobarbital can therefore be considered in patients who lack intravenous access and will not require administration of contrast medium; however, the presence of intravenous access is preferred if at all possible in children with CHD even if the oral route of administration is chosen for sedation.

Potential side effects of barbiturates include dose-related central respiratory depression with decreased minute ventilation, and hypotension due to peripheral vasodilation and decreased sympathetic outflow.[45] Cardiovascular effects are more pronounced in hypovolemic patients. Decreased venous return is seen secondary to venous dilation and pooling.[46] Unlike benzodiazepines and opioids there is no specific antidote or reversal agent for barbiturates. Dysphoric or paradoxic reactions are occasionally seen in some children.

Benzodiazepines: midazolam

Benzodiazepines are a mainstay of sedation in pediatric patients as they provide sedation, amnesia, and anxiolysis, and have hypnotic, muscular relaxation, and anticonvulsant properties. Midazolam is short-acting and water-soluble, and is the most commonly used benzodiazepine for premedication and procedural sedation in children. It may be administered by multiple routes: nasal, oral, intravenous, or intramuscular. Although nasal administration can provide rapid and effective onset of sedation,[47,48] it is generally avoided due to the resultant burning and irritation of the nasal mucosa.[49] Time to onset of action after intravenous administration of midazolam is 2 to 3 minutes, with a duration of action of 45 to 60 minutes followed by a short elimination half-life and metabolism by the liver. If necessary, midazolam may be administered orally in doses of 0.25 to 0.75 mg/kg (maximum dose 20 mg) to allay anxiety in children before placement of intravenous access. Although midazolam is extremely effective as an anxiolytic and amnestic drug, it rarely suffices alone even for short and painless imaging procedures; it is therefore most often used in combination with other sedative or analgesic drugs.[50] Caution should be used when combining midazolam with opioids, as adverse cardiovascular and respiratory effects are more likely to be seen in this circumstance.

Although effective as an anxiolytic in most patients, midazolam can elicit paradoxic reactions in certain patients, particularly when rapidly administered by the intravenous route.[51] Respiratory depression, although rare, can also be seen, especially when opioids have been concurrently administered. Flumazenil, a benzodiazepine antagonist, can quickly reverse sedative and dysphoric effects of midazolam. As the half-life of flumazenil is less than that of midazolam, however, the potential for resedation exists and repeat dosing may be necessary. Negative effects of flumazenil include lowering of the seizure threshold and sympathetic stimulation.[52]

Propofol

Propofol (2,6-diisopropylphenol), a potent hypnotic drug with sedative and amnestic properties, was initially described in 1977 as an agent for induction of general anesthesia.[53] Now the most frequently used drug for induction of general anesthesia in the United States, propofol has also gained immense popularity for provision of sedation in environments outside the operating room due to its rapid onset, short duration of action, short recovery time, and antiemetic properties.[54] In addition, it can be administered either by bolus doses of 1 to 2 mg/kg (yielding 3–5 minutes of sedation) or by titratable infusion for longer procedures, such as MR studies, with either method allowing rapid postprocedural recovery.

Like other sedative/hypnotic agents, propofol can cause significant cardiovascular and respiratory depression. Propofol can have significant hemodynamic effects, which must be considered carefully in more fragile patients. Williams and colleagues[55] compared the hemodynamic effects of propofol in 30 children with CHD, with propofol initially administered as a 2 mg/kg bolus and then continued as an infusion. Systemic mean arterial pressure and systemic vascular resistance decreased significantly, whereas systemic blood flow increased. In patients with cardiac shunts this yielded an increase in right-to-left shunt flow, resulting in clinically important decreases in $PaCO_2$ and SpO_2 in cyanotic patients. Two patients with unrepaired tetralogy of Fallot (TOF) and left-to-right shunting exhibited reversal of shunt flow after administration of propofol. Propofol should be used with caution in patients whose pulmonary blood flow (PBF) depends on balancing their systemic and PVRs and in patients who cannot tolerate systemic afterload reduction. Severe respiratory depression or apnea can be observed after bolus doses of propofol, whereas maintenance infusions reduce minute ventilation by decreases in tidal volume and respiratory rate. Other adverse effects associated with administration of propofol include pain on injection, which can be profound with small intravenous lines, and myoclonus.

Although many series have advocated the use of propofol (alone or in combination with other drugs) by nonanesthesiologists in nonoperating room locations,[56–58] this practice remains extremely controversial, as many, if not most, patients who receive propofol for sedation cross the line differentiating deep sedation and general anesthesia.[59] A recent study by Zgleszewski and colleagues[60] comparing the use of propofol to intravenously administered pentobarbital in infants undergoing diagnostic CT found a significantly higher incidence of adverse respiratory events and need for airway manipulations in the group receiving propofol, even though anesthesia providers administered the propofol. The authors therefore strongly endorse the 2006 ASA statement advising that only practitioners qualified to administer general anesthesia, or appropriately supervised anesthesia professionals, should be granted privileges to administer deep sedation,[7] and further believe that this is particularly true regarding the care of children with CHD and the use of propofol.

Etomidate

Etomidate, an imidazole-derived sedative-hypnotic agent, is an ultrashort-acting drug that may be used for sedation or induction of general anesthesia. It has a rapid onset of action (5–15 seconds) and minimal cardiovascular effects, making it an extremely useful agent in critically ill patients undergoing short procedures. Due to its side effects of pain on injection, myoclonus, incidence of postoperative nausea and vomiting, and possible adrenocorticoid suppression, its use had remained selective but has recently increased, particularly in the emergency department setting. Although prolonged use or multiple doses of etomidate may cause adrenal suppression, single doses of 0.3 mg/kg in children have not been shown to decrease cortisol levels below the lower limits of normal.[61,62] In a study examining the effects of etomidate on failing and non-failing human cardiac tissue it was further shown that etomidate does not cause myocardial depression at clinically relevant concentrations,[63] making etomidate an excellent alternative to propofol for intravenous sedation or induction of anesthesia in children with marginal cardiac reserve.

The use of etomidate for sedation has been well described in the emergency department and for imaging studies. Baxter and colleagues compared the use of intravenous pentobarbital (with or without midazolam) and etomidate for CT sedation in healthy pediatric patients between 6 months and 6 years old, and found that the quality of sedation was superior with etomidate. Moreover, the time to recovery with etomidate sedation was significantly lower, as were the number of adverse events.[64] Apnea may occasionally occur with bolus doses of etomidate; this is more likely if etomidate is given in conjunction with opioids and as always the ability to assist or control the patient's ventilation should be assured before drug administration.

Alpha-2 Adrenergic Agonist: Dexmedetomidine

Dexmedetomidine (Precedex) is a highly selective α_2-adrenoreceptor agonist with sedative, anxiolytic, and mild analgesic properties. Although it does not have US Food and Drug Administration (FDA) approval for use in children, the use of dexmedetomidine in infants and children in multiple settings including the intensive care unit (ICU), the operating suite, cardiac catheterization laboratory, and radiology has been well described. It has been used in a variety of ways including sedative agent, anesthetic adjuvant, premedicant, and for prevention of withdrawal syndromes due to opioid or benzodiazepine usage.[65] Initially approved in 1999 by the FDA only for use in intubated, mechanically ventilated adult patients for up to 24 hours of use, approval was granted in 2008 for use in nonintubated patients requiring sedation before or during surgical and other procedures.

Dexmedetomidine is most commonly administered as a loading dose (0.5–1 µg/kg) for 10 minutes followed by an infusion (0.2–2 µg/kg/h). Major advantages of dexmedetomidine include its rapid redistribution and elimination half-lives, minimal risk of respiratory depression, and relative lack of cardiovascular effects. Decreases in heart rate and mean arterial blood pressure, usually limited to a reduction of less than 15% below baseline, are the most common cardiovascular side effects seen with administration of bolus or infusion doses of dexmedetomidine, but hypertension can occasionally occur with rapid administration of the drug due to peripheral α_{2B} receptor stimulation resulting in vasoconstriction. In most cases of hypotension or bradycardia no treatment other than a decrease in infusion rate or cessation of the infusion is necessary.

Dexmedetomidine has been successfully used for pediatric CT and MR sedation, although Mason and colleagues[66,67] noted the need for higher infusion rates in children undergoing MR compared with CT. Koroglu and colleagues studied a population of 60 ASA PS 1 and two children undergoing MRI examinations, comparing loading doses and infusions of dexmedetomidine with loading doses and infusions of propofol. Although propofol provided a faster onset of action and time to recovery than dexmedetomidine, it also resulted in more frequent episodes of hypotension and oxygen desaturation.[68] A similar study in patients undergoing MRI compared dexmedetomidine and midazolam administered by loading dose followed by infusion and found the quality of sedation to be better with dexmedetomidine.[69] Barton and colleagues described the use of bolus doses of dexmedetomidine in six young children with CHD undergoing a variety of more invasive procedures including central line placement, fiberoptic bronchoscopy, and chest tube insertion. Three of the children required small additional doses of ketamine for supplemental analgesia, but all patients remained hemodynamically stable and breathed spontaneously throughout the procedure.[70] The successful use of ketamine in combination with dexmedetomidine for cardiac catheterization has also been described in several studies.[71,72]

The use of dexmedetomidine should be avoided in cardiac patients with preexisting bradyarrhythmias or atrioventricular block and those who are receiving negative chronotropic drugs.[73] Chrysostomou and colleagues described the use of dexmedetomidine by bolus dosage or infusion as either primary treatment or rescue therapy in 14 cardiac intensive care patients experiencing atrial or junctional tachyarrhythmias. Although rhythm control was achieved in 93% of patients, adverse effects included hypotension (three patients), need for transient pacing (nine patients), and brief atrioventricular block in one patient.[74] Dexmedetomidine is considered to be contraindicated in patients who are receiving digoxin, as it has been associated with bradycardia and cardiac arrest in that subset of patients.[75,76]

RECOVERY

Infants and children who have originated from an intensive care setting may return there for recovery from sedation. All others should be taken to an appropriately staffed and equipped, dedicated postanesthesia or postsedation recovery area where they can awaken before return to the ward or discharge home. Full monitoring, including noninvasive blood pressure, ECG, and pulse oximetry, should be maintained until the child is awake. Discharge criteria should include a return to baseline mental status and level of consciousness along with stable respiratory and cardiovascular status. If being discharged home, a responsible adult must be available to accompany the patient, watch for any complications, and administer any necessary scheduled cardiac medications. Written instructions for diet, medication, and activity should be provided as well as a contact number in case of complications or emergency.

SUMMARY

The number of pediatric patients requiring sedation for procedures performed outside the operating room environment continues to grow yearly, as does the number of patients surviving to adulthood with the residua and sequelae of CHD. The ongoing efforts of the AAP and the ASA, as well as others, to develop and implement guidelines to enhance the safety of these pediatric sedative encounters have resulted in great strides in the prevention of adverse events. In addition, the Society for Pediatric Sedation, associated with the Pediatric Sedation Research Consortium, provides an important forum for practitioner education and the promotion of safe care for infants and children undergoing sedative experiences. Within the larger population of pediatric patients the subset of patients with CHD or pulmonary hypertension remains especially demanding to care for even in the best of circumstances. The additional safety challenges posed by transport to, and care in, remote locations makes the highest level of vigilance essential when planning and performing sedation for these children.

REFERENCES

1. Welke KF, Diggs BS, Karamlou T, et al. Comparison of pediatric cardiac surgical mortality rates from national administrative data to contemporary clinical standards. Ann Thorac Surg 2009;87:216–23.

2. American Academy of Pediatrics. Guidelines for the elective use of conscious sedation, deep sedation and general anesthesia in pediatric patients. Committee on drugs, section on anesthesiology. Pediatrics 1985;76(2):317–21

3. Cote CJ, Wilson S. The Work Group on Sedation. Guidelines for monitoring and management of pediatric patients during and after sedation for diagnostic and therapeutic procedures: an update. Pediatrics 2006;118:2587–602.

4. American College of Emergency Physicians Policy Statement. The use of pediatric sedation and analgesia. Ann Emerg Med 2008;52:595–6.

5. Joint Commission on Accreditation of Healthcare Organizations. Comprehensive accreditation manual for hospitals. Oakbrook Terrace (IL): Joint Commission on Accreditation of Healthcare Organizations; 2005.

6. American Society of Anesthesiologists Task Force on Sedation and Analgesia by Non-Anesthesiologists. Practice guidelines for sedation and analgesia by non-anesthesiologists. Anesthesiology 2002;96:1004–17.

7. Statement on granting privileges to nonanesthesiologist practitioners for personally administering deep sedation or supervising deep sedation by individuals who are not anesthesia professionals. American Society of Anesthesiologists House of Delegates, October 18, 2006.

8. Cote CJ. Strategies for preventing sedation accidents. Pediatr Ann 2005;34: 625–33.

9. Cravero JP, Beach ML, Blike GT, et al. The incidence and nature of adverse events during pediatric sedation/anesthesia with propofol for procedures outside the operating room: a report from the Pediatric Sedation Research Consortium. Anesth Analg 2009;108:795–804.

10. Cote CJ, Karl HW, Notterman DA, et al. Adverse sedation events in pediatrics: analysis of medications used for sedation. Pediatrics 2000;106:633–44.

11. Robbertze R, Posner KL, Domino KB. Closed claims review of anesthesia for procedures outside the operating room. Curr Opin Anaesthesiol 2006;19:436–42.

12. Wilson W, Taubert KA, Gewitz M, et al. Prevention of infective endocarditis: recommendations by the American Heart Association Rheumatic Fever, Endocarditis and Kawasaki Disease Committee, Council on Cardiovascular Disease in the Young, and the Council on Clinical Cardiology, Council on Cardiovascular Surgery and Anesthesia, and the Quality of Care and Outcomes Research Interdisciplinary Working Group. Circulation 2007;116:1736–54.

13. Practice guidelines for preoperative fasting and the use of pharmacologic agents to reduce the risk of pulmonary aspiration: application to healthy patients undergoing elective procedures: a report by the American Society of Anesthesiologists Task Force on Preoperative Fasting. Anesthesiology 1999;90:896–905.

14. Cook-Sather SD, Litman RS. Modern fasting guidelines in children. Best Pract Res Clin Anaesthesiol 2006;20:471–81.

15. Agrawal D, Manzi S, Gupta R, et al. NPO status and adverse events in children undergoing procedural sedation and analgesia in a pediatric emergency department. Ann Emerg Med 2003;42:636–46.

16. Roback MG, Bajaj L, Wathen JE, et al. Preprocedural fasting and adverse events in procedural sedation and analgesia in a pediatric emergency department: are they related? Ann Emerg Med 2004;44:454–9.

17. Anderson JL, Junkins E, Pribble C, et al. Capnography and depth of sedation during propofol sedation in children. Ann Emerg Med 2007;49:9–13.

18. Lightdale JR, Goldmann DA, Feldman HA, et al. Microstream capnography improves patient monitoring during moderate sedation: a randomized, controlled trial. Pediatrics 2006;117:e1170–8.

19. Cote CJ, Wax DF, Jennings MA, et al. Endtidal carbon dioxide monitoring in children with congenital heart disease during sedation for cardiac catheterization by nonanesthesiologists. Paediatr Anaesth 2007;17:661–6.
20. Glass PS, Bloom M, Kearse L, et al. Bispectral analysis measures sedation and memory effects of propofol, midazolam, isoflurane, and alfentanil in healthy volunteers. Anesthesiology 1997;86:836–47.
21. Rosow C, Manberg PJ. Bispectral index monitoring. Anesthesiol Clin North America 2001;19:947–66.
22. Rosen DA, et al. Is the BIS monitor vital in children undergoing cardiothoracic surgery [abstract]. Anesthesiology 1999;V91:A1244.
23. Hering W, Geisslinger G, Kamp HD, et al. Changes in the EEG power spectrum after midazolam anaesthesia combined with racemic or S-(+) ketamine. Acta Anaesthesiol Scand 1994;38:719–23.
24. Overly FL, Wright RO, Connor FA Jr, et al. Bispectral analysis during pediatric procedural sedation. Pediatr Emerg Care 2005;21:6–11.
25. Baysal A, Polat TB, Yalcin Y, et al. Can analysis of the bispectral index prove helpful when monitoring titration of doses of midazolam and ketamine for sedation during paediatric cardiac catheterization. Cardiol Young 2008;18:51–7.
26. Dahaba AA. Different conditions that could result in the bispectral index indicating an incorrect hypnotic state. Anesth Analg 2005;101:765–73.
27. White PF, Way WL, Trevor AJ. Ketamine – its pharmacology and therapeutic uses. Anesthesiology 1982;56:119–36.
28. Christ G, Mundigler G, Merhaut C, et al. Adverse cardiovascular effects of ketamine infusion in patients with catecholamine-dependent heart failure. Anaesth Intensive Care 1997;25:255–9.
29. Stoelting RK, Hillier SC. Nonbarbiturate intravenous anesthetic drugs. In: Stoelting RK, Hiller SC, editors. Pharmacology and physiology in anesthetic practice. 4th edition. Philadelphia: Lippincott Williams & Wilkins; 2006. p. 115–78.
30. Lin C, Durieux ME. Ketamine and kids: an update. Paediatr Anaesth 2005;15:91–7.
31. Marshal BE, Longnecker DE. General anesthetics. In: Hardman JG, Limbird LE, editors. Goodman & Gilman's the pharmacological basis of therapeutics. 9th edition. New York: McGraw-Hill Health Professions Division; 1996. p. 307–30.
32. Strayer RJ, Nelson LS. Adverse events associated with ketamine for procedural sedation in adults. Am J Emerg Med 2008;26:985–1028.
33. Green SM, Roback MG, Krauss B et al. Predictors of airway and respiratory adverse events with ketamine sedation in the emergency department: an individual patient meta-analysis of 8,282 children. Ann Emerg Med, in press.
34. Brown L, Christian-Kopp S, Sherwin TS, et al. Adjunctive atropine is unnecessary during ketamine sedation in children. Acad Emerg Med 2008;15:314–8.
35. Williams GD, Philip BM, Chu LF, et al. Ketamine does not increase pulmonary vascular resistance in children with pulmonary hypertension undergoing sevoflurane anesthesia and spontaneous ventilation. Anesth Analg 2007;105:1578–84.
36. Reisine T, Pasternak G. Opioid analgesics and antagonists. In: Hardman JG, Limbird LE, editors. Goodman & Gilman's the pharmacological basis of therapeutics. 9th edition. New York: McGraw-Hill Health Professions Division; 1996. p. 521–55.
37. Bailey PL, Pace NL, Ashburn MA, et al. Frequent hypoxemia and apnea after sedation with midazolam and fentanyl. Anesthesiology 1990;73(5):826–30.
38. Ackerman WE, Phero JC, Theodore GT. Ineffective ventilation during conscious sedation due to chest wall rigidity after intravenous midazolam and fentanyl. Anesth Prog 1990;37(1):46–8.

39. Glick C, Evans OB, Parks BR. Muscle rigidity due to fentanyl infusion in the pediatric patient. South Med J 1996;89:1119–20.
40. MacGregor DA, Bauman LA. Chest wall rigidity during infusion of fentanyl in a two-month-old infant after heart surgery. J Clin Anesth 1996;8:251–4.
41. Singer AJ, Stark MJ. Pretreatment of lacerations with lidocaine, epinephrine, and tetracaine at triage: a randomized double-blind trial. Acad Emerg Med 2000;7: 751–6.
42. Mahisekar UL, Callan CM, Derasari M, et al. Infusion of large particles of thiopental sodium during anesthesia induction. J Clin Anesth 1994;6:55–8.
43. Polavarapu N, Sullivan J, Wall K, et al. Age-related effects of pentobarbital for non-invasive pediatric procedural sedation. Crit Care Med 2005;33:A177 [abstract supplement].
44. Mason KP, Zurakowski D, Connor L, et al. Infant sedation for MR imaging and CT: oral versus intravenous pentobarbital. Radiology 2004;233:723–8.
45. Todd MM, Drummond JC, U HS. The hemodynamic consequences of high-dose thiopental anesthesia. Anesth Analg 1985;64:681–7.
46. Eckstein JW, Hamilton WK, McCammond JM. The effect of thiopental on peripheral venous tone. Anesthesiology 1961;22:525–8.
47. Yildirim SV, Guc BU, Bozdogan N, et al. Oral versus intranasal midazolam premedication for infants during echocardiographic study. Adv Ther 2006;23: 719–24.
48. Tschirch FT, Gopfert K, Frohlich JM, et al. Low-dose intranasal versus oral midazolam for routine body MRI of claustrophobic patients. Eur Radiol 2007;17: 1403–10.
49. Kogan A, Katz J, Efrat R, et al. Premedication with midazolam in young children: a comparison of four routes of administration. Paediatr Anaesth 2002; 12:685–9.
50. Moro-Sutherland DM, Algren JT, Louis PT, et al. Comparison of intravenous midazolam with pentobarbital for sedation for head computed tomography imaging. Acad Emerg Med 2000;7:1370–5.
51. Massanari M, Novitsky J, Reinstein LJ. Paradoxical reactions in children associated with midazolam use during endoscopy. Clin Pediatr 1997;36:681–4.
52. Shannon M, Albers G, Burkhart K, et al. Safety and efficacy of flumazenil in the reversal of benzodiazepine-induced conscious sedation. J Pediatr 1997;131: 582–6.
53. Kay B, Rolly G. I.C.I. 35868, a new intravenous induction agent. Acta Anaesthesiol Belg 1997;28:303–16.
54. Borgeat A, Wilder-Smith OH, Suter PM. The nonhypnotic therapeutic applications of propofol. Anesthesiology 1994;80:642–56.
55. Williams GD, Jones TK, Hanson KA, et al. The hemodynamic effects of propofol in children with congenital heart disease. Anesth Analg 1999;89:1411–6.
56. Green SM, Krauss B. Propofol in emergency medicine: pushing the sedation frontier. Ann Emerg Med 2003;42:792–7.
57. Barbi E, Gerarduzzi T, Marchetti F, et al. Deep sedation with propofol by nonanesthesiologists: a prospective pediatric experience. Arch Pediatr Adolesc Med 2003;157:1097–103.
58. Tosun Z, Aksu R, Guler G. Propofol-ketamine vs propofol-fentanyl for sedation during pediatric upper gastrointestinal endoscopy. Paediatr Anaesth 2007;17: 983–8.
59. Reeves ST, Havidich JE, Tobin DP. Conscious sedation of children with propofol is anything but conscious. Pediatrics 2004;114:e74–6.

60. Zgleszewski SE, Zurakowski D, Fontaine PJ. Is propofol a safe alternative to pentobarbital for sedation during pediatric diagnostic CT? Radiology 2008;247: 528–34.

61. Donmez A, Kaya H, Haberal A, et al. The effect of etomidate induction on plasma cortisol levels in children undergoing cardiac surgery. J Cardiothorac Vasc Anesth 1998;12:182–5.

62. Schenarts CL, Burton JH, Riker RR. Adrenocortical dysfunction following etomidate induction in emergency department patients. Acad Emerg Med 2001;8:1–7.

63. Sarkar M, Laussen PC, Zurakowski D, et al. Hemodynamic responses to etomidate on induction of anesthesia in pediatric patients. Anesth Analg 2005;101: 645–50.

64. Baxter AL, Mallory MD, Spandorfer PR, et al. Etomidate versus pentobarbital for computed tomography sedations. Pediatr Emerg Care 2007;23:690–5.

65. Phan H, Nahata MC. Clinical uses of dexmedetomidine in pediatric patients. Paediatr Drugs 2008;10:49–69.

66. Mason KP, Zgleszewski SE, Prescilla R, et al. Hemodynamic effects of dexmedetomidine sedation for CT imaging studies. Paediatr Anaesth 2008;18:393–402.

67. Mason KP, Zurakowski D, Zgleszewski SE, et al. High dose dexmedetomidine as the sole sedative for pediatric MRI. Paediatr Anaesth 2008;18:403–11.

68. Koroglu A, Teksan H, Sagir O, et al. A comparison of the sedative, hemodynamic, and respiratory effects of dexmedetomidine and propofol in children undergoing magnetic resonance imaging. Anesth Analg 2006;103:63–7.

69. Koroglu A, Demirbilek S, Teksan H, et al. Sedative, hemodynamic and respiratory effects of dexmedetomidine in children undergoing magnetic resonance imaging examination: preliminary results. Br J Anaesth 2005;94:821–4.

70. Barton KP, Munoz R, Morell VO, et al. Dexmedetomidine as the primary sedative during invasive procedures in infants and toddlers with congenital heart disease. Pediatr Crit Care Med 2008;9:612–5.

71. Munro HM, Tirotta CR, Felix DE, et al. Initial experience with dexmedetomidine for diagnostic and interventional cardiac catheterization in children. Paediatr Anaesth 2007;17:109–12.

72. Mester R, Easley RB, Brady KM, et al. Monitored anesthesia care with a combination of ketamine and dexmedetomidine during cardiac catheterization. Am J Ther 2008;15:24–30.

73. Hammer GB, Drover DR, Cao H, et al. The effects of dexmedetomidine on cardiac electrophysiology in children. Anesth Analg 2008;106:79–83.

74. Chrysostomou C, Beerman L, Shiderly D, et al. Dexmedetomidine: a novel drug for the treatment of atrial and junctional tachyarrhythmias during the perioperative period for congenital cardiac surgery: a preliminary study. Anesth Analg 2008; 107:1514–22.

75. Berkenbosch JW, Tobias JD. Development of bradycardia during sedation with dexmedetomidine in an infant concurrently receiving digoxin. Pediatr Crit Care Med 2003;4:203–5.

76. Ingersoll-Weng E, Manecke GR, Thistlethwaite PA. Dexmedetomidine and cardiac arrest. Anesthesiology 2004;100:738–9.

Anesthesia and Hemoglobinopathies

Paul G. Firth, MBChB[a,b],*

KEYWORDS

• Sickle cell disease • Thalassemia • Hemoglobin
• Hemoglobinopathies • Anesthesia • Surgery

Hemoglobinopathies are diseases involving abnormalities of the structure or production of hemoglobin. This group of disorders poses many challenges to the anesthesiologist, both in the questions they raise about basic physiology and in the practical issues of assisting patients through a wide variety of surgical procedures. Hemoglobinopathies may present to the anesthesiologist as the primary cause of a surgical procedure, as an incidental complicating factor of a surgical patient, or with a problem arising from the disease itself. An understanding of the disease process, the potential complicating issues, and the evidence surrounding management principles is key to helping people with this group of diseases. This article reviews the common types of hemoglobinopathies, presents a basic summary of pathophysiology relevant to anesthesia, and outlines current perioperative management.

STRUCTURE AND GENETICS OF HEMOGLOBIN

With the exception of embryonic hemoglobins present in early fetal life, hemoglobin is a tetrameric protein consisting of two alpha (α) and two nonalpha polypeptide chains attached to four iron-containing heme complexes. All normal hemoglobins of adult life contain two α chains, with different types of hemoglobin varying in the structure of the nonalpha chain pairs. These types of chains include epsilon ε (embryonic hemoglobins), gamma γ (fetal hemoglobin F), beta β (hemoglobin A), and delta δ (hemoglobin A2).

Adult red cells contain mixes of hemoglobin A ($\alpha_2\beta_2$, approximately 95%–98%), hemoglobin A2 ($\alpha_2\delta_2$, about 2%–3%), and hemoglobin F ($\alpha_2\gamma_2$, less than 2%). In the neonate, the predominant hemoglobin is hemoglobin F, with the proportion of

Administrative funding was provided by the Department of Anesthesia, Massachusetts General Hospital, Boston, MA.

[a] Department of Anesthesia and Critical Care, Massachusetts General Hospital, 55 Fruit Street, Boston, MA 02114, USA
[b] Harvard Medical School, Boston, MA, USA
* Corresponding author. Department of Anesthesia and Critical Care, Massachusetts General Hospital, 55 Fruit Street, Boston, MA 02114.
E-mail address: pfirth@partners.org

hemoglobin A superseding that of hemoglobin F during early infancy. In adults, hemo-globin F is usually limited to a population of erythrocytes known as F cells.

The alleles coding for the polypeptides are codominant, so chain production is the result of the combined expression of all alleles. Genetic coding for the alpha chains is stored in four codominant alleles paired on chromosome 16. The nonalpha chains are coded by two codominant alleles located in a cluster of beta-genes on chromosome 11, the various genes within this cluster coding for different non-alpha chains. The four hemoglobin polypeptides are thus encoded by six alleles, two nonalpha and four alpha alleles.

HEMOGLOBIN FUNCTION

Most oxygen in the blood is transported by hemoglobin, with only a small proportion in solution in the plasma. Hemoglobin binds and releases oxygen in an elegant and finely controlled manner. At high oxygen concentrations typical in the pulmonary capillaries, oxygen binds to the iron of the heme group in the ferrous Fe^{2+} state; at low concen-trations found in the peripheral circulation, the oxygen is released. The binding of oxygen to the iron of one heme subunit induces a conformational or structural change in the whole hemoglobin molecule, producing an increased affinity for oxygen in the other subunits. The binding of oxygen is thus a cooperative process.

The oxyhemoglobin dissociation curve traces the relationship of the partial pressure of oxygen in the plasma with the affinity and hence saturation of hemoglobin with oxygen. The curve is roughly sigmoid, the abrupt change in hemoglobin affinity between the oxygen tensions in the lungs and the peripheries reflecting the coopera-tive binding to oxygen. By contrast, a dissociation plot of noncooperative binding would trace a normal hyperbolic curve. The upper portion of the sigmoid curve repre-sents the affinity of hemoglobin at oxygen tensions typical in the lung. The flatter shape of the curve at these tensions reflects that small changes in oxygen tensions in the pulmonary capillaries have little effect on oxygen uptake, because the hemoglobin has a high affinity for oxygen. The steepness of the lower section of the curve repre-sents the rapid release of oxygen that occurs with only a small drop in capillary oxygen pressure.[1,2]

The oxygen affinity of hemoglobin, and hence the dissociation curve, is affected by several factors. The Bohr effect is the change caused by alterations in hydrogen ion concentration. A right shift in the curve, reflecting a decreased affinity for oxygen, occurs with the increase in hydrogen ion concentration at levels typically present in peripheral tissue. The offloading of oxygen into the tissues is therefore facilitated by this physiologic function. Increases in 2,3-diphosphoglycerate, temperature, or carbon dioxide tension also shift the curve right and promote oxygen release.[1,2] A left shift reflects an increased affinity and decreased unloading at a given tension.

Although the oxygen-carrying function of hemoglobin has long been recognized, the role of hemoglobin in the transport and release of nitric oxide has attracted intense study only in recent years. Nitric oxide is a key messenger involved in vasodilation, vascular wall modeling, endothelial activation, platelet aggregation, and leukocyte adhesion.[3,4] As high-affinity binding to many organic molecules inactivates the phys-iologic actions of nitric oxide, means of transport of bioactive forms of nitric oxide from the lung to sites of action in the peripheries must exist. Nitric oxide is transported to the peripheries as a variety of nitric oxide products, directly by binding to proteins or indirectly by secondary reactions with oxygen, to form nitrosating species that in turn bind to organic molecules.[5,6]

Nitric oxide interacts with hemoglobin in a variety of ways: the reversible binding to the heme iron, the irreversible oxidation to nitrate after reaction with bound oxygen, and the formation of S-nitrosothiol hemoglobin.[7,8] S-Nitrosothiol is a cysteine residue at position 93 on the hemoglobin β chain. Because the affinity of this site is affected by the conformational oxygen state of hemoglobin, it has been suggested that this reaction can deliver bioavailable nitric oxide to the peripheries.[5,8] However, nitric oxide has a short half-life measured in seconds, with many physiologically active metabolites.[9] Determining the in vivo peripheral delivery and biologic effects of the various metabolites of nitric oxide is therefore technically difficult, and has not yet been definitively delineated. Hemoglobin seems to play a role in the pulmonary uptake and systemic release of nitric oxide, but the precise physiologic mechanisms remain incompletely understood.[10–12]

The intricate structure of hemoglobin thus allows not only for the uptake, transport, and release of oxygen but also may affect the blood flow, vascular structure, inflammation, coagulation, and cell adhesiveness through nitric oxide signaling mechanisms.

HEMOGLOBINOPATHIES

Hemoglobin is a large and complex protein. Several hundred variants have been discovered. Most are benign or are of minimal significance, whereas other variants produce disease or are incompatible with life. Sickle cell disease and the thalassemias are the largest and most significant groups of hemoglobinopathies. Whereas hemoglobinopathies have long been viewed largely within the paradigm of oxygen delivery, more recent views approach these diseases as a broader consequence of oxygen and nitric oxide transport dysfunction.[13–15] These diseases have a wide range of clinical expression, even between individuals with identical hemoglobin genotypes. Symptoms are therefore a product not simply of the primary genetic defect, but rather of the complex interactions of multiple other genes.[16]

Sickle Cell Disease

Sickle cell disease results from the inheritance of a mutant β-globin gene that codes for a variant of hemoglobin A called hemoglobin S. Various genotypes produce disease states. Paired inheritance of the mutant gene results in exclusive expression of hemoglobin S and the most severe form of the disease, known as sickle cell anemia. The heterozygous inheritance of a mutant and a normal gene results in the largely benign carrier state, sickle cell trait, with erythrocytes containing hemoglobin S and hemoglobin A. The heterozygous inheritance of the β^S-allele and a thalassemia mutation that codes for impaired or absent hemoglobin A production also produces symptoms. The coexpression of hemoglobin S and hemoglobin C, a variant of hemoglobin A that does not afford protection against hemoglobin S, also results in a disease phenotype. The coinheritance of hemoglobin S with other rare mutants such as hemoglobin O-Arab, hemoglobin D-Punjab, or hemoglobin Lepore-Boston can also result in disease.[13] Sickle cell disease is thus a group of disorders with similar genotypes and phenotypes, all characterized by the inheritance of hemoglobin S.

Approximately 8% of African Americans are heterozygous and have sickle cell trait, and roughly 1 in 600 has some form of sickle cell disease.[17] The carrier state of sickle cell trait provides some protection against severe forms of malaria, believed to be the reason for the evolutionary persistence and high incidence of the mutant allele.[18] There are believed to have been at least five separate spontaneous mutations of the allele occurring in human history, four in Africa and one in south-east Asia, areas where malaria has historically been prevalent.[19] The African mutations are common in equatorial Africa, the eastern Mediterranean littoral, and western Saudi Arabia, whereas the Asian mutation is prevalent in the Gulf region and parts of India. With global migration, these mutations are now distributed worldwide.

The point mutation of a single nucleotide substitution, guanine-adenine-guanine for guanine-thymine-guanine, results in the substitution of the negatively charged glutamic acid by the nonpolar valine in the β chain.[20] This has at least three interrelated effects on hemoglobin function: the hemoglobin S molecule is unstable and degrades more rapidly, the deoxygenated form is insoluble and precipitates out of solution in the cytosol, and, indirectly, the expression of hemoglobin F is upregulated.

The instability of hemoglobin is associated with widespread vascular inflammation, related to the release of iron and disturbances in nitric oxide physiology. In the intact hemoglobin molecule, the iron-containing heme moieties are contained within a hydrophobic pocket formed by the polypeptide chains. This constrains the reactivity of iron with oxygen, allowing for reversible binding in the ferrous Fe^{2+} form rather than in the ferric Fe^{37+} form. The accelerated disintegration of hemoglobin releases the iron moieties from this protective encasing, exposing the cell membrane to oxidative damage from the iron. Subsequent hemolysis releases free iron into the circulation, both consuming free nitric oxide and exposing the vascular endothelium to oxidant damage. Loss of intracellular intact hemoglobin may also impair normal physiologic transport of nitric oxide within the erythrocyte. People with sickle cell disease may, therefore, be in a chronic state of nitric oxide deficiency based on impaired nitric oxide transport and increased scavenging of nitric oxide by free plasma iron.[15] This contributes to a chronic inflammatory vasculopathy.

The second and associated consequence is the insolubility of the deoxygenated hemoglobin. Hemoglobin is normally in solution in the cytosol. On deoxygenation, hemoglobin S tends to crystallize and precipitate out of solution into a gel. The precipitation and polymerization of hemoglobin deforms the cell; the distortions include the characteristic "sickle" shape that gives the disease its name. This process is time dependent, with most red cells transiting the circulation and reoxygenating before widespread precipitation and cell deformation occurs.[21] Only a small proportion of cells sickle reversibly during normal circulation. The polymerization process is exquisitely sensitive to the concentration of the hemoglobin.[22] Extensive cell membrane damage associated with the accelerated hemoglobin breakdown results in pathologic cell dehydration and consequently an increased intracellular hemoglobin concentration. As a terminal result in the accelerated aging process, concentration increases to the point whereby a small proportion of pathologically dehydrated cells sickle reversibly, before deteriorating to an irreversibly sickled state. Cell sickling results therefore not just from the insolubility of deoxyhemoglobin S but also from the pathologic cellular dehydration due to membrane damage associated with the breakdown of the unstable hemoglobin S. There is therefore no specific hemoglobin oxygen saturation at which sickle cells universally start to sickle but rather a spectrum of responses related to cell membrane health. The responses range from cells that do not sickle during the physiological circulation time, to cells that circulate in a permanent and irreversible sickled state, irrespective of oxygenation.[22]

A third associated effect on hemoglobin is an increased expression of hemoglobin F, which has a protective effect. Compared with the African haplotypes, the Asian mutation has a more benign course associated with high levels of hemoglobin F.[23]

Clinical Picture

Sickle cell disease is characterized clinically by a shortened life span, chronic hemolytic anemia, extensive vascular disease, progressive end organ damage, and acute exacerbations.[24,25] The two most common acute complications are pain crises and acute chest syndrome. Pain crises or vaso-occlusive crises can loosely be defined as an acute episode of pain not attributable to pathology other than sickle cell disease.[13] Bone pain most commonly presents following marrow infarction of the lumbar spine, femoral shaft, or knee, is often present in multiple areas, and is sometimes symmetrically distributed.[26] Abdominal pain may arise from gastrointestinal dysfunction, splenic or liver infarction, or be referred from the ribs. The acute chest syndrome is an acute lung injury specific to sickle cell disease, although overlap with other pulmonary syndromes may occur. The syndrome consists of a new pulmonary infiltrate involving at least one lung segment on chest radiography, together with chest pain, fever of greater than 38.5°C, tachypnea, wheezing, or cough.[15,27] Three probable precipitants of the syndrome include pulmonary infection, bone marrow fat embolism following a pain crisis, and occasionally pulmonary sequestration and entrapment of erythrocytes leading to lung injury and infarction.

In attempting to tease out the relative contributions of the insolubility and instability of hemoglobin S to the end clinical picture, a comparison with other diseases yields some interesting insights. The thalassemias are a group of hemoglobinopathies that are also characterized by accelerated breakdown of hemoglobin, heightened oxidative stress, nitric oxide disruption, and widespread vascular damage. Clinical features common to sickle cell disease and the thalassemias include a chronic hemolytic anemia, pulmonary damage, stroke, arterial occlusion, leg ulcers, and shortened life expectancy. Other hereditary chronic hemolytic anemias, such as hereditary spherocytosis, also develop vascular damage and similar complications associated with marked hemolysis. Much of the clinical picture of sickle cell disease also found in other hemoglobinopathies or hemolytic diseases may be accounted for by the instability and breakdown of the hemoglobin.[14,15]

By contrast, the pathognomic features of sickle cell disease, the pain crisis and some types of acute chest syndrome, might be related to the unique feature of hemoglobin S: the insolubility and polymerization of the deoxygenated molecule. Experimental and observational studies also provide some interesting data. Experimental exposure to acute severe hypoxia does not seem to trigger pain crises or pulmonary problems. One study exposed 17 subjects to hypoxic gas mixes, and induced hypoxemia of 33.1 ± 6.9 mmHg and arterial oxygen saturation of $62.4\% \pm 3.5\%$ (mean and standard deviation).[28] Despite this severe hypoxemia, there were no acute complications. Other small early studies exposed a total of five people with symptoms of sickle cell disease to hypoxia, without significant problems.[29,30] The uneventful use of occlusive arterial orthopedic tourniquets has been described in series totaling 37 patients.[31–33] Prolonged survival with coexisting cyanotic heart disease and right-to-left communication, such as tetralogy of Fallot, is possible.[34–38] As some symptom complexes of sickle cell disease are unique to the disease, the unique feature of hemoglobin S presumably plays a significant role in the pathology. However, these studies suggest that hemoglobin polymerization and cell sickling are not the sole precipitants of complications.

Perioperative Management

Management of sickle cell disease includes the confirmation of a preoperative diagnosis, a clinical assessment, anesthetic management appropriate to the procedure and clinical status of the patient, and the prevention and management of postoperative complications.[13] The quoted incidence of complications varies widely, and may relate to the type of procedure, disease activity and severity, patient age, and preexisting organ dysfunction. A retrospective study of 1079 procedures noted an incidence of acute sickle cell exacerbations of 0% for tonsillectomy, 2.9% for hip surgery, 3.9% for myringotomy, 7.8% for intra-abdominal nonobstetric surgery, 16.9% for cesarean section and hysterectomy, and 18.6% for dilation and curettage.[39]

Preoperative Assessment and Workup

The appropriate preoperative screening for sickle cell disease is unclear. In the United States and parts of Western Europe, neonatal screening for hemoglobinopathies is widespread. Most patients or families in these parts of the world will know if they or their children have the disease. For patients from countries with a higher incidence of sickle cell disease but no universal screening, such as tropical African countries, the Caribbean, or some Mediterranean countries, the decision to request a screening test in younger children is ill defined. Children who reach the age of 10 years and have no symptoms are unlikely to have a clinically severe form of the disease that manifests for the first time in the perioperative period. Reports of universal or targeted preoperative screening programs including younger children have noted zero or clinically insignificant detection rates.[40–43]

For those with established disease, the history and examination should identify the frequency, pattern, and severity of recent sickle exacerbations, and the presence and extent of organ damage.[13] The lungs, kidneys, and brain are most commonly affected. Additional investigations may be indicated based on an assessment of the patient's disease severity and the planned procedure. A hemoglobin level, a chest radiograph, and urine dipstick are inexpensive investigations that are easily obtained. Pulmonary function tests, arterial blood gas, electrocardiogram, or neurologic imaging may be indicated in more severe individual cases. Although the expression of hemoglobin S and hemoglobin F vary widely, there is little practical clinical use in determining hemoglobin S levels preoperatively.[13]

Hydration

Perioperative hydration is often suggested as an important issue in sickle cell disease. This assumption is based on the fact that hemoglobin polymerization is closely related to intracellular concentration,[22,44] blood containing hemoglobin S has greater viscosity than hemoglobin A, the presence of urine-concentrating defects in many sicklers, and published statements that dehydration causes acute complications. However, as noted previously, pathologic cellular dehydration is produced by cell membrane damage,[21,22] not passive osmotic gradients. Whether minor alterations in intravascular volume significantly alter intracellular hydration, whether this alters sickling rates in vivo, and if so, whether this is of clinical relevance, is unclear. Most sicklers are anemic with stable hemoglobin levels in the range of 5 to 10 g/dL.[25] At this level, blood viscosity as measured in vitro is actually less than or similar to normal hemoglobin A blood. To achieve in vivo hemoconcentration to levels at which the in vitro measurement of sickle erythrocyte viscosity starts to increase exponentially would require profound dehydration not typically seen in surgical patients. The relevance of mild concentrating defects to perioperative fluid management has not been studied.

Dehydration is suggested as a cause of acute complications, but there is a paucity of clinical accounts to clearly substantiate this statement.[13,14] In recent years, preoperative fasting guidelines have been shortened to allow for oral intake of clear fluid up to 2 hours preoperatively. There is also an increased awareness of the complications of invasive intravascular monitoring, such as central line infection. Whereas the clinical effects of fluid shifts in the sickle cell population have not been studied, there is a lack of evidence to support admission for intravenous hydration during preoperative fasting, aggressive hydration, or invasive monitoring beyond that appropriate for the surgical procedure and the degree of renal dysfunction.

Transfusion

Erythrocyte transfusion may be indicated to augment oxygen-carrying capacity, or to prevent acute exacerbations of sickle cell disease. Sickle cell disease is characterized by chronic anemia, increased minute ventilation, increased cardiac output, decreased peripheral vascular resistance, and increased 2,3-diphosphoglycerate. Hemoglobin levels are typically in the range of 5 to 10 g/dL, although values are somewhat higher in sickle cell-hemoglobin C disease.[25] Replacement of blood loss should be individualized based on a patient's baseline hematocrit, end organ pathology, and surgical losses.[13] Autologous transfusion and the use of cell-saver blood have been reported in case literature.

The efficacy of transfusion to dilute the sickle cells and prevent acute exacerbations remains controversial.[45,46] A prospective randomized trial involving 604 patients compared the use of an aggressive transfusion protocol designed to reduce the proportion of hemoglobin S to less than 30% with one designed to achieve a hematocrit of 30%.[47] There was no significant difference in postoperative sickle exacerbations. The group that received more transfusions due to the aggressive protocol had a higher incidence of transfusion complications such as alloimmunization, the development of new non-ABO antibodies. This result suggested that aggressive transfusion protocols to dilute hemoglobin S were no more effective than the correction of anemia in preventing complications. However, there are no prospective randomized trials comparing outcome following transfusion with no transfusion. Two retrospective studies of children undergoing minor procedures without transfusion found low rates of acute sickle complications.[48,49] The investigators concluded that transfusion could be avoided in low-risk cases. By contrast, another retrospective study found higher complication rates in nontransfused patients than in transfused patients undergoing minor procedures.[39] Recent nonrandomized or retrospective studies comparing transfused and nontransfused patients undergoing moderate-risk procedures such as abdominal or orthopedic procedures have had varied results.[39,50,51] Interpretation is confounded by small group sizes and uncontrolled additional risk factors. The effectiveness of prophylactic transfusion is therefore not clearly established at present.

If blood is transfused, extensive crossmatching for minor blood groups should be preformed.[13] Sickle cell patients have a high incidence of alloimmunization, which may lead to life-threatening or fatal hemolytic transfusion reactions.[52]

Oxygenation

Although hypoxia and an increase in sickling are traditionally considered to be a trigger of perioperative sickle exacerbations,[47,53] there are no definitive clinical accounts in the anesthetic or surgical literature to demonstrate this.[13,14] Avoidance of acute hypoxia is a basic standard of anesthetic care in any patient population, as in sickle cell patients. However, there is no direct evidence to support hyperoxygenation or prolonged oxygen supplementation beyond the levels needed to support the patient's baseline oxygen saturation. Pulse oximetry tends to underestimate true hemoglobin oxygen saturation by about 2% because of the high concentration of coexisting methemoglobin.[54]

Thermoregulation

Hypothermia causes a left shift in the oxygen dissociation curve, and thus in isolation would tend to retard sickling. Patients have suggested that skin cooling may be a precipitant of acute complications occurring in community settings,[26,55] but the relevance of this to anesthetic-induced hypothermia is unclear. Maintenance of normothermia is a basic anesthetic aim in the general population, and therefore presumably should be the goal in sickle patients.[13,14] Uneventful hypothermia during cardiopulmonary bypass has been reported.

Acid-Base Regulation

Acidosis has been suggested as precipitant of complications,[47] but it is difficult to separate the effects of acidemia from an underlying pathologic condition. It seems unlikely that minor fluctuations in acid-base status are a potent trigger of acute problems.[13,14]

Regional Anesthesia

A retrospective study of 1079 anesthetics noted a higher incidence of postoperative complications associated with regional anesthesia compared with general anesthesia, but this finding was confounded by obstetric anesthetics.[39] Later studies did not detect an association of increased complications with neuroaxial anesthesia.[50,56] Neuroaxial anesthesia is commonly used for orthopedic and obstetric indications, as well as the treatment of pain crises.[56–58] Sickle cell children report more pain and use more morphine postoperatively than nonsickle children,[59] so regional anesthesia may be an effective alternative for postoperative pain management.

Specific Procedures

Outpatient surgery may be appropriate for selected patients and procedures. The baseline health of the patient, the type of procedure, and the rapid access to health care should problems arise are factors to be considered.[13]

Since cholelithiasis associated with high erythrocyte turnover is common, cholecystectomy is a frequent surgical procedure.[39,50] The incidence of perioperative sickle complications is approximately 10% to 20%.[39,51,60] Laparoscopic techniques are now typically used in preference to open cholecystectomy.

There is an increased incidence of spontaneous abortion, intrauterine growth retardation, antepartum hospitalization, premature labor, and postpartum infection in parturients with sickle cell disease.[61–63] Complications of sickle cell disease increase during pregnancy. The incidence of pregnancy complications is higher in homozygous hemoglobin S parturients than in those with hemoglobin SC. Pregnancy, outcome is unaffected by sickle cell trait. The reported incidence of postoperative complications is 14% to 19% following dilation and curettage, and 11% to 17% after cesarean section and hysterectomy.[39] Rates of adverse birth outcomes and neonatal complications in infants with sickle cell disease are similar to rates for normal infants.[62] The predominant neonatal hemoglobin is fetal hemoglobin F, which contains γ chains rather than the mutant β^S chain.

Orthopedic procedures to treat sickle cell complications, such as drainage of bone infection, joint replacement, or correction of musculoskeletal deformities, are frequent indications for anesthesia. In a study comparing sickle cell and control patients undergoing hip surgery, the onset time of atracurium was delayed, although total duration of action was unchanged; the investigators suggested this was due to the increased intravascular volume of sickle cell disease.[64] The reported incidence of sickle complications after hip surgery ranges from 0% to 19%.[51]

Arterial cerebrovascular disease is a common and often devastating complication of sickle cell disease, leading to multiple thrombosis or hemorrhagic strokes, neurologic impairment, and death.[24] Anesthesia is often needed for neurovascular imaging, and for radiological or surgical ablation of intracranial aneurysms.[65] Moyamoya disease, an unstable neovascularization, is another complication that can be treated surgically. Modern nonionic contrast dyes seem to be safe for use with sickle cell disease. Although historically aggressive transfusion has been used for these procedures, more recent management involves the avoidance or conservative use of blood transfusion.

There is a large case literature of cardiopulmonary bypass in sickle cell patients. Most involve reports of the correction of congenital anomalies in young children.[13,14] Although earlier reports described the use of exchange transfusion, more recently there are reports of bypass being performed without transfusion.[66,67] Children can survive with right-to-left shunts,[34–38] so the rationale of interventions to minimize sickling in an artificial circuit designed to repair a natural circuit that allows circulation of sickled cells is unclear.[14] Whereas cardiopulmonary bypass can be performed without specific alterations to standard practice, the optimal management of this patient group is not established. Sickle cell trait does not seem to affect outcome after cardiopulmonary bypass and specific alterations to management are not indicated.[68]

Management of Complications

Painful crises are a common complication, and often present difficult management problems. The relative roles of psychological vulnerability, exacerbation of the pain experience by recurrent exposure to opioids, acquired tolerance to analgesics, and the variability of each attack are not clearly defined. There are few controlled trials of pain management, perhaps due to the wide variability in the presentation of pain and the difficulty of objective assessment.

Pain crises may be mild, and treatable with oral analgesics in an outpatient setting. Conversely, pain may be severe enough to require admission and prolonged treatment with high doses of multiple analgesics.[25] Pain should be closely assessed and measured using a pain scale. A randomized comparison of intravenous infusion and oral sustained-release morphine showed no benefit from intravenous administration. However, intravenous administration of opioids is commonly used, as a continuous infusion or with patient-controlled analgesia.[69] This is a more effective regime than scheduled dosing with optional supplementation. Additional analgesics such as acetaminophen and nonsteroidal anti-inflammatory drugs are often used. Ketamine in low doses may be a useful accessory drug, and is currently undergoing investigation. Regional anesthesia for localized sites of pain is an effective analgesic technique.[57,58]

Other factors are important. Reassurance, empathy, and support are essential. A search should be made for occult infection, a potential precipitant of complications. As the acute chest syndrome may complicate painful crises,[27] the lungs should be examined regularly. Incentive spirometry decreases atelectasis and may prevent further pulmonary problems.[70] Supplemental oxygen does not affect pain duration or analgesic use.[71] Erythrocyte transfusion is not indicated during uncomplicated pain crises. Aggressive hydration is often used, although the benefits of this are not clearly established.[72]

The acute chest syndrome is a frequent postoperative problem. In a study of 604 surgical patients, symptoms typically presented 3 days after surgery and lasted for 8 days.[73] Early incentive spirometry, bronchodilator therapy, supplemental oxygen, adequate analgesia, and broad-spectrum antibiotics are recommended treatment.[27] Correction of anemia with transfusion can improve oxygenation,[27] although the effect on outcome has not been clearly established. The outcome following mechanical ventilation for respiratory failure is usually good.

Thalassemias

The thalassemias are a broad group of hemoglobinopathies characterized by a disruption of the normal 1:1 ratio of the α- and β-polypeptide chains. The disease was initially described in children of Mediterranean ethnic origin; the word thalassemia derives from the Greek word for sea, *thalassa*. The thalassemias are commonest in people of Mediterranean, African, and South-east Asian descent. As with sickle cell disease, carrier states give some protection against severe forms of malaria.

Thalassemias are classified by whether the α- or β-chain production is affected. The α-thalassemias result from a deficiency or deletion of one or more of the quartet of α-1 and α-2 genes. The clinical severity varies with the differing genotypes that produce the disease. When all genes are abnormal, hemoglobin Bart hydrops fetalis syndrome results with demise in utero or shortly after birth. Hemoglobin Bart is a γ-chain tetramer produced in the absence of α chains. When three of the four genes are dysfunctional, hemoglobin H disease results. This condition is characterized by severe anemia, hepatosplenomegaly, jaundice, and vascular damage. Hemoglobin H is an abnormal hemoglobin made of four β chains, in the setting of severe underproduction of α chains. Thalassemia caused by two missing or damaged copies of the α gene has a mild anemia, whereas a single aberrant copy of the gene may result in a clinically silent carrier state. The β-thalassemias arise from the absence (β-0 thal) or reduction (β+ thal) of the synthesis of β-globin chains. Homozygous or coinheritance of two mutant alleles results in thalassemia intermedia or thalassemia major, a clinical classification based on the severity of the symptoms. The inheritance of a single mutant gene results in the carrier state, characterized by a mild microcytic, hypochromic anemia and a slightly elevated concentration of hemoglobin A2. Coinheritance of thalassemia mutations with hemoglobin S will produce sickle cell disease, whereas coinheritance of hemoglobin E leads to symptoms of thalassemia.

The disruption of the normal balance of α- and β-chain production produces unstable hemoglobin, rapid breakdown, release of iron complexes, and damage to the erythrocyte membrane. As in sickle cell disease, the chronic hemolysis and disturbed nitric oxide physiology are associated with progressive vascular damage, pulmonary hypertension, and activation of coagulation. Ineffective erythropoiesis results in accelerated apoptosis, disruption of erythroid maturation, and marked erythroid marrow expansion. Extramedullary erythropoietic tissue expansion in the thorax, head, and paraspinal regions can lead to deformation of the face and skull, demineralization/osteopenia, and fractures. Anemia, splenomegaly, and increased plasma volume due to shunting through expanded marrow are other sequelae. Iatrogenic iron overload and hemochromatosis are complications of chronic transfusion therapy.

Common indications for anesthesia include cholecystectomy, splenectomy, vascular access needed for frequent transfusions, osteotomies of bony deformities, or repair of fractured demineralized bone. The anesthetic literature is scant; reported issues include airway access and hemodynamic control of a vasculopathic population. Bony abnormalities of the maxillofacial area may occasionally complicate airway access, making intubation difficult.[74,75] Laparoscopic techniques have been successfully used for cholecystectomy and splenectomy,[76] although perioperative hypertension may be a problem.[77] Blood loss can be managed with cell salvage, avoiding the chronic complications of repeated transfusion.[78,79] Successful cardiopulmonary bypass with cautious use of sodium nitroprusside in two patients with hemoglobin H disease has been reported.[80]

Hemoglobin C and E

Hemoglobin C, a β-chain variant, is commonest in people of West African descent whereas another β-hemoglobinopathy, hemoglobin E, is commonest in South-east Asia. Homozygous inheritance of either mutant allele causes a mild hemolytic anemia and mild to moderate splenomegaly.[81] The combination with another mutation, for example hemoglobin SC disease or hemoglobin E β-thalassemia, produces disease symptoms of sickle cell disease or thalassemia, respectively.

Other Congenital Hemoglobinopathies

A small number of other hemoglobinopathies have been reported to affect anesthetic management. The central issue is the accuracy and interpretation of pulse oximetry in the presence of an abnormal hemoglobin.[82–88] Pulse oximeters rely on the principle of spectrophotometry, based on the Beer-Lambert law.[1] Using two absorption spectra, the degree of oxygen binding is calculated from the differences in absorption spectra of oxygenated and deoxygenated hemoglobin. Dyshemoglobins, such as methemoglobin, carboxyhemoglobin, or sulfhemoglobin, have different absorption spectra or oxygen affinities. The presence of large quantities of these hemoglobins can make oximetry calculations and assumptions about oxygen delivery inaccurate. Some hemoglobinopathies similarly have differing absorption spectra, and the usefulness of pulse oximetry may be limited. Co-oximetry uses multiple waveforms, allowing analysis of multiple hemoglobins, and may provide a more accurate picture than pulse oximetry.[88] As an alternative, measurement of arterial blood gas can be used as an estimate of arterial oxygenation and delivery.

Several hemoglobinopathies, designated hemoglobin M variants, closely resemble methemoglobin but have slightly different absorption spectra.[1] This group of hemoglobinopathies has an altered oxygen affinity that results in a cyanosis that is usually asymptomatic. Methemoglobin is produced by the oxidation of ferrous iron (Fe^{2+}) to ferric iron (Fe^{3+}). Typical levels of less than 1% are abnormally raised when the enzyme responsible for reducing methemoglobin, reduced nicotinamide adenine dinucleotide (NADH)-cytochrome $b5$ reductase, is congenitally deficient or disabled by a drug. By contrast, the oxygen affinity of the iron in hemoglobin M variants is abnormal due to amino acid substitutions in the α and β chains close to the heme groups. These may variously produce increased auto-oxidation to methemoglobin, or altered absorption spectra to pulse oximetry.

Hemoglobin M$_{Iwate}$ is an unstable hemoglobin with an accelerated auto-oxidation into the ferric methemoglobin form.[88] The oxygenated form has a similar absorption spectrum to methemoglobin. The high levels of methemoglobin and altered absorption spectrum of the oxygenated form make pulse oximetry ineffectual. Hemoglobin$_{Cheverley}$ (B45 Phe→Ser) and Hemoglobin$_{Hammersmith}$ (B42 Phe→Ser) similarly produce low readings that preclude use of the oximetry to monitor arterial oxygenation.[85] By contrast, Hb$_{Kohn}$, a hemoglobin with an abnormal a chain, has an increased oxygen affinity. Despite the left-shifted oxygen dissociation curve, however, pulse oximetry readings are paradoxically low.[82,83] In these settings, knowledge of the limitations of conventional oximetry, attention to detail, increased vigilance, and alternative monitoring such as arterial blood gas analysis, co-oximetry, and end-tidal oxygen concentration may assist the delivery of a safe and uncomplicated anesthetic.[85,87]

SUMMARY

Hemoglobinopathies are a large and diverse group of disorders that present many interesting and challenging situations. Common problems relating to the instability of the hemoglobin molecule are often present in these diseases. Close communication and collaboration between the surgeon, anesthesiologist, and hematologist are essential to ensure the safe and optimum management of people with these disorders.

REFERENCES

1. Moyle JTB. Pulse oximetry. London: BMJ Publishing Group; 1994.
2. Nunn JF. Nunn's respiratory physiology. Oxford: Butterworth-Heinemann; 1997.
3. Steudel W, Hurford WE, Zapol WM. Inhaled nitric oxide: basic biology and clinical applications. Anesthesiology 1999;91(4):1090–121.
4. Wang T, El Kebir D, Blaise G. Inhaled nitric oxide in 2003: a review of its mechanisms of action. Can J Anaesth 2003;50(8):839–46.
5. Crawford JH, Isbell TS, Huang Z, et al. Hypoxia, red blood cells, and nitrite regulate NO-dependent hypoxic vasodilation. Blood 2006;107(2):566–74.
6. Nagasaka Y, Fernandez BO, Garcia-Saura MF, et al. Brief periods of nitric oxide inhalation protect against myocardial ischemia-reperfusion injury. Anesthesiology 2008;109(4):675–82.
7. Gow AJ. The biological chemistry of nitric oxide as it pertains to the extrapulmonary effects of inhaled nitric oxide. Proc Am Thorac Soc 2006;3(2):150–2.
8. McMahon TJ, Doctor A. Extrapulmonary effects of inhaled nitric oxide: role of reversible S-nitrosylation of erythrocytic hemoglobin. Proc Am Thorac Soc 2006;3(2):153–60.
9. Robinson JM, Lancaster JR Jr. Hemoglobin-mediated, hypoxia-induced vasodilation via nitric oxide: mechanism(s) and physiologic versus pathophysiologic relevance. Am J Respir Cell Mol Biol 2005;32(4):257–61.
10. Isbell TS, Sun CW, Wu LC, et al. SNO-hemoglobin is not essential for red blood cell-dependent hypoxic vasodilation. Nat Med 2008;14(7):773–7.
11. Stamler JS, Singel DJ, Piantadosi CA. SNO-hemoglobin and hypoxic vasodilation. Nat Med 2008;14(10):1008–9 [author reply: 1009–10].
12. Palmer LA, Doctor A, Gaston B. SNO-hemoglobin and hypoxic vasodilation. Nat Med 2008;14(10):1009 [author reply: 1009–10].
13. Firth PG, Head CA. Sickle cell disease and anesthesia. [see comment]. Anesthesiology 2004;101(3):766–85.
14. Firth PG. Anaesthesia for peculiar cells – a century of sickle cell disease. Br J Anaesth 2005;95(3):287–99.
15. Gladwin MT, Vichinsky E. Pulmonary complications of sickle cell disease. N Engl J Med 2008;359(21):2254–65.
16. Powars D, Chan LS, Schroeder WA. The variable expression of sickle cell disease is genetically determined. Semin Hematol 1990;27(4):360–76.
17. Uddin DE, Dickson LG, Brodine CE. Screening of military recruits for hemoglobin variants. JAMA 1974;227(12):1405–7.
18. Allison AC. Protection afforded by sickle-cell trait against subtertian malarial infection. Br Med J 1954;1(4857):290–4.
19. Antonarakis SE, Boehm CD, Serjeant GR, et al. Origin of the beta S-globin gene in blacks: the contribution of recurrent mutation or gene conversion or both. Proc Natl Acad Sci U S A 1984;81(3):853–6.
20. Marotta CA, Forget BG, Cohne-Solal M, et al. Human beta-globin messenger RNA.I. Nucleotide sequences derived from complementary RNA. J Biol Chem 1977;252(14):5019–31.
21. Mozzarelli A, Hofrichter J, Eaton WA. Delay time of hemoglobin S polymerization prevents most cells from sickling in vivo. Science 1987;237(4814):500–6.

22. Eaton WA, Hofrichter J. Hemoglobin S gelation and sickle cell disease. Blood 1987;70(5):1245–66.
23. Wood WG, Pembrey ME, Serjeant GR, et al. Hb F synthesis in sickle cell anaemia: a comparison of Saudi Arab cases with those of African origin. Br J Haematol 1980;45(3):431–45.
24. Platt OS, Brambilla DJ, Rosse WF, et al. Mortality in sickle cell disease. Life expectancy and risk factors for early death. N Engl J Med 1994;330(23): 1639–44.
25. Steinberg MH. Management of sickle cell disease. N Engl J Med 1999;340(13): 1021–30.
26. Serjeant GR, Ceulaer CD, Lethbridge R, et al. The painful crisis of homozygous sickle cell disease: clinical features. Br J Haematol 1994;87(3):586–91.
27. Vichinsky EP, Neumayr LD, Earles AN, et al. Causes and outcomes of the acute chest syndrome in sickle cell disease. National Acute Chest Syndrome Study Group. N Engl J Med 2000;342(25):1855–65.
28. Sproule BJ, Halden ER, Miller WF. A study of cardiopulmonary alterations in patients with sickle cell disease and its variants. J Clin Invest 1958;37(3):486–95.
29. Klinefelter KM. The heart in sickle cell anemia. Am J Med Sci 1942;203:34–51.
30. Henderson AB, Thornell HE. Observations on the effect of lowered oxygen tension on sicklemia and sickle cell anemia amongst military flying personnel. J Lab Clin Med 1946;31:769–76.
31. Stein RE, Urbaniak J. Use of the tourniquet during surgery in patients with sickle cell hemoglobinopathies. Clin Orthop Relat Res 1980;151:231–3.
32. Adu-Gyamfi Y, Sankarankutty M, Marwa S. Use of a tourniquet in patients with sickle-cell disease. Can J Anaesth 1993;40(1):24–7.
33. Oginni LM, Rufai MB. How safe is tourniquet use in sickle-cell disease? Afr J Med Med Sci 1996;25(1):3–6.
34. Harris LC, Haggard ME, Travs LB. The coexistence of sickle cell disease and congenital heart disease: a report of three cases, with repair under cardiopulmonary by-pass in two. Pediatrics 1964;33:562–70.
35. Pearson HA, Schiebler GL, Krovetz J, et al. Sickle-cell anemia associated with tetralogy of Fallot. N Engl J Med 1965;273(20):1079–83.
36. O'Keefe JD, LePere R, Britton HA. Blalock-Taussig shunt for tetralogy of Fallot in a patient with sickle cell anemia. A case report. JAMA 1967;200(3):252–4.
37. Szentpetery S, Robertson L, Lower RR. Complete repair of tetralogy associated with sickle cell anemia and G-6-PD deficiency. J Thorac Cardiovasc Surg 1976;72(2):276–9.
38. Hudson RL, Castro O, Spivak JL, et al. Sickle cell anemia and transposition of the great vessels. Am J Dis Child 1978;132(2):149–51.
39. Koshy M, Weiner SJ, Miller ST, et al. Surgery and anesthesia in sickle cell disease. Cooperative Study of Sickle Cell Diseases. Blood 1995;86(10):3676–84.
40. Baraka A, Haddock G, Roussis X, et al. An audit of sickle cell screening in a paediatric hospital population. Scott Med J 1994;39(3):84–5.
41. Mason C, Porter SR, Mee A, et al. The prevalence of clinically significant anaemia and haemoglobinopathy in children requiring dental treatment under general anaesthesia: a retrospective study of 1000 patients. Int J Paediatr Dent 1995; 5(3):163–7.
42. Pemberton PL, Down JF, Porter JB, et al. A retrospective observational study of pre-operative sickle cell screening. Anaesthesia 2002;57(4):334–7.
43. Crawford MW, Galton S, Abdelhaleem M. Preoperative screening for sickle cell disease in children: clinical implications. Can J Anaesth 2005;52(10):1058–63.

44. Bookchin RM, Balazs T, Landau LC. Determinants of red cell sickling. Effects of varying pH and of increasing intracellular hemoglobin concentration by osmotic shrinkage. J Lab Clin Med 1976;87(4):597–616.

45. Goodwin SR, Haberkern C, Crawford M, et al. Sickle cell and anesthesia: do not abandon well-established practices without evidence. Anesthesiology 2005; 103(1):205 [author reply: 205–7].

46. Firth PG. Pulmonary complications of sickle cell disease. N Engl J Med 2009; 360(10):1044 [author reply: 1044–5].

47. Vichinsky EP, Haberkern CM, Neumayr L, et al. A comparison of conservative and aggressive transfusion regimens in the perioperative management of sickle cell disease. The Preoperative Transfusion in Sickle Cell Disease Study Group. N Engl J Med 1995;333(4):206–13.

48. Griffin TC, Buchanan GR. Elective surgery in children with sickle cell disease without preoperative blood transfusion. J Pediatr Surg 1993;28(5):681–5.

49. Fu T, Corrigan NJ, Quinn CT, et al. Minor elective surgical procedures using general anesthesia in children with sickle cell anemia without pre-operative blood transfusion. Pediatr Blood Cancer 2005;45(1):43–7.

50. Haberkern CM, Neumayr LD, Orringer EP, et al. Cholecystectomy in sickle cell anemia patients: perioperative outcome of 364 cases from the National Preoperative Transfusion Study. Preoperative Transfusion in Sickle Cell Disease Study Group. Blood 1997;89(5):1533–42.

51. Vichinsky EP, Neumayr LD, Haberkern C, et al. The perioperative complication rate of orthopedic surgery in sickle cell disease: report of the National Sickle Cell Surgery Study Group. Am J Hematol 1999;62(3):129–38.

52. Petz LD, Calhoun L, Shulman IA, et al. The sickle cell hemolytic transfusion reaction syndrome. Transfusion 1997;37(4):382–92.

53. Shapiro ND, Poe MF. Sickle-cell disease: an anesthesiological problem. Anesthesiology 1955;16(5):771–80.

54. Fitzgerald RK, Johnson A. Pulse oximetry in sickle cell anemia. Crit Care Med 2001;29(9):1803–6.

55. Murray N, May A. Painful crises in sickle cell disease—patients' perspectives. BMJ 1988;297(6646):452–4.

56. Camous J, N'da A, Etienne-Julan M, et al. Anesthetic management of pregnant women with sickle cell disease—effect on postnatal sickling complications. Can J Anaesth 2008;55(5):276–83.

57. Yaster M, Tobin JR, Billett C, et al. Epidural analgesia in the management of severe vaso-occlusive sickle cell crisis. Pediatrics 1994;93(2):310–5.

58. Finer P, Blair J, Rowe P. Epidural analgesia in the management of labor pain and sickle cell crisis—a case report. Anesthesiology 1988;68(5):799–800.

59. Crawford MW, Galton S, Naser B. Postoperative morphine consumption in children with sickle-cell disease. Paediatr Anaesth 2006;16(2):152–7.

60. Wales PW, Carver E, Crawford MW, et al. Acute chest syndrome after abdominal surgery in children with sickle cell disease: is a laparoscopic approach better? J Pediatr Surg 2001;36(5):718–21.

61. Powars DR, Sandhu M, Niland-Weiss J, et al. Pregnancy in sickle cell disease. Obstet Gynecol 1986;67(2):217–28.

62. Brown AK, Sleeper LA, Pegelow CH, et al. The influence of infant and maternal sickle cell disease on birth outcome and neonatal course. Arch Pediatr Adolesc Med 1994;148(11):1156–62.

63. Smith JA, Espeland M, Bellevue R, et al. Pregnancy in sickle cell disease: experience of the Cooperative Study of Sickle Cell Disease. Obstet Gynecol 1996;87(2):199–204.

64. Dulvadestin P, Gilton A, Hernigou P, et al. The onset time of atracurium is prolonged in patients with sickle cell disease. Anesth Analg 2008;107(1):113–6.
65. Firth PG, Peterfreund RA. Management of multiple intracranial aneurysms: neuroanesthetic considerations of sickle cell disease. J Neurosurg Anesthesiol 2000; 12(4):366–71.
66. Metras D, Coulibaly AO, Ouattara K, et al. Open-heart surgery in sickle-cell haemoglobinopathies: report of 15 cases. Thorax 1982;37(7):486–91.
67. Frimpong-Boateng K, Amoah AG, Barwasser HM, et al. Cardiopulmonary bypass in sickle cell anaemia without exchange transfusion. Eur J Cardiothorac Surg 1998;14(5):527–9.
68. Djaiani GN, Cheng DC, Carroll JA, et al. Fast-track cardiac anesthesia in patients with sickle cell abnormalities. Anesth Analg 1999;89(3):598–603.
69. Robieux IC, Kellner JD, Coppes MJ, et al. Analgesia in children with sickle cell crisis: comparison of intermittent opioids vs. continuous intravenous infusion of morphine and placebo-controlled study of oxygen inhalation. Pediatr Hematol Oncol 1992;9(4):317–26.
70. Bellet PS, Kalinyak KA, Shukla R, et al. Incentive spirometry to prevent acute pulmonary complications in sickle cell diseases. N Engl J Med 1995;333(11):699–703.
71. Zipursky A, Robieux IC, Brown EJ, et al. Oxygen therapy in sickle cell disease. Am J Pediatr Hematol Oncol 1992;14(3):222–8.
72. Pegelow CH. Survey of pain management therapy provided for children with sickle cell disease. Clin Pediatr (Phila) 1992;31(4):211–4.
73. Vichinsky EP, Styles LA, Colangelo LH, et al. Acute chest syndrome in sickle cell disease: clinical presentation and course. Cooperative Study of Sickle Cell Disease. Blood 1997;89(5):1787–92.
74. Orr D. Difficult intubation: a hazard in thalassaemia. A case report. Br J Anaesth 1967;39(7):585–6.
75. Mak PH, Ooi RG. Submental intubation in a patient with beta-thalassaemia major undergoing elective maxillary and mandibular osteotomies. Br J Anaesth 2002; 88(2):288–91.
76. Katz R, Goldfarb A, Muggia M, et al. Unique features of laparoscopic cholecystectomy in beta thalassemia patients. Surg Laparosc Endosc Percutan Tech 2003;13(5):318–21.
77. Suwanchinda V, Tengapiruk Y, Udomphunthurak S. Hypertension perioperative splenectomy in thalassemic children. J Med Assoc Thai 1994;77(2):66–70.
78. Waters JH, Lukauskiene E, Anderson ME. Intraoperative blood salvage during cesarean delivery in a patient with beta thalassemia intermedia. Anesth Analg 2003;97(6):1808–9.
79. Perez Ferrer A, Ferrazza V, Gredilla E, et al. Bloodless surgery in a patient with thalassemia minor. Usefulness of erythropoietin, preoperative blood donation and intraoperative blood salvage. Minerva Anestesiol 2007;73(5):323–6.
80. Rowbottom SJ, Sudhaman DA. Haemoglobin H disease and cardiac surgery. Anaesthesia 1988;43(12):1033–4.
81. Olson JF, Ware RE, Schultz WH, et al. Hemoglobin C disease in infancy and childhood. J Pediatr 1994;125(5 Pt 1):745–7.
82. Gottschalk A, Silverberg M. An unexpected finding with pulse oximetry in a patient with hemoglobin Koln. Anesthesiology 1994;80(2):474–6.
83. Katoh R, Miyake T, Arai T. Unexpectedly low pulse oximeter readings in a boy with unstable hemoglobin Koln. Anesthesiology 1994;80(2):472–4.
84. Chisholm DG, Stuart H. Congenital methaemoglobinaemia detected by preoperative pulse oximetry. Can J Anaesth 1994;41(6):519–22.

85. Hohl RJ, Sherburne AR, Feeley JE, et al. Low pulse oximeter-measured hemoglobin oxygen saturations with hemoglobin Cheverly. Am J Hematol 1998;59(3):181–4.
86. Aravindhan N, Chisholm DG. Sulfhemoglobinemia presenting as pulse oximetry desaturation. Anesthesiology 2000;93(3):883–4.
87. Holbrook SP, Quinn A. An unusual explanation for low oxygen saturation. Br J Anaesth 2008;101(3):350–3.
88. Kuji A, Satoh Y, Kikuchi K, et al. The anesthetic management of a patient with hemoglobin M(Iwate). Anesth Analg 2001;93(5):1192–3.

Blood Conservation Strategies in Pediatric Anesthesia

Shilpa Verma, MBBS[a],*, Michael Eisses, MD[a,b],
Michael Richards, BM, MRCP, FRCA[a,b]

KEYWORDS

- Blood • Coagulation • Management • Pediatric
- Anesthesia • Surgery

It is widely accepted in modern medical practice that the use of blood products is an integral part of many aspects of patient care. Even with advances in the knowledge of blood cross-matching, there remains a small but significant risk of morbidity and mortality associated with any form of blood product administration. Because coagulation is inherently intertwined with blood conservation, a good understanding of the options to manipulate the coagulation pathways is an integral aspect of the following discussion.

There are undoubtedly certain specific aspects of pediatric physiology that present their own distinct challenges to the management of transfusion in children. Through this article, the authors aim to highlight the challenges that the pediatric anesthesiologist may face when encountering a situation requiring blood transfusion and to address some of the modalities available to minimize the necessity and frequency of blood product use.

WHY SHOULD WE GIVE BLOOD AND BLOOD PRODUCTS?

The replacement of blood or blood products in a patient who is deficient in blood cells or protein complexes seems a natural goal; however, there are little or no data to define the absolute benefit. The practice of transfusion was adopted long before the advent of randomized trials. As with many advances in medicine, the widespread adoption of transfusion occurred during a time of conflict; the use of blood products undoubtedly saved many lives before the risks associated with it were identified.[1] In

The authors have no external funding interests.

[a] Department of Anesthesiology and Pain Medicine, University of Washington, Box 356540BB-1469 Health Sciences, 1959 NE Pacific Street, Seattle, WA, USA

[b] Seattle Children's Hospital, 4800 Sandpoint Way NE, PO Box 5371/W9824, Seattle, WA 98105-0371, USA

* Corresponding author. Department of Anesthesiology and Pain Medicine, University of Washington, Box 356540BB-1469 Health Sciences, 1959 NE Pacific Street, Seattle, WA.

E-mail address: shilpa.verma@seattlechildrens.org (S. Verma).

Anesthesiology Clin 27 (2009) 337–351
doi:10.1016/j.anclin.2009.05.002
1932-2275/09/$ – see front matter © 2009 Elsevier Inc. All rights reserved.

simplistic terms, the following rationale cannot be debated: Red blood cells contain hemoglobin, which is used to transport oxygen. If a patient is deficient in red cells, then oxygen delivery is impaired; by increasing the concentration of red cells, the oxygen carrying capacity of blood and hence oxygen delivery can be increased.

In vivo blood contains the primary components of the coagulation cascade; when these become depleted, they can only be replaced by synthesis or transfusion. Synthesis is limited by the speed of production; transfusion allows rapid resolution of coagulation deficiencies in a state of ongoing blood loss.

With blood loss, the intravascular volume becomes depleted. There are many intravascular volume expanders; however, none of them have an intravascular life span of more than a few hours. Red blood cells have a far greater longevity in the intravascular space and are therefore much more effective in volume replacement therapy than any other product available.

WHY SHOULD WE AVOID BLOOD PRODUCTS WHEN POSSIBLE?

Although in recent years the mainstream media have extensively covered the risks associated with human immunodeficiency virus (HIV) transmission from blood transfusion, there are many other blood-borne diseases, specifically the hepatitides,[2,3] that have a higher incidence of transmission through transfusion and arguably a greater impact on morbidity and mortality.

The potential immunologic consequences of transfusion are also a major cause of morbidity. In particular, the immunomodulation associated with the exposure of the critically ill patient to non–leukocyte-reduced transfusions has been shown to significantly worsen outcome data on intensive care units,[4] whereas transfusion-related acute lung injury is probably the most common cause (1 in 2000 patients) of major organ dysfunction secondary to blood product administration.[5]

WHY IS THE PEDIATRIC PATIENT DIFFERENT?

The neonate is born with a predominance of hemoglobin (Hb) F, a variable but usually high hemoglobin level (about 16 g/dL), an oxygen dissociation curve that is shifted to the left as a consequence of existing in a hypoxic environment for the previous 9 months, and an immature coagulation system.

From the hemoglobin perspective, most authorities treat children older than 4 months as adults, with regard to transfusion guidelines.[6] For children younger than this age, there are very little data to support any guidelines.[7,8] In the situation of ongoing blood loss, then, the decision to transfuse is obvious; however, when transfusion should be triggered is a moot point. During the 10 weeks after delivery, the hemoglobin falls to 11 g/dL; however, by this age, virtually all hemoglobin is Hb A. So, although the decrease in hemoglobin concentration reduces oxygen delivery, the Hb A enhances oxygen extraction at the tissue level.

The coagulation system of the neonate is immature and does not reach a level comparable with the adult coagulation cascade until at least 6 months of age.[9] The key differences are the vitamin K–dependent factors (II, VII, IX, and X) that are less than 70% of adult levels, the inhibitors of coagulation (including antithrombin III and proteins C and S) that are 50% of adult levels, and platelets, whose numbers are at a similar level to that of adults but take 2 weeks to develop adult levels of reactivity.[10]

All the factors briefly highlighted earlier leave us in a quandary; there is no conclusive evidence as to what, how, or when blood and blood products should be used in children, particularly in neonates. There are inherent risks associated with use of blood products; however, it is unlikely that there will ever be definitive guidelines based on irrefutable evidence. What physicians can do is have a good awareness of the under-lying physiology and developmental changes that occur within the child and try to coor-dinate management to maintain the patient's physiology as close to normal as possible.

Through the rest of this article, the authors try to identify patients who are at high risk of requiring blood products, and they review the options available for prophylaxis against blood loss, which help to minimize the need for blood products. They also examine some of the strategies for acute management of blood loss and look at which blood products should be administered, including discussion of transfusion thresholds.

THE HIGH-RISK PATIENT

In determining that a patient is at significant risk of transfusion, there are 4 factors that should be considered: patient-, drug-, physician-, and procedure-related risk.

Patient-Related Risk

Concurrent pathology and current physiologic status can have profound implications on patients' potential for blood loss during any form of surgical procedure. Increased bleeding potential, either from direct means such as thrombocytopenia or indirectly from pathology such as renal impairment–induced platelet dysfunction, needs to be recognized. Preoperative anemia will limit the patient's reserve to deal with intraoper-ative blood loss.

Something that should be mentioned at this juncture is a patient's moral choice not to receive blood products. This can provide a challenging ethical problem that is made all the more difficult with children, when one has to determine who has the "right" to make such decisions: the parent or guardian, the child (a minor), the medical practi-tioner, or a court of law. It is imperative that every establishment that deals with children in a situation such as this, where medical, moral, ethical, and religious beliefs may produce disagreement and conflict, institute a well-publicized, legally approved protocol for patient management, which is transparent and easily available for both health care practitioners and families.

Drug-Related Risk

In pediatric practice, the two major categories of drugs that are likely to be encoun-tered that increase the likelihood of intra- and postoperative bleeding are antiplatelet agents (nonsteroidal antiinflammatory drugs [NSAIDs]) and anticoagulants (heparin and warfarin). NSAIDs (used for either acute or chronic indications) act by reversibly inhibiting cyclooxygenase, thereby inhibiting platelet activity. They require an adequate lag time of 5 to 7 days from cessation of therapy until platelet function is restored, which needs to be considered; however, the urgency of the surgical proce-dure may eliminate NSAIDs as a prophylactic option.

Heparin enhances the effects of antithrombin III and inhibits platelet aggregation. When used intravenously, it has a half-life of 90 minutes with clinical effects persisting for 4 to 6 hours; hence it can almost invariably be stopped appropriately before a surgical procedure. The advent of prophylactic and therapeutic treatment with low–molecular weight heparin has made management slightly more complicated with its longer half-life of 2 to 4 times that of standard heparin, independent of dosage. Most authorities would advocate, if time permits, waiting at least 12 hours for prophy-lactic and 24 hours for therapeutic treatment to normalize. In the eventuality of emer-gency, both normal and low–molecular weight heparin can be reversed with protamine sulfate, which forms an inert complex with circulating heparin.[11]

Warfarin competes with vitamin K in the synthesis of factors II, VII, IX, and X and has a half-life of 30 hours. The dosage is adjusted according to coagulation studies. Although careful scheduling and institution of alternate anticoagulation usually allow for straightforward management of patients receiving warfarin, clinical urgency may override this situation. In this circumstance, the effects of warfarin can be reversed with fresh frozen plasma (FFP) to replace the absent coagulation factors or by cautious titration of intravenous vitamin K. There have also been reports of activated factor VII being used to shorten the prothrombin time.[12]

In the pediatric population, other drugs that provoke an increased risk of bleeding, such as antithrombotics and thrombolytics, may rarely be encountered. In most cases, these can be stopped after appropriate discussion with the primary prescriber or surgical team. However, when the ongoing use of these drugs is considered to be in the patient's best interests, appropriate preoperative counseling of the increased risk is necessary. At this juncture, it is worth mentioning the increasing use of herbal remedies within the general public; some of these have been implicated as modulators of the clotting pathway and others have been noted to have a significant impact on the metabolism of particularly procoagulant drugs that medical practitioners use.

Physician-Related Risk

Individual physicians and even institutions have dramatically different blood product use and blood product transfusion protocols that vary enormously, nationally and internationally. This variation is because of personal and institutional preference rather than national and international guidelines. Adherence to guidelines is of course at the individual's discretion. Within surgery per se, there is also significant inter-individual surgical practice that undoubtedly exists. Some surgeons are "more bloody" than others while performing the same procedure; that is not to say that they are worse or better, just that their practice involves greater blood loss to get to the same end result, hence greater use of blood products.

Procedure-Related Risk

Although it may seem to be stating the obvious that different procedures have different risks for the requirement for blood product administration, there is considerable variation with what seems superficially to be the same procedure. A single surgical description can cover a multitude of impending actual procedures that, depending on the patient in question, can have enormous variation in time duration, physiologic and anatomic upheaval, and subsequent circulatory compromise. For example, a patient listed for a "craniosynostosis repair" could represent a repair of one suture, or many sutures and therefore have significantly different blood-loss potential. Any reoperations should give rise to extreme caution because of the inevitable adhesions that need to be addressed at the primary operative site.

As is the essence to the majority of clinical practice, the most important aspect of preoperative preparedness involves a team approach, with adequate discussion with the surgical practitioner and research into the patient's preoperative physiologic condition. This should allow the perioperative physician to be prepared for the expected, and a healthy degree of caution allows the physician to be prepared for the unexpected.

STRATEGIES FOR BLOOD TRANSFUSION PROPHYLAXIS

Strategies to avoid intraoperative administration of blood or blood products can be divided into preoperative and intraoperative interventions.

Preoperative Interventions

These options are useful when one anticipates a high degree of blood loss in surgical procedures that are elective in nature.

Recombinant erythropoietin

Erythropoietin (EPO) is an endogenous hormone produced in the kidney. It has a high affinity for the erythropoietin receptor expressed on the surface of erythroid cells. It is necessary for the survival of developing erythroid progenitor cells and controls the proliferation and differentiation of these cells. The recombinant alfa form of EPO has been available in the United States since 1997. EPO's role to increase red blood cell mass in pediatric patients has precedence through its use to treat anemia associated with end-stage renal disease, malignancies, and also anemia of prematurity. As a result, its safety profile has been well evaluated.

There are several case reports and reviews exploring the use of EPO preoperatively to avoid, or at least minimize, allogeneic blood transfusions in children. Jadhav and colleagues[13] administered EPO with iron supplementation 3 times a week for 6 weeks to 3 children scheduled for major elective surgery who were Jehovah's Witnesses. There was a rise in hemoglobin by a mean of 4.1 g/dL and hematocrit by a mean of 14%, and none required allogeneic blood products intraoperatively or postoperatively, demonstrating that red blood cell mass can increase considerably just weeks before scheduled surgery. There are also studies demonstrating EPO's role as an adjunct with other blood conservation techniques. In a retrospective review[14] of 19 patients, 10 patients, with a mean age between 11 and 13 months, received EPO and iron for several weeks before craniosynostosis repair and oral vitamin K the previous night. Coupled to that strategy was intraoperative aprotinin, acute normovolemic hemodilution (ANH), and controlled hypotension. Patients receiving EPO increased their red cell mass within 4 weeks by an average of 28% (hematocrit 34.9%–44.5%). Compared with those not receiving EPO, the incidence of transfusion and total volume of blood products were lower. Although many blood conservation strategies were used in conjunction with EPO, clouding the individual contribution of EPO, the investigators did find an increase in allowable blood loss measurements having used EPO preoperatively. To them, this represented an advantage to preoperative EPO administration by allowing more patients to qualify for ANH.

With EPO administration, the rate of hematocrit increase varies in patients and may be dose dependent;[15] therefore consultation with a hematologist to guide candidacy of intervention, response to dosage, and potential side effects is advisable. The first sign that EPO has taken effect is an increase in reticulocyte count within 10 days, whereas a clinically significant increase in hematocrit should be visible by 2 weeks. Iron supplementation is necessary to provide for increased requirements during expansion of red cell mass secondary to marrow stimulation by EPO.

Preoperative autologous blood donation

When considering preoperative autologous donation (PAD) as another preoperative blood conservation strategy, the differences between adults and children must be noted. Each donation results in a significant alteration in intravascular volume, which through oral rehydration can easily be compensated for in adults by increasing left ventricular stroke volume and heart rate. Children older than 4 years have adult-like cardiovascular physiology[16] and demonstrate a similar compensatory mechanism to blood loss. Infants do not have this buffer because of their immature myocardial infrastructure, which results in a limited ability to increase stroke volume in response to hypovolemia. Without supplementation of iron, it can take 3 months to naturally replenish iron stores after one autologous donation.[17] However, if one takes into consideration the weight and estimated blood volume of the child and allows for appropriate intravascular volume replacement, PAD can successfully be tolerated by the pediatric patients without hemodynamic consequences. Longatti and colleagues[18] report PAD in patients as young as 3 months and weighing as little as 6.7 kg.

One important advantage to PAD is the potential for a decreased incidence in alloimmunization, which can have a huge impact on future blood transfusion, pregnancy, and organ transplantation. Autologous programs may increase the donor pool because many autologous donors subsequently become allogeneic donors and, at the same time, decrease the demand for allogeneic blood.

The principle concern regarding PAD use is that accurate prediction of blood loss is necessary to maintain its advantage of reducing allogenic blood product exposure. In a study by Letts and colleagues,[19] surgeons were asked to predict the number of autologous units required for a given procedure to determine the volume of blood needed for predonation; the reported accuracy was 53.8%. PAD does not prevent septicemia from a bacterially contaminated unit. It does not avoid clerical or laboratory error leading to transfusion of a wrong unit. The scheduling of surgery may have to be altered to permit donation or avoid wastage of the predonated autologous blood. The cost of a blood unit obtained via PAD is higher than that which is obtained via a random donor. Given these concerns, the potential benefits in a carefully chosen population may outweigh the risks.

Similar transfusion thresholds should be used as with administering allogeneic blood. EPO and iron supplementation are useful in helping to offset preoperative anemia associated with the technique. Successful programs address the psychosocial issues of the predonation process and have a deep commitment to the multidisciplinary team approach.

Intraoperative Interventions

Acute normovolemic hemodilution

ANH involves the removal of whole blood from the patient shortly before the anticipated surgical blood loss and the restoration of the circulating blood volume with a crystalloid or colloid solution to maintain normovolemia. The premise is that the blood lost during the surgery will consist of blood with a lower hematocrit and, hence, proportionately less of the patient's red blood cell mass is lost. The oxygen carrying capacity can then be restored by administering the previously withdrawn blood, once the major blood loss has abated.

There are a few potential concerns when instituting ANH in pediatric patients. Infants younger than 4 months have a higher Hg F concentration. Hg F has a decreased ability to unload oxygen to the tissues, which would be undesirable in a situation where there is already a reduced oxygen supply (dilutional anemia). Children younger than 4 years may not tolerate hypovolemia well because of their limited ability to increase stroke volume and a predominant reliance on increases in heart rate to maintain cardiac output. Although there are very few studies addressing ANH in infants less than 6 months, Friesen and colleagues[20] showed benefits in limiting blood loss when ANH was used before cardiac surgery, where the replacement fluids included the banked blood already used to prime the cardiopulmonary bypass (CPB) pump. In general though, caution is advised in using this technique in the younger infant.

There are many alternate algorithms that calculate the amount of blood that is drawn from the donating patient and also how one cares for the drawn blood. The option of keeping the donated blood warm allows for the preservation of the maximum level of platelet function; however, if there is significant delay before readministration, then the blood should be refrigerated.

ANH in spinal fusion surgeries have shown to be beneficial especially if combined with other blood conserving strategies. Pouliquen-Evrard and colleagues[21] retrospectively examined four groups of children who underwent orthopedic surgery, for allogeneic blood use. The groups included (1) patients solely using allogeneic blood transfusions, (2) patients using ANH only, (3) patients using PAD and ANH, and (4) patients using PAD, ANH, and controlled hypotension. The hemoglobin target for hemodilution was 8 g/dL, and transfusion was dependent on both clinical indications and hemoglobin with lower limit of 7 g/dL. Overall, 98%, 46%, 19%, and 5% blood loss was replaced by allogeneic blood transfusion in the first, second, third, and fourth groups, respectively. This study demonstrated that ANH can significantly reduce allogeneic blood transfusion, especially when used in conjunction with additional blood conservation techniques.

In craniosynostosis surgeries, ANH has been less successful. Reasons suggested for this include a smaller pediatric population and a smaller volume of red cells, which in turn limit the volumes of whole blood being harvested before a postdilutional hematocrit level is reached.[6] In a study[22] in which infants undergoing craniosynostosis surgery were randomly assigned to receive ANH or standard fluid management, the combined intraoperative blood loss and postoperative blood loss was large enough in the ANH group that the volume of reinfused blood was inadequate to avoid allogeneic transfusion in the majority of patients. If preoperative hematocrit level had been higher, more blood could have been obtained and used for reinfusion. Therefore, the use of preoperative EPO and iron combined with ANH can potentially prove beneficial.

Cell salvage

Cell salvage is a technique by which blood lost during a procedure is processed in a way that can be given safely back to the patient in the form of fresh platelet-free autologous packed red cells with normal oxygen affinity; however, it has no clotting factor potential.

Early models of cell salvage devices required large shed-blood volumes before processing for reinfusion, making their use technically difficult in pediatric populations. Newer models use smaller processing reservoirs, making this issue less of a problem, therefore extending their usability to smaller patients. Some have argued that at least 2 units of blood needed to be recovered for cost-effectiveness.[23] However, a study by Nicolai and colleagues[24] found that cell saving technique was extremely beneficial in children with cerebral palsy undergoing acetabuloplasty; they found allogeneic blood transfusion was avoided in 82% of patients. Similarly, cell salvage was found useful in limiting allogeneic blood transfusion in infants undergoing surgical correction of craniosynostosis.[25,26] Concerns about renal injury, coagulopathy, and cytokine activation with unwashed red cell reinfusion are the same for children as for adults.[6]

Deliberate hypotension

Deliberate hypotension (DH) is the technique of purposely lowering the blood pressure through the use of intravenous agents or inhaled anesthetic agents leading to less blood loss. Concerns regarding impaired oxygen delivery to tissues during hypotension are not as significant in children compared with adults with preexisting atherosclerotic disease of the heart, brain, or kidney. However, caution still must be taken in the pediatric population. According to Gibson,[27] DH can obscure the findings of spinal cord monitoring during surgical correction of scoliosis secondary to spinal cord hypoperfusion. To avoid spinal cord hypoperfusion, there is now less reliance on DH and an emphasis on proper patient positioning and the use of antifibrinolytics in patients undergoing scoliosis repair. However, as with other blood conservation techniques, DH has its application in a chosen population undergoing specific surgeries. It has been found to significantly reduce blood loss and surgery time and to improve surgical operative conditions by enhancing visualization and allowing better delineation and dissection of lesions and structures.[28,29] Dolman and colleagues[30] compared DH to normotension in a randomized, double-blind, controlled study in patients scheduled to have Le Fort I osteotomies. They found that the quality of the surgical field was improved, and there was a significant reduction in blood loss.

Contraindications to DH in children are similar to those in adults: any pathology involving significant reduction in the availability of oxygen to the tissues, including decreased oxygen saturation, cardiac output, or anemia; cardiac, cerebral, or renal disease; and increased intracranial pressure. Factors enhancing the safety of the technique include the proper selection of cases, maintenance of near-normal acid-base balance, accurate monitoring of pressure, maintenance of high arterial oxygen tension, and avoidance of hyperventilation, as this may significantly reduce cerebral blood flow.[28] Of all the hemodynamic variables, mean arterial pressure correlates best to the degree of blood-loss reduction.[14]

Pharmacologic agents: aprotinin, ε-aminocaproic acid and tranexamic acid

In discussions of pharmacologic agents to reduce bleeding, the drug aprotinin usually receives significant attention. However, because of newer studies, especially the BART study[31] from 2008, which raised serious safety concerns, aprotinin has been removed from the market by its maker, Bayer. It can only be used for investigational purposes according to the Food and Drug Administration (FDA).[32] Its use in children for reducing blood loss in a variety of procedures has been mixed; many of its beneficial effects with respect to bleeding were reported in studies involving adults only.

ε-Aminocaproic acid and tranexamic acid are synthetic lysine analogs that competitively inhibit activation of plasminogen to plasmin, thus serving as alternatives to aprotinin. Tranexamic acid has a longer half-life, is 7 to 10 times more potent, and is more active in tissue than aminocaproic acid, with no greater toxicity.[15] Studies on aminocaproic acid and tranexamic acid in children have been promising. Chauhan and colleagues[33] compared the efficacy of aminocaproic acid and tranexamic acid in reducing postoperative blood loss and blood and blood product requirements in children with cyanotic congenital heart disease. Children from age 2 months to 14.5 years (150 total) underwent corrective surgery on CPB. Patients were randomized into 3 groups based on receiving aminocaproic acid, tranexamic acid, or no antifibrinolytic (control). The control group had the maximum blood loss at 24 hours and maximum requirements of blood products. There was no significant difference in postoperative blood loss or blood product requirement in the two groups given antifibrinolytics; however, both agents were equally effective compared with controls. Similar beneficial effects have been shown in noncardiac surgery. Studies in scoliosis surgery,[34,35] despite different dosing between studies, demonstrated a reduction in blood loss and allogeneic blood transfusion requirements in pediatric patients. A Cochrane systematic review of antifibrinolytic agents[36] concluded similarly.

Surgical technique

Surgical technique is an integral component of both blood loss and blood conservation. There are well-established and seemingly obvious aspects of surgical technique that have had a profound impact on blood component usage for years, such as electrocautery and the application of tourniquets. Some newer developments such as fibrin sealants have also significantly changed surgical practice. Fibrin sealant is prepared from two plasma-derived protein fractions: a fibrinogen-rich concentrate and a thrombin concentrate.[37] Mixing fibrinogen and thrombin mimics the last step of the blood coagulation cascade, resulting in formation of a fibrin clot that adheres to the application site and acts as a fluid-tight sealing agent able to stop bleeding. Resorption of the clot is achieved within days to weeks following application. It has been used to successfully reduce the amount of clotting factor replacement in children with hemophilia A undergoing circumcision.[38] As this product is derived from donor plasma, one must keep in mind the potential for transmission of infection. The fibrinogen and thrombin fractions are exposed to several robust viral inactivation steps, such as solvent-detergent, pasteurization, vapor-heat treatment, and nanofiltration. However, there have been case reports of possible transmission of parvovirus B19 (B19V) by 1 commercial product identified in Japan. Implementation of nucleic acid tests to screen for B19V may reduce this risk.[37]

Temperature control
Infants, particularly the neonate, are highly susceptible to hypothermia in the operating room environment. There is a fairly high rate of heat loss in proportion to heat production in the infant; this is caused by an immature thermoregulatory mechanism, a relatively thin layer of subcutaneous brown fat for insulation,[39] and extensive superficial circulation that facilitates rapid dissipation of heat from the body. Studies dating back to the 1970s have demonstrated the effect of hypothermia on coagulation in the newborn. Chadd and Gray[40] found that infants whose temperature was allowed to drift to 34°C and below had a reduced platelet count and prolonged thrombin times. Hypothermia-related coagulation disorders are caused by anomalies in clotting factor enzyme function, platelet function, and fibrinolytic activity.[41]

TRANSFUSION TRIGGERS

There is little evidence to suggest absolute levels at which one should transfuse blood products to patients. However, there are certain "accepted" levels or "triggers," as reported in the latest American Society of Anesthesiologists (ASA) Practice Guidelines.[42] Although these guidelines were targeted for adult patients and not infants or neonates, these recommendations, for lack of other evidence, are often extrapolated to younger patient groups. When discussing transfusion triggers surrounding surgery, findings in the medical history, physical examination, and preoperative testing will likely have significant impact. For example, one's threshold for red cell transfusion may be different for the cyanotic patient versus the acyanotic patient. Also, a patient with certain religious preferences (eg, Jehovah's Witness) may persuade one to consider a lower trigger than in patients without such preferences. These types of factors, and thus the preoperative evaluation and preparation, cannot be ignored when discussing transfusion triggers. A good understanding of factors affecting thresholds for transfusion can lead to better use of blood products and therefore conservation.

Red Cells and Whole Blood

Transfusion of red cells, whether in the form of packed red blood cells or whole blood, is intended to increase the red cell mass within the bloodstream, with potential benefits to blood pressure, viscosity, and oxygen carrying capacity. Generally, most practitioners use the hemoglobin or hematocrit to determine when such a transfusion should occur. As stated earlier, the absolute level at which this should occur has not been well established. However, according to the latest practice guidelines from the ASA Task Force on perioperative blood transfusion and adjuvant therapies, a hemoglobin level less than 6 g/dL generally requires red cell transfusion, and a hemoglobin level greater than 10 g/dL generally does not require red cell transfusion.[42] Within that range, whether one administers red cells to the infant or child patient will depend on their vital signs, adequacy of oxygenation and perfusion, acuity and degree of blood loss, and other physiologic and surgical factors. Above that range, the decision to administer red blood cells to a neonate or infant should take into account a high baseline concentration of hemoglobin, high oxygen consumption, and high affinity of residual fetal hemoglobin for oxygen. In addition, the patient's absolute blood volume (85 mL/kg in full-term neonate, 100 mL/kg in preterm neonate) should also be considered, especially in procedures where considerable blood loss is expected, and initial vigorous replacement with crystalloid followed by red cell transfusion rather than just red cell replacement may be unfavorable from the standpoint of volume status.

Therefore, the threshold for red cell transfusion in a healthy neonate may be much higher than that outlined in the Task Force guidelines, especially in nonhealthy neonates, for example, those with significant lung disease requiring mechanical ventilation, cyanotic congenital heart disease and/or heart failure, or chronic lung disease.[43,44] For the preterm infant, one must keep in mind that the risks of hypovolemia, hypotension, acidosis, and postoperative apnea may be amplified in the setting of operative blood loss and anemia.

Platelet Concentrates

Transfusion of platelet concentrates, whether in the form of single whole blood platelets, pooled platelet units, or apheresis units, is designed to increase the platelet volume, which is necessary for primary hemostasis. Consensus committees have reviewed platelet concentrate use and report similar guidelines: generally, platelet counts less than $50 \times 10^9/L$ will require platelet transfusion in the perioperative period, whereas platelet counts greater than $100 \times 10^9/L$ usually do not.[8,45] Within that range, the decision to transfuse platelets depends on the patient's underlying condition, prior platelet transfusions, surgical bleeding, and all other factors that may affect platelet function and turnover. Procedure-related effects (eg, CPB) may warrant even higher transfusion thresholds. Consideration of medication effects on platelet function may also encourage higher thresholds in the setting of surgical bleeding, especially for patients still on aspirin or nonsteroidal antiinflammatory medications. Sevoflurane and propofol have demonstrated platelet inhibition properties in vitro that may show to be deleterious in vivo and therefore may play a role in the decision to transfuse platelets.[46]

Fresh Frozen Plasma and Cryoprecipitate

Transfusion of FFP in the setting of coagulation is designed to increase primary clotting factors in the blood, whereas cryoprecipitate is designed to increase fibrinogen levels and factor VIII and vonWillebrand factor, all of which are necessary for normal clotting function. The guidelines for FFP transfusion state that generally FFP is indicated when correcting microvascular bleeding in the presence of a prothrombin time greater than 1.5 times normal or an international normalized ratio over 2.0.[42] It may also be necessary for acute warfarin reversal or heparin resistance (antithrombin III deficiency).

Cryoprecipitate transfusion is considered appropriate with fibrinogen counts less than 100 mg/dL in the presence of microvascular bleeding. It may also be useful in patients with vonWillebrand disease, where specific concentrates are unavailable for treatment. Transfusion of cryoprecipitate may be necessary at higher fibrinogen levels, when bleeding persists despite replacement of both FFP and platelets.

Transfusion Algorithms

Implementation of algorithms based on guidelines for transfusion thresholds have shown a reduction in blood replacement in some settings. Mallett and colleagues,[47] in an audit of their transfusion practices, revealed that there were several instances where blood transfusion was instituted with hemoglobin levels greater than 10 g/dL. After implementing a simple protocol of measuring a hemoglobin concentration before transfusion coupled with a transfusion algorithm based on patient ASA status, they demonstrated a 43% reduction in red cell transfusions for several types of noncardiac surgery, with no change in outcomes. In another study by Brevig and colleagues,[48] the use of a Blood Conservation Coordinator, whose job was to optimize cardiac patients' preoperative conditions, especially anemia (eg, checking iron stores), led to a decrease in red cell transfusions from 43% to 18% during a 4-year period. Conservation techniques were not only limited to preoperative optimization but were also coupled with standardization of surgical and postoperative techniques. Modifying variable transfusion practices based on reasonable thresholds for transfusion of blood products should remain a significant blood conservation strategy.

Recombinant Factor VIIa

Recombinant activated factor VIIa (NovoSeven; Novo Nordisk, Copenhagen, Denmark) is a drug approved for use in patients bleeding from complications of hemophilia. It is increasingly being used "off-label" for the treatment of acute hemorrhage resulting from non-hemophilia–related events, such as surgery and trauma. It remains attractive for these indications because of its supposedly "local" response to bleeding. Normally, activated factor VII (VIIa) interacts with exposed tissue factor (TF) at endothelial disruption sites, creating a complex that readily converts factor X to its activated form, which serves to convert prothrombin to thrombin, the main substance needed for clot formation. The recombinant form of factor VII (rVIIa) acts in the same way as endogenous VIIa, leading to significant thrombin generation. Therefore, it needs to complex with exposed TF to initiate its effects of thrombin formation. Because of its "supposed" local response, complications rates of thromboembolism have been considered to be low by many. However, there remain very few data to support this notion, because most of its off-label use has been reported in case reports and retrospective reviews in adult populations.

Despite the scarcity of data, one can hypothesize how rVIIa could potentially serve as a means for improved blood conservation. Jen and Shew[49] report their review of 32 nonhemophiliac infants who received rVIIa at their institution in critical bleeding situations. They demonstrated a significant reduction in red cell transfusion during the 8 hours after receiving rVIIA by around 36 mL/kg compared with the previous 8 hours. They also showed significant reductions in platelet and cryoprecipitate transfusions. Although none of the patients in their group who required extracorporeal circulation support had any signs of clots, there were 4 other patients of the 32 (13%) who did have "spontaneous" thromboembolism complications after receiving rVIIa. However, they claimed it was not related to the number or size of the doses. The overall survival of the 32 patients was around 34%.

In one of the few randomized controlled trials that compared rVIIa in its off-label use in pediatrics, Ekert and colleagues[50] looked at its usefulness in infant cardiac surgery patients to significantly reduce blood usage. As opposed to the previous study that looked at critically ill patients with significant ongoing bleeding, this study chose patients at risk of bleeding and chose to use rVIIa prophylactically. Doses of rVIIa were given after patients separated from cardiopulmonary bypass and had been reversed from the effects of heparin with protamine. In this study, there were no differences in the amount of red cell or platelet transfusions. Despite a significantly decreased prothrombin time in the rVIIa group compared with placebo, the time to chest closure was actually longer in the rVIIa group. The case reports and retrospective studies certainly suggest rVIIa as potentially playing a role in blood conservation for certain situations in pediatrics; however, this randomized study keeps the debate open.

THE CARDIAC PATIENT

Patients undergoing congenital cardiac surgery represent a unique population with regards to blood conservation. Certainly, most of the techniques described thus far in this review apply to this population; however, there are aspects of these surgeries that bear further mention. One of the unique aspects of these cases is the use of CPB to facilitate surgical exposure and repair. A consequence of CPB is the requirement for anticoagulation to prevent clots forming in the CPB pump. Heparin is the predominant anticoagulant during CPB; however, patients with allergy or immune reactions to heparin will require the use of direct thrombin inhibitors. One of the benefits of heparin is that there is an agent to "reverse" its effects, namely protamine, which is not the case with direct thrombin inhibitors. Furthermore, CPB also has systemic effects that essentially disrupt the normal regulatory pathways of coagulation. The mechanism of this disruption is still under debate and is clearly multifactorial in nature.

Much of the research into the mechanisms of blood loss in these surgeries has centered on specific interventions, such as using antifibrinolytic agents, using biocompatible surfaces in the CPB pump tubing to reduce activation of hemostatic processes, reducing the reinfusion of shed blood during the surgery, and reducing the degree of hemodilution (especially true for children), to name a few. It is becoming clearer that combining several of these interventions may be necessary to significantly affect bleeding and promote blood conservation.[51]

SUMMARY

There is little doubt that management of bleeding in the neonate, infant, or child presents its own set of dilemmas and challenges. One of the primary problems that perioperative pediatric physicians have to deal with is the lack of good scientific evidence regarding the best management strategies for children rather than for adults; this scenario is unlikely to change dramatically in the near future. This leaves us reliant on extrapolated adult data, and we are all too aware that children are not just small adults.

The key to success in the predicament is firstly to ensure that the physician has a clear understanding of the underlying normal physiology of the young child's hematologic status. Then by adding knowledge of the abnormal pathology that is being presented, the physician can at least understand what anomalies he or she is facing. Once all the available information has been well digested—concerning the patient's clinical condition and the options available—a multidisciplinary approach allows the optimal use of all available resources. Good teamwork, understanding, and communication between all vested parties allows for a synergistic relationship to enhance patient care and to give the best available end result.

REFERENCES

1. Ferraris VA, Ferraris SP, Saha SP, et al. The Society of Thoracic Surgeons & the Society of Cardiovascular Anesthesiologists. Perioperative blood transfusion and blood conservation in cardiac surgery: clinical practice guideline. Ann Thorac Surg 2007;83:S27–86.
2. Goodnough LT, Shander A, Breccher ME. Transfusion medicine: looking to the future. Lancet 2003;361:161–9.
3. AuBuchon JP, Birkmeyer JD, Busch MP. Safety of the blood supply in the United States: opportunities and controversies. Ann Intern Med 1997;127:904–9.
4. Bilgin YM, van de Watering LM, Eijsman L, et al. Double-blind randomized controlled trial on the effect of leukocyte-depleted erythrocyte transfusions in cardiac valve surgery. Circulation 2004;109:2755–60.
5. Siliman CC, Paterson AJ, Dickey WO, et al. The association of biologically active lipids with the development of transfusion-related acute lung injury: a retrospective study. Transfusion 1997;37:719–26.
6. Weldon CB. Blood conservation in pediatric anesthesia. Anesthesiol Clin North America 2005;23:347–61.
7. Hume HA, Limoges P. Perioperative blood transfusion therapy in pediatric patients. Am J Ther 2002;9:396–405.
8. Gibson BE, Todd A, Roberts I, et al. The British Committee for Standards in Haematology. Transfusion guidelines for neonates and older children. Br J Haematol 2004;124:433–53.
9. McEwan A. Aspects of bleeding after cardiac surgery in children. Paediatr Anaesth 2007;17:1126–33.
10. Williams MD, Chalmers EA, Gibson BE. The investigation and management of neonatal haemostasis and thrombosis. Br J Haematol 2002;119:295–309.
11. Monagle P, Michelson A, Bovil E, et al. Antithrombotic therapy in children. Chest 2001;119(1 Suppl):344S–70S.
12. Goodnough LT, Shander AS. Recombinant factor VIIa: safety and efficacy. Curr Opin Hematol 2007;14(5):504–9.
13. Jadhav MN, Lobdell D, Stanitski D, et al. Use of preoperative erythropoietin in children undergoing major surgery to reduce the need for allogenic blood transfusions [abstract]. Pediatr Res 1998;43(2 Suppl):134.
14. Meara JG, Smith EM, Harshbarger RJ, et al. Blood-conservation techniques in craniofacial surgery. Ann Plast Surg 2005;54:525–59.
15. Auer IK. The role of pharmacologic agents in blood conservation. AACN Clin Issues 1996;7:260–76.
16. Streitz SL, Hickey PR. Cardiovascular physiology and pharmacology in children: normal and diseased pediatric cardiovascular systems. In: Cote, Ryan, Todres, editors. A practice of anesthesia for infants and children. 2nd edition. Philadelphia: WB Saunders; 1993. p. 271–89.
17. Murto KT, Splinter WM. Perioperative autologous blood donation in children. Transfus Sci 1999;21:41–62.
18. Longatti PL, Paccagnella F, Agostini S, et al. Autologous hemodonation in the corrective surgery of craniostenosis. Childs Nerv Syst 1991;7:40–2.
19. Letts M, Perng R, Luke B, et al. An analysis of a preoperative pediatric autologous blood donation program. Can J Surg 2000;43(2):125–9.
20. Friesen, Perryman KM, Weigers KR, et al. A trial of fresh autologous whole blood to treat dilutional coagulopathy following cardiopulmonary bypass in infants. Paediatr Anaesth 2006;16(4):429–35.

21. Pouliquen-Evrard M, Mangin F, Pouliquen JC, et al. Autotransfusion and hemodilution in orthopaedic surgery in children. Rev Chir Orthop Reparatrice Appar Mot 1981;67:609–15.
22. Hans P, Collin V, Bonhomme V, et al. Evaluation of acute normovolemic hemodilution for surgical repair of craniosynostosis. J Neurosurg Anesthesiol 2000;12(1): 33–6.
23. Goodnough LT, Mont TG, Sicard G, et al. Intraoperative salvage in patients undergoing elective abdominal aortic aneurysm repair; an analysis of cost and benefit. J Vasc Surg 1996;24:213–8.
24. Nicolai P, Leggetter PP, Glithero PR, et al. Autologous transfusion in acetobuloplasty in children. J Bone Joint Surg Br 2004;86:110–2.
25. Jimenez DF, Barone CM. Intraoperative autologous blood transfusion in the surgical correction of craniosynostosis. Neurosurgery 1995;37:1075–9.
26. Fearon JA. Reducing allogeneic blood transfusions during pediatric cranial vault surgical procedures: a prospective analysis of blood recycling. Plast Reconstr Surg 2004;113:1126–30.
27. Gibson PR. Anaesthesia for correction of scoliosis in children [Review]. Anaesth Intensive Care 2004;32(4):548–59.
28. Salem MR, Wong AY, Bennett EJ, et al. Deliberate hypotension in infants and children. Anesth Analg 1974;53:975.
29. Diaz JH, Lockhart CH, et al. Deliberate hypotension for craniectomies in infancy. Br J Anaesth 1979;51:233.
30. Dolman RM, Bentley KC, Head TW, et al. The effect of hypotensive anesthesia on blood loss and operative time during Le Fort I osteotomies. J Oral Maxillofac Surg 2000;58(8):834–9.
31. Fergusson DA, Hébert PC, Mazer CD, et al. A comparison of aprotinin and lysine analogues in high-risk cardiac surgery. N Engl J Med 2008;358(22):2319–31.
32. Available at: http://www.fda.gov/CDER/DRUG/infopage/aprotinin/default.htm. Accessed May, 2008.
33. Chauhan S, Das SN, Bisoi A, et al. Comparison of epsilon aminocaproic acid and tranexamic acid in pediatric cardiac surgery. J Cardiothorac Vasc Anesth 2004; 18(2):141–3.
34. Senthna NF, Zurakowski D, Brustowicz RM, et al. Tranexamic acid reduces intraoperative blood loss in pediatric patients undergoing scoliosis surgery. Anesthesiology 2005;102:727–32.
35. Neilipovitz DT, Murto K, Hall L, et al. A randomized trial of tranexamic acid to reduce blood transfusion for scoliosis surgery. Anesth Analg 2001;93:82–7.
36. Tzortzopoulou A, Cepeda MS, Schumann R, et al. Antifibrinolytic agents for reducing blood loss in scoliosis surgery in children. Cochrane Database Syst Rev 2008;3:CD006883.
37. Burnouf T, Radosevich M, Goubran HA. Local hemostatic blood products: fibrin sealant and platelet gel. Treatment of Hemophilia 2004;36:1–7.
38. Kavakli K, Kurugol Z, Goksen D, et al. Should haemophiliac patients be circumcised? Pediatr Hematol Oncol 2000;17(2):149–53.
39. Phillips NF, Berry EC, Kohn ML et al. Room technique; 2003. p. 123.
40. Chadd MA, Gray OP. Hypothermia and coagulation defects in the newborn. Arch Dis Child 1972;47(255):819–21.
41. Doufas AG. Consequences of inadvertent perioperative hypothermia. Best Pract Res Clin Anaesthesiol 2003;17:535–49.
42. American Society of Anesthesiologists Task Force on Perioperative Blood Transfusion and Adjuvant Therapies. Practice guidelines for perioperative blood

transfusion and adjuvant therapies: an updated report by the American Society of Anesthesiologists Task Force on Perioperative Blood Transfusion and Adjuvant Therapies. Anesthesiology 2006;105(1):198–208.

43. Simon TL, Alverson DC, AuBuchon J, et al. Practice parameter for the use of red blood cell transfusions: developed by the Red Blood Cell Administration Practice Guideline Development Task Force of the College of American Pathologists. Arch Pathol Lab Med 1998;122(2):130–8.

44. Gibson BE, Todd A, Roberts I, et al. Transfusion guidelines for neonates and older children. Br J Haematol 2004;124(4):433–53.

45. Samama CM, et al. Perioperative platelet transfusion: recommendations of the Agence française de sécurité sanitaire des produits de santé (AFSSaPS) 2003. Can J Anaesth 2005;52(1):30–7.

46. Dogan IV, Ovali E, Eti Z, et al. The in vitro effects of isoflurane, sevoflurane, and propofol on platelet aggregation. Anesth Analg 1999;88(2):432–6.

47. Mallett SV, Peachey TD, Sanehi O, et al. Reducing red blood cell transfusion in elective surgical patients: the role of audit and practice guidelines. Anaesthesia 2000;55(10):1013–9.

48. Brevig J, McDonald J, Zelinka ES, et al. Blood transfusion reduction in cardiac surgery: multidisciplinary approach at a community hospital. Ann Thorac Surg 2009;87(2):532–9.

49. Jen H, Shew S. Recombinant activated factor VII use in critically ill infants with active hemorrhage. J Pediatr Surg 2008;43(12):2235–8.

50. Ekert H, Brizard C, Eyers R, et al. Elective administration in infants of low-dose recombinant activated factor VII (rFVIIa) in cardiopulmonary bypass surgery for congenital heart disease does not shorten time to chest closure or reduce blood loss and need for transfusions: a randomized, double-blind, parallel group, placebo-controlled study of rFVIIa and standard haemostatic replacement therapy versus standard haemostatic replacement therapy. Blood Coagul Fibrinolysis 2006;17(5):389–95.

51. Eisses MJ, Seidel K, Aldea GS, et al. Reducing hemostatic activation during cardiopulmonary bypass: a combined approach. Anesth Analg 2004;98(5):1208–16.

BONUS ARTICLE:
Monitoring Endocrine Function

Vivek Moitra, MD, Robert N. Sladen, MB, ChB, MRCP, FRCP, FCCM

Edited by Stanley H. Rosenbaum, MD

Monitoring Endocrine Function

Vivek Moitra, MD, Robert N. Sladen, MB, ChB, MRCP, FRCP, FCCM*

KEYWORDS

- Monitoring • Endocrine • Diabetes • Thyroid disease
- Adrenal disease • Pheochromocytoma • Carcinoid

DIABETES MELLITUS

Diabetes mellitus is a systemic disorder characterized by absolute or relative lack of insulin, resulting in abnormal carbohydrate metabolism, hyperglycemia, and diffuse vasculopathy. The underlying comorbidity and consequences of poor perioperative glycemic control present unique challenges in the monitoring of the surgical patient with diabetes. Perioperative glycemic control is impeded by multiple factors that affect blood sugar and pancreatic function, including surgical stress, acute illness, anorexia and fasting, and the masking of hypoglycemic signs and symptoms by β-blockade and anesthetics.

Glycosylated Hemoglobin: A Monitor of Long-term Glucose Control

Hemoglobin undergoes continuous nonenzymatic glycation by glucose at the N-terminal valine residue of the β chain, resulting in a series of glycohemoglobins, the most prevalent of which is hemoglobin A1c (HbA1c). Cation-exchange chromatography can be used to measure HbA1c levels. The concentration of HbA1c provides a measurement of long-term glycemic control, and may be helpful in the early detection of diabetes mellitus.

The American Diabetes Association currently recommends a target HbA1c of less than 7% for patients with type 2 diabetes. Studies support the theory that lower levels of HbA1c are associated with a reduction in microvascular and neuropathic complications. In a large retrospective meta-analysis, an increase in HbA1c was associated with a greater risk of cardiovascular events;[1] elevation of HbA1c was associated with cardiac morbidity and mortality independent of a diagnosis of diabetes. These results suggest that the risk for coronary heart disease correlates with glucose control regardless of whether a patient is diabetic.[2]

In the management of intracranial hypertension, cerebral perfusion pressure may be decreased by increasing cerebral vascular tone through induced mild hypocapnia. In

Division of Critical Care, Department of Anesthesiology, PH 527-B, College of Physicians and Surgeons of Columbia University, 630 West 168th St, New York, NY 10032, USA
* Corresponding author.
E-mail address: rs543@columbia.edu (R.N. Sladen).

Anesthesiology Clin 27 (2009) 355–364
doi:10.1016/j.anclin.2009.05.005   **anesthesiology.theclinics.com**

patients with diabetes the vasomotor response to carbon dioxide, as measured by transcranial Doppler, is impaired, and the degree of impairment correlates with the levels of HbA1c.[3] This finding implies that long-term glucose control may play a role in the regulation of cerebral vasoreactivity in patients with diabetes. Abnormalities from autonomic neuropathy of the enteric nervous system are common among patients with diabetes.[4] Short-term hyperglycemia and poor long-term glycemic control delay gastric emptying,[5] resulting in increased gastric fluid volume and risk of aspiration at anesthetic induction. Routine use of preoperative promotility agents such as metoclopramide is advocated in practice guidelines for patients with diabetes to reduce pulmonary aspiration.[6] However, a recently conducted prospective trial demonstrated that after 8 hours of fasting, gastric fluid volumes are small and clinically inconsequential in patients with type 1 and type 2 diabetes. The investigators concluded that prokinetic therapy may be essential only for patients with poorly controlled diabetes and HbA1c values greater than 9%.[7]

When glycemic control is poor, serum and tissue proteins are glycosylated, and abnormal collagen is deposited in connective tissues and joints. Patients with diabetes with a history of chronic hyperglycemia may consequently develop stiff joint syndrome, resulting in impaired joint mobility. When the cervical and atlanto-occipital joints are involved, airway exposure and laryngoscopy may become difficult. The risk of limited joint mobility increases as HbA1c values increase, but there are currently no data to show that poor glycemic control is predictive of difficult airway management.[8]

Hyperglycemia: A Monitor of Illness Severity

Observational studies of surgical patients suggest that hyperglycemia is associated with increased hospital stay, admission to the intensive care unit, postoperative infections, neurologic events, and the risk of in-hospital mortality.[9,10] Patients with newly diagnosed hyperglycemia, which likely represented undiagnosed diabetes, prediabetes, or stress-induced hyperglycemia, had a higher in-hospital mortality than patients with known diabetes and hyperglycemia. Blood glucose values were not statistically different in both groups.[10]

Hyperglycemia has emerged as an outcome marker in diverse settings. Several studies have demonstrated a correlation between blood glucose and the development of congestive heart failure in patients with and without diabetes after a myocardial infarction.[11–13] After ischemic stroke, the presence of hyperglycemia is associated with reduced functional capacity, decreased penumbral salvage, and increased final infarction size.[14,15] Trauma patients without diabetes who have hyperglycemia on admission have a greater risk for longer hospital stay, and increased infection rate and mortality.[16] Although an elevated blood glucose level often reflects the severity of illness and the stress response, it may itself contribute to organ injury and should be regarded as a reversible, treatable, and independent determinant of outcome.

Perioperative Glycemic Monitoring

There is considerable evidence that poor intraoperative glucose control may increase postoperative morbidity and exacerbate postoperative complications such as wound infection or sternal dehiscence after cardiac surgery.[17,18] However, there is no well-established parameter for intraoperative "normoglycemia." The demonstration that postoperative tight glucose control (80–110 mg/dL) can dramatically decrease morbidity and long-term mortality[19] has received an enormous amount of attention. However, surgical stress makes it difficult to maintain intraoperative normoglycemia, even with carefully controlled anesthesia. This situation is exacerbated during nonphysiologic circulatory states such as cardiopulmonary bypass (CPB). The secretion of large quantities of counterregulatory hormones such as epinephrine, glucagons, and cortisol establishes a state of relative glucose intolerance and insulin resistance. High doses of insulin may be required to induce normoglycemia, but soon after surgery the levels of these hormones rapidly decline and patients may be at increased risk for hypoglycemia.[20]

Nonetheless, several protocols have been offered for intraoperative glucose management that predictably and safely achieve strict glucose control.[17,18,21,22] These have ranged from simple, cost-effective glucose-insulin protocols to achieve normoglycemia in low-risk patients with diabetes scheduled for elective surgery[22] to more complex glucose-insulin-potassium regimens that have improved outcome in cardiac surgery patients.[17] The "glucose clamp" (hyperinsulinemic normoglycemic clamp technique) is an alternative approach to overcome insulin resistance during CPB, in which the dose of the insulin infusion is fixed, and a dextrose infusion is titrated to achieve normoglycemia.[21]

Preoperative hyperglycemia and renal failure may predict difficulty in intraoperative glucose control. Intraoperative normoglycemia is especially difficult in patients with diabetes with initial blood glucose values of more than 300 mg/dL, and glucose control in advance of surgery can facilitate intraoperative management.[23] A low insulin infusion rate and frequent glucose monitoring may prevent intraoperative hypoglycemia in patients with compromised renal function.[23]

THYROID DISORDERS

Patients with thyroid dysfunction who require urgent or elective surgery represent a particular challenge to anesthesiologists. An understanding of the physiology and pathophysiology of the hypothalamic-pituitary axis is a prerequisite for effective monitoring of thyroid function. The hypothalamus synthesizes thyrotropin-releasing hormone (TRH), which regulates thyroid stimulating hormone (TSH) secretion by the anterior pituitary gland. TSH stimulates the synthesis and secretion of triiodothyronine (T3) and thyroxine (T4) by the thyroid gland. T3 and T4 provide a negative feedback loop through their suppression of TRH.

Perioperative Outcomes: The Systemic Effects of Thyroid Dysfunction

Hypothyroidism and hyperthyroidism are associated with increased perioperative morbidity and mortality.[24] In the hyperthyroid patient, cardiac output and heart rate increase, pulse pressure widens, and systemic vascular resistance decreases.[25] Thyrotoxicosis is associated with a high incidence of atrial fibrillation and warrants vigilant electrocardiac monitoring during the perioperative period.[24] Close respiratory monitoring is essential because oxygen consumption (VO_2) and carbon dioxide production (VCO_2) are increased, and may coexist with ventilatory muscle weakness, decreased lung volume, and dyspnea.[26,27] Patients are extremely susceptible to hypopnea or apnea with sedative or anesthetic agents.

In the hypothyroid patient, heart rate, myocardial contractility, and cardiac output decrease.[28,29] Muscle weakness results in hypoventilation and an impaired response to hypoxia and hypercapnia.[30,31] Successful treatment of overt thyroid dysfunction has been associated with an improvement in survival. Some studies have suggested that patients with mild to moderate thyroid disease are not at a greater risk of major perioperative complications.[32,33] However, when thyroid dysfunction is severe, surgery and stress can precipitate myxedema coma or thyroid storm.[29]

Monitoring Thyroid Function

Thyroid function assays can be a useful tool to evaluate patients with thyroid disorders and to identify patients at risk for morbidity. They may be less useful or misleading with entities such as the "euthyroid sick syndrome"; subclinical hyperthyroidism (abnormal TSH levels with normal levels of free T3 and free T4); alterations in protein binding; and administration of medications such as dopamine, amiodarone, and glucocorticoids. Under these conditions, clinical, metabolic, and end organ measures may be helpful in the assessment of thyroid function.[25]

Although the prevalence of thyroid disorders remains high, there is little evidence to support the routine screening of asymptomatic patients without risk factors for thyroid disease.[34] The assessment of a patient's thyroid function begins with an evaluation of the hypothalamic pituitary axis. In patients with an intact axis and steady-state physiology, TSH levels can be used to monitor thyroid function. Small changes in thyroid hormone concentration lead to large inverse changes in TSH concentration. Current guidelines suggest using sensitive assays that can detect a TSH level of 0.02 mU/L.[35] Relying on the TSH alone can be misleading if patients have been treated recently for thyrotoxicosis or have pituitary disease, nonthyroidal illness, or thyroid hormone resistance.[36] Total T3 and T4 assays measure free (biologically active) and protein-bound (biologically inactive) hormone concentrations. Numerous drugs and systemic pathologies affect the degree of protein binding, and measurement of total thyroid hormone concentrations has been largely replaced by measurement of free hormone concentrations (ie, free T3 and T4).

Monitoring Thyroid Function in the Critically Ill or Hospitalized Patient

Evaluation of thyroid function in patients who are hospitalized is difficult and controversial. Current guidelines suggest that thyroid function tests should not be ordered for seriously ill patients unless there is a strong suspicion of thyroid disease. A TSH level alone is inadequate to assess thyroid function in the critically ill patient. Critical illness is associated with biphasic alterations in the thyroid axis irrespective of a history of thyroid disease.[37] During the first phase of stress, peripheral conversion of T4 to T3 is decreased and TSH levels increase. The initial decrease in T3 levels is related to the severity of illness.[38] During the prolonged phase of critical illness, hypothalamic stimulation is impaired and T3 and T4 decrease without an increase in TSH; indeed an increase in TSH in the critically ill patient may indicate recovery from severe illness.[39]

Treatment of Hypothyroidism and Hyperthyroidism

The primary treatment of hypothyroidism is thyroid hormone replacement therapy. In primary hypothyroidism, TSH concentrations can be used to monitor this treatment. Free T4 is an insensitive indicator and may be within the normal range when TSH is inhibited. However, measurement of free T4 is warranted in secondary hypothyroidism when TSH release is impaired. The treatments for hyperthyroidism are antithyroid drugs, radioiodine, or surgery. TSH levels are useful for the diagnosis of hyperthyroidism, but not for determining its degree of severity. Therefore, measuring free T3 and T4 is necessary to assess the efficacy of treatment. Once steady state is achieved, TSH can be used to assess the efficacy of therapy.

PARATHYROID DISORDERS

Parathyroid hormone (PTH) regulates the extracellular calcium concentration through its actions on the bone, kidney, and intestine; in turn, the extracellular calcium concentration is the major determinant of PTH secretion.[40]

Monitoring Hypoparathyroidism

Patients may develop hypoparathyroidism and hypocalcemia after thyroidectomy or removal of a parathyroid adenoma. Hypoparathyroidism may also result from renal resistance to parathyroid hormone. Ionized serum and urine calcium should be monitored at regular intervals preoperatively. Severe hypocalcemia may be associated with prolonged QT interval and a predisposition to ventricular arrhythmias, notable Torsades des Pointes.[40] It may also impair cardiac contractility and vascular tone, but levels are seldom low enough to interfere with coagulation.

Monitoring Hyperparathyroidism

Primary hyperparathyroidism, a common cause of hypercalcemia, is most often associated with parathyroid adenomas. Surgical candidates present with several risk factors. They are more likely to be taking antihypertensive medications; exhibit T-wave abnormalities and ST-segment depressions on ECG, and have a history of congestive heart failure, thromboembolic disease, stroke, or diabetes.[41] Hypercalcemia enhances digitalis toxicity.[40]

Preoperative imaging of patients undergoing parathyroid surgery includes ultrasonography or sestamibi scanning of the parathyroid glands to facilitate an operative approach.[42] Traditionally, successful parathyroidectomy depended on inspection of all four parathyroid glands with a complete neck dissection. This procedure increases the risk of inadvertent recurrent laryngeal nerve damage.[43] The use of intraoperative PTH assays can ensure complete parathyroid extirpation without a complete neck dissection, thus decreasing patient morbidity and the incidence of persistent postoperative hypercalcemia.[42,44]

PHEOCHROMOCYTOMA

Pheochromocytomas are catecholamine-secreting tumors composed of chromaffin tissue derived from the embryonic neural crest.[45,46] Manipulation of the pheochromocytoma during surgical resection releases boluses of catecholamines that may induce significant hemodynamic perturbation, morbidity, and even mortality. Persistent hemodynamic fluctuations are also possible after tumor removal.[47] Improvements in perioperative outcomes and reductions in mortality have been associated with improvements in preoperative and intraoperative monitoring.[46]

Preoperative Monitoring

The improvement in perioperative outcomes for patients undergoing pheochromocytoma resection has been attributed in part to more effective preoperative α- and β-adrenergic blockade.[48] This facilitates preoperative intravascular volume repletion and attenuates the catecholamine surges associated with intraoperative tumor manipulation. Preoperative monitoring of cardiac function starts with careful history taking and physical examination focusing on the presence of a catecholamine-induced cardiomyopathy. Preoperative α- and β-adrenergic blockade can also improve cardiac function and reverse catecholamine-induced cardiomyopathy.[46,49] Echocardiography may be a useful tool for detecting cardiac dysfunction and assessing the efficacy of α-adrenergic blockade. The preoperative electrocardiogram may show prolonged Q-Tc intervals and an elevated QRS complex reflecting ventricular hypertrophy;[50] ST-segment and T-wave changes may suggest ischemia. These abnormalities can resolve in the postoperative period.[51] Recommendations have been made for monitoring the adequacy of preoperative pharmacologic therapy.

The adequacy of preoperative α-adrenergic blockade is established by a blood pressure consistently less than 160/90 mmHg, orthostatic hypotension, resolution of ST-segment abnormalities, and infrequent premature ventricular contractions.[52]

Intraoperative Monitoring

Adverse perioperative events are more likely to occur with large tumors and prolonged duration of anesthesia, and elevations in urinary vanillylmandelic acid, epinephrine, norepinephrine, and metanephrine have been implicated. Despite the use of α- and β-adrenergic blockade, patients who were premedicated continued to manifest significant intraoperative hemodynamic lability.[48] Because catecholamine surges are expected with laryngoscopy and intubation, an intra-arterial catheter should be placed before induction of anesthesia and together with a central venous catheter will facilitate the titration of rapidly acting vasodilators and vasopressors throughout the operation. Arrhythmias and hypertension may result from skin incision or during tumor manipulation. Profound hypotension requiring norepinephrine infusion may occur because of persistent α-adrenergic blockade, inadequate volume repletion, and low plasma norepinephrine after tumor removal, in the face of α-receptor downregulation. Blood glucose levels should be monitored frequently because elevated catecholamine levels depress insulin release and cause hyperglycemia.[46]

ADRENAL INSUFFICIENCY

An intact hypothalamic-pituitary-adrenal axis (HPA) responds to the stress of surgery, trauma, and infection by increasing adrenal output of glucocorticoids. Endogenous glucocorticoids modulate the effect of catecholamines on vascular tone, and glucocorticoid deficiency results in vasodilation and hypotension.

Monitoring Adrenal Insufficiency

Primary adrenal insufficiency is uncommon, and occurs as a consequence of autoimmune adrenalitis, tuberculosis, and HIV.[53] Electrolyte abnormalities such as hyponatremia and hyperkalemia may arise from aldosterone deficiency. Suppression of the HPA axis and adrenal insufficiency is most commonly iatrogenic in nature, induced by chronic steroid therapy for conditions such as Crohn disease, chronic obstructive pulmonary disease, asthma, and rheumatoid arthritis.

However, it has been more recently recognized that acute adrenal insufficiency may be induced in elderly or debilitated patients with acute sepsis. Provocative testing with an adrenocorticotropic hormone (ACTH) analogue (cosyntropin) can detect relative or absolute adrenal insufficiency. In patients who were septic and critically ill, with hypotension unresponsive to fluids, an increase in plasma cortisol of more than 9 μg/dL 30 minutes after cosyntropin stimulation identified those who benefited from supplemental corticosteroid therapy.[54,55] Wider application of preoperative cosyntropin testing might be useful in identifying those patients who would most benefit from perioperative adrenal support with corticosteroids.

CARCINOID TUMORS

Carcinoid tumors are rare and neuroendocrine in origin, arising from chromaffin cells in the gastrointestinal (GI) tract, and occasionally in the bronchi or lung. Carcinoid syndrome results from the release of vasoactive mediators such as serotonin, bradykinin, histamine, gastrin, and substance P.[56–58] Mediators released from carcinoid tumors in the GI tract enter the portal venous circulation and are usually metabolized by the liver before they reach the systemic circulation. Therefore, carcinoid syndrome is more likely to be discovered with metastatic GI tumors or primary tumors outside of the GI tract. Serotoninergic manifestations include hypertension induced by vasoconstriction, and increased GI motility with associated diarrhea, high gastric output, and hyperglycemia.[56] High serotonin levels have been implicated in the development of carcinoid heart disease, characterized by endocardial fibrosis of right-sided heart valves, with tricuspid regurgitation and pulmonic stenosis.[56,59] Carcinoid tumors are associated with multiple endocrine neoplasia type 1, and the presence or absence of parathyroid, pancreatic, and pituitary disease should be identified preoperatively.

Preoperative Monitoring

Preoperative monitoring of the surgical patient with a carcinoid tumor should focus on the systemic manifestations and location of the tumor. Measurement of 24-hour urinary 5-hydroxyindoleacetic acid (5-HIAA) helps to confirm carcinoid syndrome. Although 5-HIAA levels cannot predict the physiologic response to surgical manipulation of the tumor, in the presence of carcinoid heart disease, elevated 5-HIAA levels are associated with increased perioperative morbidity and mortality.[60] A full panoply of imaging studies including chest radiography, CT scans, MRI, and radionucleotide scans may be necessary to properly identify the location of the primary tumor and metastasis.[58] Bronchoscopy is indicated if a bronchial site is suspected.[57] An echocardiogram should be performed to evaluate the pulmonary and tricuspid valves.

Intraoperative Monitoring

Intraoperative monitoring should include an invasive arterial line to monitor hemodynamic changes during carcinoid crises or blood loss from resection of a vascular tumor. Central venous access is helpful for the rapid titration of vasoactive drugs, but central venous pressure monitoring must be interpreted in the context of possible right-sided valvular lesions.[56]

REFERENCES

1. Selvin E, Marinopoulos S, Berkenblit G, et al. Meta-analysis: glycosylated hemoglobin and cardiovascular disease in diabetes mellitus. Ann Intern Med 2004;141: 421–31.
2. Selvin E, Coresh J, Golden S, et al. Glycemic control and coronary heart disease risk in persons with and without diabetes. Ann Intern Med 2005;165:1910–6.
3. Kadoi Y, Hinohara H, Kunimoto F, et al. Diabetic patients have an impaired cerebral vasodilatory response to hypercapnia under propofol anesthesia. Stroke 2003;34:2399–403.
4. Dyck PJ, Kratz KM, Kaines JL, et al. The prevalence of staged severity of various types of diabetic neuropathy, retinopathy, and nephropathy in a population based cohort: the Rochester Diabetic Neuropathy Study. Neurology 1993;43:817–24.
5. Fraser RJ, Horowitz M, Maddox AF, et al. Hyperglycemia slows gastric emptying in type I diabetes mellitus. Diabetologia 1990;33:675–80.
6. Warner MA, Caplan RA, Epstein BS, et al. Practice guidelines for preoperative fasting and the use of pharmacologic agents to reduce the risk of pulmonary aspiration: application to healthy patients undergoing elective procedures. Anesthesiology 1999;90:896–905.
7. Jellish WS, Kartha V, Fluder E, et al. Effect of metoclopramide on gastric fluid volumes in diabetic patients who have fasted before elective surgery. Anesthesiology 2005;102:904–9.

8. Silverstein JH, Gordon G, Pollock BH, et al. Long-term glycemic control influences the onset of limited joint mobility in type 1 diabetes. J Pediatr 1998;132: 944–7.

9. Pomposelli J, Baxter J, Babineau T, et al. Early postoperative glucose control predicts nosocomial infection rate in diabetic patients. JPEN J Parenter Enteral Nutr 1998;22:77–81.

10. Umpierrez GE, Isaacs SD, Bazargan N, et al. Hyperglycemia: an independent marker of inhospital mortality in patients with undiagnosed diabetes. J Clin Endocrinol Metab 2002;87:978–82.

11. Bolk J, van der Ploeg T, Cornel JH, et al. Impaired glucose metabolism predicts mortality after a myocardial infarction. Int J Cardiol 2001;79:207–14.

12. Capes SE, Hunt D, Malmberg K, et al. Stress hyperglycaemia and increased risk of death after myocardial infarction in patients with and without diabetes: a systemic overview. Lancet 2000;355:773–8.

13. Malmberg K, Norhammar A, Wedel H, et al. Glycometabolic state of admission: important risk marker of mortality in conventionally treated patients with diabetes mellitus and acute myocardial infarction: long term results from the Diabetes and Insulin-Glucose Infusion in Acute Myocardial Infarction (DIGAMI) Study. Circulation 1999;99:2626–32.

14. Capes SE, Hunt D, Malmberg K, et al. Stress hyperglycemia and prognosis of stroke in non-diabetic and diabetic patients: a systematic overview. Stroke 2001;32:2426–30.

15. Parsons MW, Barber A, Desmond PM, et al. Acute hyperglycemia adversely affects stroke outcome: a magnetic resonance imaging and spectroscopy study. Ann Neurol 2002;52:20–8.

16. Sung J, Bochicchio GV, Joshi M, et al. Admission hyperglycemia is predictive of outcome in critically ill trauma patients. J Trauma 2005;59:80–3.

17. Lazar HL, Chipkin SR, Fitzgerald CA, et al. Tight glycemic control in diabetic coronary artery bypass graft patients improves perioperative outcomes and decreases recurrent ischemic events. Circulation 2004;109:1497–502.

18. Ouattara A, Lecomte P, Le Manach Y, et al. Poor intraoperative blood glucose control is associated with a worsened hospital outcome after cardiac surgery in diabetic patients. Anesthesiology 2005;103:687–94.

19. van den Berghe G, Wouters P, Weekers F, et al. Intensive insulin therapy in the critically ill patients. N Engl J Med 2001;345:1359–67.

20. Chaney MA, Nikolov MP, Blakeman BP, et al. Attempting to maintain normoglycemia during cardiopulmonary bypass with insulin may initiate postoperative hypoglycemia. Anesth Analg 1999;89:1091–5.

21. Carvalho G, Moore A, Qizilbash B, et al. Maintenance of normoglycemia during cardiac surgery. Anesth Analg 2004;99:319–24.

22. Miriam A, Korula G. A simple glucose insulin regimen for perioperative blood glucose control: the Vellore regimen. Anesth Analg 2004;99:598–602.

23. Smith CE, Styn NR, Kalhan S, et al. Intraoperative glucose control in diabetic and nondiabetic patients during cardiac surgery. J Cardiothorac Vasc Anesth 2005; 19:201–8.

24. Boelaert K, Franklyn JA. Thyroid hormone in health and disease. J Endocrinol 2005;187:1–15.

25. Klein I. Clinical, metabolic, and organ-specific indices of thyroid function. Endocrinol Metab Clin North Am 2001;30:415–27, ix.

26. Ayres J, Rees J, Clark TJ, et al. Thyrotoxicosis and dyspnoea. Clin Endocrinol (Oxf) 1982;16:65–71.

27. Kahaly G, Hellermann J, Mohr-Kahaly S, et al. Impaired cardiopulmonary exercise capacity in patients with hyperthyroidism. Chest 1996;109:57–61.
28. Klein I, Ojamaa K. Thyroid hormone and the cardiovascular system: from theory to practice. J Clin Endocrinol Metab 1994;78:1026–7.
29. Woeber KA. Thyrotoxicosis and the heart. N Engl J Med 1992;327:94–8.
30. Ladenson PW, Goldenheim PD, Ridgway EC. Prediction and reversal of blunted ventilatory responsiveness in patients with hypothyroidism. Am J Med 1988;84: 877–83.
31. Siafakas NM, Salesiotou V, Filaditaki V, et al. Respiratory muscle strength in hypothyroidism. Chest 1992;102:189–94.
32. Ladenson PW, Levin AA, Ridgway EC, et al. Complications of surgery in hypothyroid patients. Am J Med 1984;77:261–6.
33. Weinberg AD, Brennan MD, Gorman CA, et al. Outcome of anesthesia and surgery in hypothyroid patients. Arch Intern Med 1983;143:893–7.
34. US Preventive Services Task Force. Screening for thyroid disease: recommendation statement. Ann Intern Med 2004;140:125–7.
35. Ladenson PW, Singer PA, Ain KB, et al. American Thyroid Association guidelines for detection of thyroid dysfunction. Arch Intern Med 2000;160:1573–5.
36. Dayan CM. Interpretation of thyroid function tests. Lancet 2001;357:619–24.
37. Fliers E, Guldenaar SE, Wiersinga WM, et al. Decreased hypothalamic thyrotropin-releasing hormone gene expression in patients with nonthyroidal illness. J Clin Endocrinol Metab 1997;82:4032–6.
38. Rothwell PM, Lawler PG. Prediction of outcome in intensive care patients using endocrine parameters. Crit Care Med 1995;23:78–83.
39. Bacci V, Schussler GC, Kaplan TB. The relationship between serum triiodothyronine and thyrotropin during systemic illness. J Clin Endocrinol Metab 1982;54: 1229–35.
40. Mihai R, Farndon JR. Parathyroid disease and calcium metabolism. Br J Anaesth 2000;85:29–43.
41. Lind L, Ljunghall S. Pre-operative evaluation of risk factors for complications in patients with primary hyperparathyroidism. Eur J Clin Invest 1995;25:955–8.
42. The American Association of Clinical Endocrinologists and the American Association of Endocrine Surgeons position statement on the diagnosis and management of primary hyperparathyroidism. Endocr Pract 2005;11:49–54.
43. Fukagawa M, Tominaga Y, Kitaoka M, et al. Medical and surgical aspects of parathyroidectomy. Kidney Int Suppl 1999;73:S65–9.
44. Sokoll LJ, Wians FH Jr, Remaley AT. Rapid intraoperative immunoassay of parathyroid hormone and other hormones: a new paradigm for point-of-care testing. Clin Chem 2004;50:1126–35.
45. Alderazi Y, Yeh MW, Robinson BG, et al. Phaeochromocytoma: current concepts. Med J Aust 2005;183:201–4.
46. Kinney MA, Narr BJ, Warner MA. Perioperative management of pheochromocytoma. J Cardiothorac Vasc Anesth 2002;16:359–69.
47. Bravo EL. Evolving concepts in the pathophysiology, diagnosis, and treatment of pheochromocytoma. Endocr Rev 1994;15:356–68.
48. Kinney MA, Warner ME, vanHeerden JA, et al. Perianesthetic risks and outcomes of pheochromocytoma and paraganglioma resection. Anesth Analg 2000;91: 1118–23.
49. Nanda AS, Feldman A, Liang CS. Acute reversal of pheochromocytoma-induced catecholamine cardiomyopathy. Clin Cardiol 1995;18:421–3.

50. Liao WB, Liu CF, Chiang CW, et al. Cardiovascular manifestations of pheochromocytoma. Am J Emerg Med 2000;18:622–5.
51. Stenstrom G, Swedberg K. QRS amplitudes, QTc intervals and ECG abnormalities in pheochromocytoma patients before, during and after treatment. Acta Med Scand 1988;224:231–5.
52. Witteles RM, Kaplan EL, Roizen MF. Safe and cost-effective preoperative preparation of patients with pheochromocytoma. Anesth Analg 2000;91:302–4.
53. Connery LE, Coursin DB. Assessment and therapy of selected endocrine disorders. Anesthesiol Clin North America 2004;22:93–123.
54. Annane D, Briegel J, Sprung CL. Corticosteroid insufficiency in acutely ill patients. N Engl J Med 2003;348:2157–9.
55. Rivers EP, Gaspari M, Saad GA, et al. Adrenal insufficiency in high-risk surgical ICU patients. Chest 2001;119:889–96.
56. Graham GW, Unger BP, Coursin DB. Perioperative management of selected endocrine disorders. Int Anesthesiol Clin 2000;38:31–67.
57. Holdcroft A. Hormones and the gut. Br J Anaesth 2000;85:58–68.
58. Modlin IM, Kidd M, Latich I, et al. Current status of gastrointestinal carcinoids. Gastroenterology 2005;128:1717–51.
59. Pellikka PA, Tajik AJ, Khandheria BK, et al. Carcinoid heart disease. Clinical and echocardiographic spectrum in 74 patients. Circulation 1993;87:1188–96.
60. Kinney MA, Warner ME, Nagorney DM, et al. Perianaesthetic risks and outcomes of abdominal surgery for metastatic carcinoid tumours. Br J Anaesth 2001;87:447–52.

Index

Note: Page numbers of article titles are in **boldface** type.

A

Acute normovolemic hemodilution. *See* Hemodilution.
Acute pain. *See* Pain, acute.
Additives, to local anesthetics for peripheral nerve blocks in children, 209
Adrenal insufficiency, endocrine monitoring in, 360
Air-Q laryngeal mask, for difficult pediatric airway management, 192–193
Airtraq, for difficult pediatric airway management, 190
Airway management, difficult pediatric, devices and techniques for, **185–195**
 flexible scopes, 193–194
 laryngeal masks, 191–193
 optical stylets, 185–187
 video/optical laryngoscopes, 187–191
Alpha-2 agonists, for acute pediatric pain, 248–249
Alvimopan, for acute pediatric pain, 247
Aminocaproic acid, ϵ-, intraoperative blood transfusion prophylaxis with, 344
Analgesia, acute pediatric pain, pharmacologic management of, **241–288**
 in therapy of pediatric traumatic brain injury, 225–226
Anatomy, brachial plexus, 198
 lumbar plexus, 203
 single ventricle and Fontan procedure, 285–288
Anesthesia, pediatric. *See* Pediatric anesthesia.
Anesthetics, effect on developing brain, 231–232
 local, for peripheral nerve blocks in children, 209
Antipyretics, for acute pediatric pain, 242–244
Apoptosis, necrosis and, in pediatric traumatic brain injury, 214–215
Aprotinin, intraoperative blood transfusion prophylaxis with, 344
Autologous blood donation, preoperative, blood transfusion prophylaxis with, 341–342
Autoregulation, cerebral blood flow and, in pediatric traumatic brain injury, 216
Axillary brachial plexus block, 200–201
Axonal injury, in pediatric traumatic brain injury, 216–217

B

Barbiturates, for sedation of child with congenital heart disease, 311–312
 in therapy of pediatric traumatic brain injury, 228
Benzodiazepines, for sedation of child with congenital heart disease, 312
Blocks, nerve. *See* Peripheral nerve blockade.
Blood conservation, strategies in pediatric patients, **337–351**
 high-risk patients, 339–340
  drug-related risk, 339–340
  patient-related risk, 339
  physician-related risk, 340

Anesthesiology Clin 27 (2009) 365–375
doi:10.1016/S1932-2275(09)00067-6
1932-2275/09/$ – see front matter © 2009 Elsevier Inc. All rights reserved.

anesthesiology.theclinics.com

Blood (*continued*)
    procedure-related risk, 340
   intraoperative interventions, 342–345
     acute normovolemic hemodilution, 342–343
     cell salvage, 343
     deliberate hypotension, 343–344
     pharmacologic, 344
     surgical technique, 344–345
     temperature control, 345
   preoperative interventions, 341–342
     autologous blood donation, 341–342
     recombinant erythropoietin, 341
   rationale for use of blood and blood products, 337–338
   reasons to avoid blood products when possible, 338
   transfusion triggers, 345–348
     algorithms, 347
     fresh frozen plasma and cryoprecipitate, 346–347
     platelet concentrates, 346
     recombinant factor VIIa, 347–348
     red cells and whole blood, 345–346
Blood donation, preoperative autologous, blood transfusion prophylaxis with, 341-342
Bonfils endoscope, for difficult pediatric airway management, 187
Brachial plexus, upper extremity blocks, ultrasound guidance for pediatric, 198–201
   anatomy, 198
   axillary brachial plexus block, 200–201
   interscalene brachial plexus block, 199
Brain, newborn, effects of anesthesia on, **269–284**
Brain injury. *See* Traumatic brain injury.

   C

Carcinoid tumors, endocrine monitoring in, 360–361
   intraoperative, 361
   preoperative, 361
Cell salvage, intraoperative blood transfusion prophylaxis with, 343
Cerebral blood flow, autoregulation and, in pediatric traumatic brain injury, 216
Cerebral perfusion pressure, in therapy of pediatric traumatic brain injury, 224–225
Cerebral swelling, in pediatric traumatic brain injury, 215–216
Cerebrospinal fluid drainage, in therapy of pediatric traumatic brain injury, 226, 230
   lumbar, 230
   ventricular, 226
Childhood, early, exposure to general anesthesia in, 275–276
Children, anesthesia in. *See* Pediatric anesthesia.
Codeine, for acute pediatric pain, 246–247
Computed tomography (CT), diagnostic, in pediatric traumatic brain injury, 219–220
Congenital heart disease, Fontan procedure, anesthetic considerations, **285–300**
  sedating child with, **301–319**
   goals of sedation and anesthesia, 303
   medications, 308–315
     alpha-2 adrenergic agonist, 314–315
     analgesic, 308–311

local anesthetics, 311
  sedative/hypnotic, 311–314
presedation assessment, 303–304
recovery, 315
sedation environment, 304–308
  equipment and resuscitation drugs, 304–305
  monitoring, 305, 308
Continuous intravenous infusion, opiate, for acute pediatric pain, 254–255
Craniectomy, decompressive, in therapy of pediatric traumatic brain injury, 228–229

D

Deliberate hypotension, intraoperative blood transfusion prophylaxis with, 343-344
Dexmedetomidine, for sedation of child with congenital heart disease, 314–315
Diabetes mellitus, monitoring endocrine function, 355–357
  glycosylated hemoglobin, 355–356
  hyperglycemia and illness severity, 356
  preoperative glycemic monitoring, 356–357
Diagnostic imaging, in pediatric traumatic brain injury, 219–220

E

Emergency department evaluation, of pediatric traumatic brain injury, 217–220
  diagnostic studies, 219–220
  physical examination, 217–219
  therapeutic options in "initial golden minutes," 220–222
Emergency surgery, in Fontan patients, 295–296
Endocarditis, bacterial, prophylaxis during Fontan procedure, 293
Endocrine function, monitoring, **355–364**
  adrenal insufficiency, 360
  carcinoid tumors, 360–361
  diabetes mellitus, 355–357
  parathyroid disorders, 358–359
  pheochromocytoma, 359–360
  thyroid disorders, 357–358
Endoscope, Bonfils, for difficult pediatric airway management, 187
Epidural analgesia, for acute pediatric pain, 255–257
Erythropoietin, recombinant, preoperative blood transfusion prophylaxis with, 341
Etomidate, for sedation of child with congenital heart disease, 313–314

F

Femoral nerve block, ultrasound guidance for pediatric, 204–205
Fentanyl, for acute pediatric pain, 246
  for sedation of child with congenital heart disease, 310–311
Fiberoptic scopes, flexible, for difficult pediatric airway management, 193–194
Flexible fiberoptic scopes, for difficult pediatric airway management, 193–194
Fluid management, during Fontan procedure, 293
Fontan procedure, single ventricle, anesthetic considerations in, **285–300**
  anatomic features and staged reconstruction, 285–288
  intraoperative management, 291–296

Fontan (*continued*)
        emergency surgery, 295–296
        fluid management/transfusion, 293
        induction and maintenance, 292–293
        laparoscopy, 294–295
        mechanical ventilation, 293
        monitoring, 291–292
        one-lung ventilation, 295
        positioning, 295
        pregnancy, 295
        special patient considerations, 294
        special surgical considerations, 294
        subacute bacterial endocarditis prophylaxis, 293
    postoperative concerns, 296–297
    preoperative assessment, 288–291
        associated defects, 289–290
        current medications, 290
        history and physical examination, 288–289
        laboratory evaluation, 290–291
        nothing by mouth status, 290
        psychosocial issues and premedication, 291
Fresh frozen plasma, transfusion of, in pediatric surgical patients, 346–347

G

Gamma-aminobutyric acid (GABA) agonists, effects on newborn brain, 271–272
    for acute pediatric pain, 249–250
GlideScope, for difficult pediatric airway management, 189
Glycemic monitoring, in diabetic patients, 355–357

H

Head position, in therapy of pediatric traumatic brain injury, 225
Heart disease, congenital, Fontan procedure, anesthetic considerations, **285–300**
    sedation of child with, **301–319**
Hemodilution, acute normovolemic, intraoperative blood transfusion prophylaxis with,
    342–343
Hemoglobin, function, 322–323
    structure and genetics, 321–322
Hemoglobin A1c, monitoring endocrine function in diabetes with, 355–356
Hemoglobin C, anesthesia in children with, 331
Hemoglobin E, anesthesia in children with, 331
Hemoglobin M variants, anesthesia in children with, 331
Hemoglobinopathies, anesthesia and, **321–336**
        hemoglobin C and F, 331
        hemoglobin function, 322–323
        hemoglobin structure and genetics, 321–322
        other congenital, 331
        sickle cell disease, 323–329
        thalassemias, 330
Herniation, in pediatric traumatic brain injury, 221–222

History, patient, prior to Fontan procedure, 288–289

Hydrocodone, for acute pediatric pain, 247

Hydromorphone, for acute pediatric pain, 245

Hyperglycemia, indicator of illness severity in diabetes, 356

Hyperosmolar therapy, for pediatric traumatic brain injury, 226–227

Hyperparathyroidism, endocrine monitoring in, 359

Hypertension, intracranial, in pediatric traumatic brain injury, guidelines for, 222–230
>   first-tier therapies, 222–228
>   second-tier therapies, 228–230

Hyperthyroidism, monitoring treatment of, 358

Hyperventilation, in therapy of pediatric traumatic brain injury, 227–228

Hypoparathyroidism, endocrine monitoring in, 359

Hypotension, deliberate, intraoperative blood transfusion prophylaxis with, 343–344

Hypothermia, in therapy of pediatric traumatic brain injury, 229

Hypothyroidism, monitoring treatment of, 358

I

Imaging, diagnostic, in pediatric traumatic brain injury, 219–220

Induction, of anesthesia, for Fontan procedure, 292–293

Infants, exposure to general anesthesia, 274–275
> with congenital heart disease, sedation of, **301–319**

Infraclavicular brachial plexus block, 199–200

Infusion, continuous intravenous, opiate, for acute pediatric pain, 254–255

Interscalene brachial plexus block, 199

Intracranial hypertension, in pediatric traumatic brain injury, guidelines for, 222–230
>   first-tier therapies, 222–228
>   second-tier therapies, 228–230

Intraoperative monitoring, in carcinoid tumors, 361

Intrathecal morphine, for acute pediatric pain, 257–258

Intravenous infusion, continuous, opiate, for acute pediatric pain, 254–255

K

Ketamine, dissociative, for sedation of child with congenital heart disease, 308–310
> for acute pediatric pain, 248

L

Laparoscopy, in Fontan patient, 294–295

Laryngeal masks, for difficult pediatric airway management, 191–193

Laryngoscopes, video/optical, for difficult pediatric airway management, 187–191
>   Airtraq, 190
>   GlideScope, 189
>   Storz, 189–190
>   Truview EVO2, 190–191

Local anesthetics, for acute pediatric pain, 250–251
> for peripheral nerve blocks in children, 209
> for sedation of child with congenital heart disease, 311

Lower extremity blocks, ultrasound guidance for pediatric, 202–208
>   femoral plexus block, 204–205
>   lumbar plexus anatomy, 203
>   lumbar plexus block, 203–204

Lower (*continued*)
    saphenous plexus block, 205–206
    sciatic nerve block, 206–208
Lumbar plexus, blockade of, ultrasound guidance for pediatric, 202–208
    femoral plexus block, 204–205
    lumbar plexus anatomy, 203
    lumbar plexus block, 203–204

M

Masks, laryngeal, for difficult pediatric airway management, 192–193
Mechanical ventilation, for Fontan procedure, 293
    one-lung, 293
Median nerve block, above elbow, ultrasound guidance for, 201–202
Methadone, for acute pediatric pain, 245–246
Methylnaltrexone, for acute pediatric pain, 247
Midazolam, for sedation of child with congenital heart disease, 312
Monitoring, during Fontan procedure, 291–292
    during sedation of child with congenital heart disease, 305, 308
    endocrine function, **355–364**
        adrenal insufficiency, 360
        carcinoid tumors, 360–361
        diabetes mellitus, 355–357
        parathyroid disorders, 358–359
        pheochromocytoma, 359–360
        thyroid disorders, 357–358
Morphine, for acute pediatric pain, 245
    intrathecal, 257–258

N

N-methyl-D-aspartate (NMDA) antagonists, effects on newborn brain, 270–271
    for acute pediatric pain, 249
Nalbuphine, for acute pediatric pain, 247
Naloxone, for acute pediatric pain, 247
Necrosis, in pediatric traumatic brain injury, 214–215
Neonates. *See* Newborns.
Nerve blocks. *See* Peripheral nerve blockade.
Neuromonitoring, in pediatric traumatic brain injury, 230–231
Neuromuscular blockade, in therapy of pediatric traumatic brain injury, 225–226
Neurotoxicity, effects of anesthesia on newborn brain, **269–284**
Newborns, effects of anesthesia on brain, **269–284**
        clinical human data, 273–277
            beneficial effects, 276–277
            early childhood exposure, 275–276
            neonatal or early infantile exposure, 273–275
            prenatal exposure, 273
        preclinical data, 270–273
            exposure effects or outcome, 273
            timing of exposure, 272–273
            type of exposures, 270–272
Nonsteroidal anti-inflammatory drugs (NSAIDs), for acute pediatric pain, 242–244

O

Opiates, for acute pediatric pain, 244–248
    for sedation of child with congenital heart disease, 310–311
Optical laryngoscopes, for difficult pediatric airway management, 187–191
Optical stylets, for difficult pediatric airway management, 185–187
        Bonfils, 187
        Shikani, 186–187
Outcomes, perioperative, systemic effects of thyroid dysfunction on, 357
Oxycodone, for acute pediatric pain, 247

P

Pain, acute pediatric, pharmacologic management of, **241–288**
        analgesic, antipyretic, anti-inflammatory drugs, 242–244
        opiate analgesics, 244–248
        other analgesics, 248–251
            alpha-2 agonists, 248–249
            gamma-aminobutyric acid (GABA) agonists, 249–250
            ketamine, 248
            local anesthetics, 250–251
            N-methyl-D-aspartate (NMDA) receptor antagonists, 249
        postoperative pain, techniques for, 251–259
            continuous intravenous opiate infusion, 254–255
            epidural analgesia, 255–257
            intrathecal morphine, 257–258
            measuring pain, 251–252
            patient-controlled analgesia, 253–254
            regional anesthesia, 258–259
            strategies for, 252–253
Parathyroid disorders, endocrine monitoring in, 358–359
        hyperparathyroidism, 359
        hypoparathyroidism, 359
Patient-controlled analgesia, pediatric, 253–254
Pediatric anesthesia, 185–351
    acute pain, pharmacologic management of, **241–288**
        analgesic, antipyretic, anti-inflammatory drugs, 242–244
        opiate analgesics, 244–248
        other analgesics, 248–251
        postoperative pain, techniques for, 251–259
    blood conservation strategies in, **337–351**
        high-risk patients, 339–340
        intraoperative interventions, 342–345
        preoperative interventions, 341–342
        rationale for use of blood and blood products, 337–338
        reasons to avoid blood products when possible, 338
        transfusion triggers, 345–348
    difficult airway management, **185–195**
        flexible scopes, 193–194
        laryngeal masks, 191–193
        optical stylets, 185–187
        video/optical laryngoscopes, 187–191

Pediatric (*continued*)
    Fontan patients, **285–300**
        anatomic features and staged reconstruction, 285–288
        intraoperative management, 291–296
        postoperative concerns, 296–297
        preoperative assessment, 288–291
    hemoglobinopathies and, **321–336**
        hemoglobin C and F, 331
        hemoglobin function, 322–323
        hemoglobin structure and genetics, 321–322
        other congenital, 331
        sickle cell disease, 323–329
        thalassemias, 330
    newborns, effects on brain, **269–284**
        clinical human data, 273–277
        preclinical data, 270–273
    peripheral nerve blockade, ultrasound guidance for, **197–212**
        local anesthetics and additives, 209
        lower extremity blocks, 202–208
        median and radial nerve block above elbow, 201
        rectus sheath block, 208–209
        trunk blocks, 208
        upper extremity blocks, 198–201
    sedating child with congenital heart disease, **301–319**
        goals of sedation and anesthesia, 303
        medications, 308–315
        presedation assessment, 303–304
        recovery, 315
        sedation environment, 304–308
    traumatic brain injury, **213–240**
        emergency department evaluation, 217–220
            diagnostic studies, 219–220
            physical examination, 217–219
            therapeutic options in "initial golden minutes," 220–222
        future directions, 230–232
            effects of anesthesia on developing brain, 231–232
            neuromonitoring, 230–231
        guidelines for intracranial hypertension, 222–230
            first-tier therapies, 222–228
            second-tier therapies, 228–230
        injury patterns, 213–214
        pathophysiology, immediate and delayed injury, cerebral blood flow
           and autoregulation, 216
            cerebral swelling, 215–216
            necrosis and apoptosis, 214–215
            traumatic axonal injury, 216–217
Perioperative monitoring, glycemic, in diabetic patients, 356
Perioperative outcomes, systemic effects of thyroid dysfunction on, 357
Peripheral nerve blockade, ultrasound guidance for pediatric, **197–212**
        local anesthetics and additives, 209
        lower extremity blocks, 202–208

femoral plexus block, 204–205
    lumbar plexus anatomy, 203
    lumbar plexus block, 203–204
    saphenous plexus block, 205–206
    sciatic nerve block, 206–208
  median and radial nerve block above elbow, 201
  rectus sheath block, 208–209
  trunk blocks, 208
  upper extremity blocks, 198–201
    anatomy, 198
    axillary brachial plexus block, 200–201
    interscalene brachial plexus block, 199
    intraclavicular brachial plexus bloc, 199–200
Pheochromocytoma, endocrine monitoring in, 359–360
    intraoperative, 360
    preoperative, 359–360
Physical examination, initial, in pediatric traumatic brain injury, 217–219
    prior to Fontan procedure, 288–289
Platelet concentrates, transfusion of, in pediatric surgical patients, 346
Postoperative care, of Fontan patient, 296–297
Postoperative pain, pediatric, strategies for management of, 252–253
Pregnancy, in Fontan patients, 295
Premedication, for Fontan procedure due to psychosocial issues, 291
Prenatal exposure, to general anesthesia, 274
Preoperative monitoring, in carcinoid tumors, 361
Prophylaxis, bacterial endocarditis, during Fontan procedure, 293
Propofol, for sedation of child with congenital heart disease, 313
Psychosocial issues, premedication for Fontan procedure due to, 291

R

Radial nerve block, above elbow, ultrasound guidance for, 201–202
Recombinant erythropoietin, preoperative blood transfusion prophylaxis with, 341
Recombinant factor VIIa, transfusion of, in pediatric surgical patients, 347–348
Rectus sheath block, ultrasound guidance for pediatric, 208–209
Red cells, transfusion of, in pediatric surgical patients, 345–346
Regional anesthesia, for acute pediatric pain, 258–259
    pediatric peripheral nerve blockade, ultrasound guidance for, **197–212**

S

Salvage, cell, intraoperative blood transfusion prophylaxis with, 343
Saphenous nerve block, ultrasound guidance for pediatric, 205–206
Sciatic nerve block, ultrasound guidance for pediatric, 206–208
Sedation, in therapy of pediatric traumatic brain injury, 225–226
  of child with congenital heart disease, **301–319**
    goals of sedation and anesthesia, 303
    medications, 308–315
      alpha-2 adrenergic agonist, 314–315
      analgesic, 308–311
      local anesthetics, 311
      sedative/hypnotic, 311–314

Sedation (*continued*)
    presedation assessment, 303–304
    recovery, 315
    sedation environment, 304–308
        equipment and resuscitation drugs, 304–305
        monitoring, 305, 308
Seizure, in therapy of pediatric traumatic brain injury, 229–230
Shikani optical stylet, for difficult pediatric airway management, 186–187
Sickle cell disease, 323–329
  acid-base regulation, 328
  anesthesia in children with, 323–329
  clinical picture, 324–325
  complications, management of, 329
  hydration, 326–327
  oxygenation, 327
  perioperative management, 325–326
  preoperative assessment and workup, 326
  regional anesthesia, 328
  specific procedures, 328–329
  thermoregulation, 327–328
  transfusion, 327
Single ventricle, Fontan procedure, anesthetic considerations, **285–300**
Storz Video Laryngoscope, for difficult pediatric airway management, 189–190
Stylets, optical, for difficult pediatric airway management, 185–187
    Bonfils, 187
    Shikani, 186–187
Swelling, cerebral, in pediatric traumatic brain injury, 215–216

T

Temperature control, intraoperative blood transfusion prophylaxis with, 345
Thalassemias, anesthesia in children with, 330
Thyroid disorders, endocrine monitoring in, 357–358
    in critically ill or hospitalized patients, 358
    perioperative outcomes and, 357
    thyroid function, 358
    treatment of hypothyroidism and hyperthyroidism, 358
Tramadol, for acute pediatric pain, 247–248
Tranexamic acid, intraoperative blood transfusion prophylaxis with, 344
Transfusion, during Fontan procedure, 293
Transfusion triggers, in pediatric surgical patients, 345–348
    algorithms, 347
    fresh frozen plasma and cryoprecipitate, 346–347
    platelet concentrates, 346
    recombinant factor VIIa, 347–348
    red cells and whole blood, 345–346
Traumatic brain injury, pediatric, **213–240**
  emergency department evaluation, 217–220
    diagnostic studies, 219–220
    physical examination, 217–219
    therapeutic options in "initial golden minutes," 220–222

future directions, 230–232
    effects of anesthesia on developing brain, 231–232
    neuromonitoring, 230–231
guidelines for intracranial hypertension, 222–230
    first-tier therapies, 222–228
    second-tier therapies, 228–230
injury patterns, 213–214
pathophysiology, immediate and delayed injury, cerebral blood flow
    and autoregulation, 216
    cerebral swelling, 215–216
    necrosis and apoptosis, 214–215
    traumatic axonal injury, 216–217
Trunk blocks, ultrasound guidance for pediatric, 208
Truview EVO2, for difficult pediatric airway management, 190–191
Tumors, carcinoid, endocrine monitoring in, 360–361

U

Ultrasound guidance, for pediatric peripheral nerve blockade, **197–212**
    local anesthetics and additives, 209
    lower extremity blocks, 202–208
        femoral plexus block, 204–205
        lumbar plexus anatomy, 203
        lumbar plexus block, 203–204
        saphenous plexus block, 205–206
        sciatic nerve block, 206–208
    median and radial nerve block above elbow, 201
    rectus sheath block, 208–209
    trunk blocks, 208
    upper extremity blocks, 198–201
        anatomy, 198
        axillary brachial plexus block, 200–201
        interscalene brachial plexus block, 199
        intraclavicular brachial plexus bloc, 199–200
Upper extremity blocks, ultrasound guidance for pediatric, 198–201
    anatomy, 198
    axillary brachial plexus block, 200–201
    interscalene brachial plexus block, 199
    intraclavicular brachial plexus bloc, 199–200

V

Ventilation, mechanical, for Fontan procedure, 293
    one-lung, 295
Ventricle, single, Fontan procedure, anesthetic considerations, **285–300**
Video laryngoscopes, for difficult pediatric airway management, 187–191

W

Whole blood, transfusion of, in pediatric surgical patients, 345–346

infant simulators, 200-202
  effect of healthcare on extracellular brain pH, 201-202
  neuroprotection, 230-234
  guidelines for intracranial hypertension, 228-230 Y
    first line therapies, 232-233
    second tier therapies, 234-230
  secondary insults, 213-214
  cerebral perfusion, intracranial and cerebral injury, cerebral blood flow
    and autoregulation, 213
  cerebral swelling, 210-212
  medical and appropriate 1-3, 3-5
  traumatic brain injury, 216-218

U
Ultrasound guidance, for bedside ... pressure, 207
Throw EVD? for difficult pediatric airway management, 190-191
fluids, can void, and adapting monitoring in ... 207

U
ultrasound guidance, for pediatric regional anesthesia, 187-212
  local anesthetics and additives, 203
  lower extremity blocks, 205-206
  femoral plexus block, 205-206
  lumbar plexus anatomy, 204
  lumbar plexus block, 205-206
  saphenous plexus block, 205-206
  sciatic nerve block, 205-206
  median and midclavicular block above clavicle, 204...
  rectus sheath block, 205-206
  trunk blocks, 206
  upper extremity blocks, 198-201
  anatomy, 198
  axillary brachial plexus block, 200-201 ...
  interscalene brachial plexus block, 198...
  infraclavicular brachial plexus block, 199-200
Upper extremity blocks, ultrasound guidance for pediatric, 198-201
  anatomy, 198
  axillary brachial plexus block, 200-201
  interscalene brachial plexus block, 198
  supraclavicular brachial plexus block, 199-200

V
Ventilation, mechanical, for Pierre Robin ... 90?
  one lung, 96
Vo (VBM) airway, simple, Rohm procedure, anesthetic management, 158-159
Vocal laryngoscope, for difficult pediatric airway management, 121-123

A
in tumor board, transformation metallic-bicarbonate, 248-256
Chinos, 4, Step procedures and air...
Intubation, flexible, 34.51-55.510

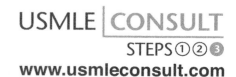

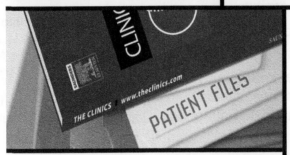